Advances in Engineering for Surgery

Advances in Engineering for Surgery

Editor: Lilly Fielden

FOSTER ACADEMICS

www.fosteracademics.com

www.fosteracademics.com

FOSTER ACADEMICS

Cataloging-in-Publication Data

Advances in engineering for surgery / edited by Lilly Fielden.
p. cm.
Includes bibliographical references and index.
ISBN 978-1-64646-557-6
1. Surgery. 2. Surgery--Case studies. 3. Medicine. I. Fielden, Lilly.
RD31.5 .S87 2023
617--dc23

Foster Academics,
118-35 Queens Blvd., Suite 400,
Forest Hills, NY 11375, USA

ISBN 978-1-64646-557-6 (Hardback)

Contents

Preface

The main aim of this book is to educate learners and enhance their research focus by presenting diverse topics covering this vast field. This is an advanced book which compiles significant studies by distinguished experts in the area of analysis. This book addresses successive solutions to the challenges arising in the area of application, along with it; the book provides scope for future developments.

The advancements in the field of engineering are applied in a wide variety of fields. One such field is surgery, where engineering innovations are used for improving patient outcomes and care. Research in this field is generally carried out within the interdisciplinary field of biomedical engineering. It involves advancements in different domains of healthcare such as diagnosis, monitoring and therapy. Some of the major advancements in this field are laparoscopic surgery and robot-assisted-surgery. Laparoscopic surgery is conducted through one or more small incisions, using small tubes, cameras and surgical instruments. Robotic surgery presents a three dimensional and magnified view to the surgeon, providing increased control and precision. This book elucidates the concepts and innovative models around prospective developments with respect to the application of engineering in the field of surgery. Those in search of information to further their knowledge will be greatly assisted by this book.

It was a great honour to edit this book, though there were challenges, as it involved a lot of communication and networking between me and the editorial team. However, the end result was this all-inclusive book covering diverse themes in the field.

Finally, it is important to acknowledge the efforts of the contributors for their excellent chapters, through which a wide variety of issues have been addressed. I would also like to thank my colleagues for their valuable feedback during the making of this book.

Editor

1

The Evolution of Tissue Engineered Vascular Graft Technologies: From Preclinical Trials to Advancing Patient Care

Yuichi Matsuzaki [1], Kelly John [1], Toshihiro Shoji [1] and Toshiharu Shinoka [1,2,3,*]

1 Center for Regenerative Medicine, Nationwide Children's Hospital, Columbus, OH 43205, USA; Yuichi.matsuzaki@nationwidechildrens.org (Y.M.); John.Kelly@nationwidechildrens.org (K.J.); Toshihiro.shoji@nationwidechildrens.org (T.S.)
2 Department of Cardiothoracic Surgery, Nationwide Children's Hospital, Columbus, OH 43205, USA
3 Department of Surgery, The Ohio State University Wexner Medical Center, Columbus, OH 43210, USA
* Correspondence: toshiharu.shinoka@nationwidechildrens.org.

Abstract: Currently available synthetic grafts have contributed to improved outcomes in cardiovascular surgery. However, the implementation of these graft materials at small diameters have demonstrated poor patency, inhibiting their use for coronary artery bypass surgery in adults. Additionally, when applied to a pediatric patient population, they are handicapped by their lack of growth ability. Tissue engineered alternatives could possibly address these limitations by producing biocompatible implants with the ability to repair, remodel, grow, and regenerate. A tissue engineered vascular graft (TEVG) generally consists of a scaffold, seeded cells, and the appropriate environmental cues (i.e., growth factors, physical stimulation) to induce tissue formation. This review critically appraises current state-of-the-art techniques for vascular graft production. We additionally examine current graft shortcomings and future prospects, as they relate to cardiovascular surgery, from two major clinical trials.

Keywords: tissue-engineered vascular grafts; biodegradable material; congenital heart surgery; arteriovenous shunts

1. Introduction

Congenital heart disease is the leading cause of neonatal death and affects almost 1% of all surviving births [1]. Almost a quarter of these patients need extensive reconstructive surgery [2]. In the adult population, cardiovascular diseases (CVD), such as aortic disease, coronary artery disease (CAD), and peripheral artery disease (PAD), are the leading cause of death worldwide [3].

Current synthetic grafts are generally made from non-biodegradable materials such as polytetrafluoroethylene (e-PTFE®) or polyethylene terephthalate (Dacron®) [4]. These grafts can be successful in large diameter surgeries, but in general, synthetic materials are not clinically suitable because they exhibit an increased risk of thrombosis, stenosis, calcification, and infection, while lacking in durability and growth potential [5]. Because synthetic materials are thrombotic in small-diameter blood vessels of 6 mm or less, the saphenous vein, internal thoracic artery, and radial arteries are often used in cases of coronary artery bypass surgery or peripheral artery bypass surgery for obstructive arteriosclerosis below the knee.

Unfortunately, in affected patient populations, there is an insufficient amount of usable native tissue, either for reasons of anatomy or use in previous operations. In order to overcome the limitations associated with autologous and synthetic graft transplantation, the concept of tissue engineering was proposed [6]. Tissue engineering is a scientific field that may solve the problems that plague current grafts. Tissue engineering is defined as an interdisciplinary field which combines engineering and biomedical principles to create materials that integrate with a patient's native tissue to restore or improve physiological function.

The classical paradigm of tissue engineering includes:

(I) Cells (i.e., progenitor cells, stem cells);
(II) Scaffolds (i.e., synthetic, decellularized extracellular matrix);
(III) Signals (growth factors, chemotactic factors) [6].

The three components are interdependent and essential to each other when attempting to form organized neotissue. Since newly created neotissue is composed of autologous tissue, these constructs would theoretically be thrombo-resistant, less prone to infection, and have growth capacity. In 1986, the first tissue engineered blood vessels were reported by Weinberg and Bell. They consisted of fibroblasts and collagen gel embedded fibers integrated with bovine endothelial cells (EC), smooth muscle cells (SMC), and Dacron mesh [7]. Since then, hundreds of tissue engineered vascular grafts (TEVGs) have been developed and evaluated in animal models but very few have progressed to human clinical trials. In fact, there are only two that are currently undergoing clinical trials in the United States. In 2001, the first clinical trial to evaluate the use of TEVGs in the venous circulation was conducted in children with congenital heart disease by Shinoka et al. [8]. In 2012, a separate clinical study conducted by Niklason et al. began to evaluate arteriovenous shunts for hemodialysis [9].

This review focuses on the traditional role of scaffolds and cells in TEVGs, the status of recent venous and arteriovenous TEVG clinical studies, and discusses their limitations and future prospects.

2. Material and Methods

The ideal scaffold is resistant to calcification, stenosis, thrombosis, and infection. From a surgical perspective, it must be easily handled, sutured, and readily available. In addition, it must have sufficient mechanical properties to withstand the hemodynamic changes of its designated system. Initially, the scaffold not only provides a TEVG's structural integrity, but also the structure to which cells attach and remodel [10]. Ultimately, the organized neotissue assumes the mechanical and structural responsibility of a TEVG as the original scaffold deteriorates. In an effort to find the ideal TEVG framework, numerous synthetic and natural materials have been proposed and evaluated. We will briefly detail some of these approaches. (Figure 1)

2.1. Biodegradable Synthetic Vascular Grafts

Biodegradable polymers often act as a temporary scaffold of a blood vessel before it is degraded by the body. Degradation of these materials is initially expressed as a loss of mechanical properties, and then followed by a decrease in their mass to volume ratio. The degradation rate of a given polymer depends on their initial molecular weight, exposed surface area, and physical state (11).

Choosing a suitable material is an important first step in scaffold design and depends on various factors, such as immunogenicity, mechanical properties, and rate of degradation.

Four of the more commonly used synthetic biodegradable materials for TEVGs are:

Poly (glycolic acid) (PGA)
Poly (lactic acid) (PLA)
Poly (ε-caprolactone) (PCL)
Poly (glycerol) sebacate (PGS)

The degradation times of these polymers have been reported to be approximately 2 to 6 weeks, 6 to 12 months, 2 to 3 years, and 4 weeks, respectively [11,12]. Below, we briefly describe each individual polymer and their use in preclinical animal studies.

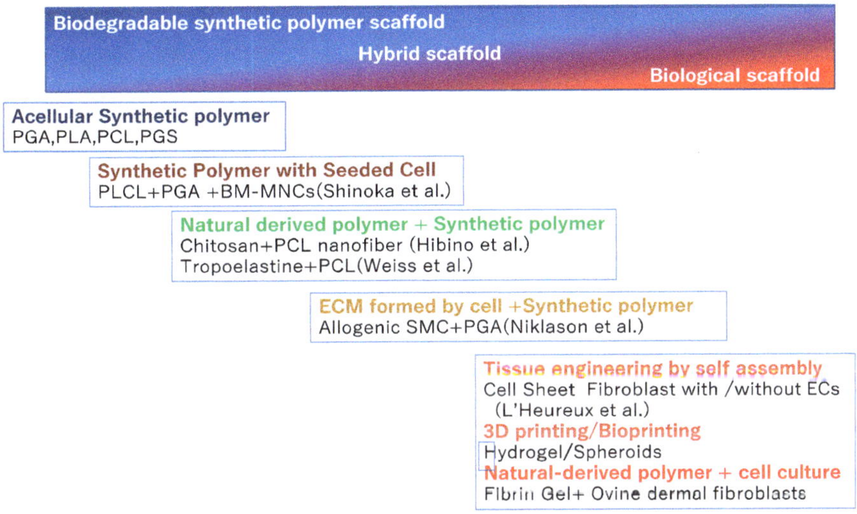

Figure 1. Graft classification by scaffold materials in animal model and clinical studies. Various combinations of biological-based scaffolds and biodegradable synthetic-based scaffolds have been developed and evaluated in large animal models and clinical studies. BM-MNCs, bone marrow mononuclear cells; EC, endothelial cell; PCL, poly (ε-caprolactone); PGA, polyglycolic acid; PLA, poly (lactic acid); PGS, poly (glycerol) sebacate; SMC, smooth muscle cells.

2.1.1. PGA

Poly (glycolic acid) (PGA) is among the most commonly used polymers in TEVGs. It was one of the first biodegradable polymers to be utilized to fabricate a scaffold. PGA degrades into glycolic acid, which is metabolized by cells and broken down into water and carbon dioxide.

Previous reports have shown that a mouse PGA inferior vena cava (IVC) interposition graft takes up to six weeks to lose its mechanical properties [13].

In an arterial model, a scaffold made of PGA alone does not have sufficient structural characteristics to withstand the arterial blood pressure. Furthermore, the rate of PGA degradation does not allow for adequate neotissue to form, often resulting in aneurysmal dilatation as the PGA begins to lose its mechanical integrity. However, the mechanical properties of PGA grafts can be improved through smooth muscle cell seeding or by being combined with other polymers [14].

PGA can be synthesized singly or as a copolymer such as PLA (PLGA). The strength, hydrophilicity, and degradation rate can be adjusted by changing the lactide: glycolide ratio in the PLGA copolymer or the D:L ratio in the lactide monomer [15]. PGA/PLGA degrade more quickly than PLA alone, and the ease with which the degradation time can be adjusted makes them clinically attractive. For this reason they are used as absorbable sutures and orthopedic implants [15,16].

2.1.2. PLA

Poly (L-lactic acid) (PLA) is another biodegradable polymer widely used in tissue engineering. PLA is more hydrophobic than PGA due to the presence of an extra methyl group. Their lower affinity to water leads to longer degradation times (6–12 months) [14]. Thus, studies have reported that PLA takes from months to years to lose its mechanical properties in vivo.

As a result of its hydrophobic characteristics, it displays a tendency towards early thrombogenicity. Therefore, researchers have tried to reduce PLA's thrombotic tendency through cell seeding and/or making chemical surface modifications. Hashi et al. investigated an electrospun, biodegradable PLA TEVG in the arterial circulation of a rat aorta [13]. They suggested that graft patency could be improved by seeding bone marrow mesenchymal cells. The same group saw a 25% improvement in patency when a PLA graft containing hirudin, a thrombin inhibiting polypeptide, was implanted in the abdominal aorta of rats [17].

Additionally, most biodegradable synthetic arterial TEVGs use electrospun nanofibers to withstand the high pressures of the arterial system. Specifically, we have shown electrospun PLA nanofiber grafts have good mechanical properties with high patency in small animal models [18].

Unfortunately, thin fibers and small pore electrospun nanofibrous scaffolds inhibit cell migration which leads to delayed neotissue formation. In contrast, thick fiber and large pore electrospun grafts can enhance the neovascularization and remodeling process by mediating macrophage polarization towards the M2 phenotype [19]. However, electrospun grafts with large pores cause significant blood leakage and exhibit premature loss of mechanical properties. Despite success in small animal models, our current application of these designs to the higher pressures of large animal models have been prone to thrombus formation and graft rupture.

2.1.3. PCL

Poly (ε-caprolactone) (PCL) is an aliphatic polyester that has been thoroughly investigated. PCL has one of the slowest degradation profiles out of all biodegradable polymers [14]. PCL is hydrophobic and exhibits a low melting point. Therefore, the PCL polymer is pliable at lower temperatures, in addition to being highly tunable and easy to fabricate [20].

A series of in vivo studies have evaluated electrospun PCL in rats at 3, 6, and 9 month timepoints. The PCL graft patency was 100% and did not display signs of thrombosis. PCL scaffolds were also found to lose 20%, 50%, and 78% of their initial molecular weight at 3, 12, and 18 month timepoints [21,22].

As a result of it's long durability and ease of handling, PCL is frequently used to create grafts suitable for arterial environments [23]. PCL demonstrates favorable mechanical properties with 70% elongation at break compared to 30% and 25% for PGA and PLA, respectively [14]. Additionally, while numerous studies on a multitude of PCL grafts have been conducted in mice and rats, the material has yet to be fully characterized because rodent lifespans expire before the material fully degrades.

In the case of Poly(l-lactic-co-ε-caprolactone)(PLCL), controlling the composition ratios and molecular weights of the individual polymers from which it is derived, allows for better control of mechanical properties and degradation rates. For example, the PLCL (LA/CL=75/25) heteropolymer is stronger than PCL individually, but manages to keep the 70% elongation at break of PCL [14]. We have confirmed the in vivo feasibility of PLA–PLCL scaffolds in high pressure, small-diameter arterial environments [24]. However, when we attempted to translate the material to a sheep carotid artery model, all grafts ruptured and thrombosed. PCL is a hydrophobic material, and without modifications, will most likely lead to a thrombotic or occluded graft.

2.1.4. PGS

Poly(glycerol sebacate) (PGS) is a soft (~300 kPa) thermoset elastomer [25] and is believed to support constructive remodeling through its rapid absorption and material properties. In vitro studies have shown that 20% of PGS mass is lost within 30 days, whereas there is 70% loss in vivo [26].

Wu et al. demonstrated rapid remodeling and good patency with PGS grafts implanted in rat arteries [26]. The grafts showed complete endothelialization and stained positive for α-SMA and major histocompatibility complex (MHC). Rats survived up to 12 months, with all postoperative failures being related to acute obstruction [27]. The neoartery showed native compliance. Perivascular innervation was observed and response to vasoactive drugs was limited. Notably, the amount of insoluble elastin was comparable to that of native arteries. Quantifying elastin is difficult, and the studies that have attempted to do so remain limited. Nevertheless, with respect to TEVGs, this remains the largest amount of elastin production reported to date. While PGS is a potentially exciting material, there are no reports that it has been successful in large animal models, most likely because of its rapid degradability and lack of strength.

2.2. *Natural Polymeric Biomaterials*

Conceptually, hybrid scaffolds are bio-based materials that enhance biocompatibility and cellular infiltration by incorporating components of a native extracellular matrix (collagen, gelatin, elastin, fibrin). In addition, naturally occurring polymers such as chitosan and silk can improve the overall structural integrity of a graft. Many biological-based scaffold materials have been investigated in small animal models [28,29].

Conceptually, hybrid scaffolds are bio-based materials that enhance biocompatibility and cellular infiltration by incorporating components of a native extracellular matrix (collagen, gelatin, elastin, fibrin). In addition, naturally occurring polymers such as chitosan and silk can improve the overall structural integrity of a graft. Many biological-based scaffold materials have been investigated in small animal models [28,29].

Scaffolds fabricated from naturally occurring polymers offer the potential of improved biocompatibility through enhanced cellular interactions and reduced likelihood of a foreign body reaction. Nevertheless, the biodegradation profiles and mechanical properties of these polymers can be less than optimal. Therefore, natural biomaterials are often combined with biodegradable synthetic polymers or are chemically modified. Of particular note to tissue engineering are elastin and chitosan.

Elastin is a primary constituent of the extracellular matrix and confers compliance to vessels, thereby ensuring smooth blood flow by the storing and releasing of elastic energy. Elastin itself is highly insoluble and a difficult material to handle when creating scaffolds [30]. Hence, there are few scaffolds composed of elastin. Instead of creating an entire scaffold made out of elastin, it is used primarily to supplement a scaffold composed of another material. Weiss et al. have reported successful results in a rabbit model with a two-layer scaffold consisting of an inner layer of recombinant human tropoelastin and an outer layer of PCL [31]. These grafts show similar mechanical strength to a human intrathoracic artery and display low thrombogenicity. The crosslinking of tropoelastin is paramount to increasing its mechanical strength, and these grafts appear promising, however further research is needed to evaluate their scaffold characteristics.

Chitosan (CS) is a natural polymer obtained from shellfish, and in addition to the ease with which it can be chemically modified, it shows good strength, a porous structure, and antibacterial characteristics. CS has been successfully used in bone, cartilage, and skin tissue engineering constructs [32].

Hibino et al. conducted a study on an electrospun PCL-chitosan nanofiber TEVG in a sheep carotid artery model which showed patency of 67% ($n = 6$) [33]. When integrated within a scaffold, rapidly degrading chitosan is thought to promote better cell invasion and neovascular remodeling due to their large pore sizes.

Another technique used to incorporate the strength of naturally occurring extracellular matrix (ECM) into a scaffold is tissue decellularization. Decellularization has been evaluated in a multitude of studies and involves removing most of the cellular and antigenic components of a tissue. The decellularized tissue would then theoretically leave an intact ECM with preserved mechanical properties. A heterologous TEVG constructed with small intestinal submucosa has been successfully transplanted into a sheep model with good results [34]. In this study, the group seeded with endothelial cells (ECs) showed good patency, but the unseeded control group occluded within 15 days. These studies indicate that decellularized vascular scaffolds will result in thrombosis unless the scaffold is endothelialized or receives additional modifications.

In addition, ECM elements can be exposed to physical and chemical stress during a decellularization process, which can adversely affect the biomechanical properties of an ECM. The disadvantages of decellularized materials include the inability to alter the content and structure of an ECM, variability between donor sources, and risk of viral transmission from animal tissues.

The most sophisticated decellularized approach has been successfully implemented by Niklason et al. Their human decellularized TEVG is prepared in vitro using allogeneic human vascular

SMCs [9]. This TEVG has undergone a multicenter clinical trial and will be further described in detail in Section 4.

2.3. *Application of Cell Biology to TEVG*

Endothelial cells and smooth muscle cells are the main components of the intima and media of a blood vessel, respectively. They were incorporated in some of the first tissue engineered graft designs given their importance in vascular function. ECs, SMCs, and fibroblasts are all essential for creating a stable intima. In addition, SMCs account for the majority of an ECM and ultimately define the mechanical properties of scaffolds. Therefore, early TEVG studies enthusiastically studied EC and SMC populations. Early TEVG studies have shown that seeding mononuclear cells on biodegradable grafts promotes rapid intima formation [35] and demonstrated physiological properties comparable to human blood vessels [36]. However, in order to avoid neointimal hyperplasia, hyperproliferation of SMCs must be controlled.

ECs are responsible for many physiological functions and the synthesis of many important regulators and growth factors [37]. It is extremely important to establish a confluent EC monolayer on the luminal surface of a TEVG to confer resistance to hyperplasia and thrombosis. There is a report that transplantation of EC-seeded ePTFE grafts resulted in a significantly higher patency rate compared to an uninoculated ePTFE control [38]. Interestingly, in another study looking at the use of Dacron seeded grafts, it has been reported that ECs in the neointima of the conduit functions at less than 10% of the physiological level found in natural vasculature [39]. Furthermore, it has been reported that 95% ECs seeded onto a graft is lost within 24 hours [39]. Although the limited number of ECs in the lumen of a TEVG may provide beneficial resistance to neointimal hyperplasia and seems to prevent acute thrombosis, the role that EC seeding has on TEVGs should be further investigated in the future.

L'Heureux et al. pioneered the tissue engineering by self assembly approach (TESA), where they cultured sheets of autologous fibroblasts, and fused these sheets via dehydration around a stainless steel mandrel [40]. Subsequently, cultured autologous ECs would be seeded onto the lumen of the scaffold followed by more culturing in a bioreactor. The TESA approach showed promising functional results in early clinical trials as the first ten patients that underwent arteriovenous shunt graft transplantation displayed a primary patency rate of 78% at 1 month (7/9) and 60% at 6 months (5/8) [41].

However, in addition to a manufacturing cost of greater than $15,000 per graft, another criticism of this approach is that it will not help patients who need rapid intervention because it can take up to 9 months to manufacture [42].

2.4. *Application of 3D Printing TEVG*

3D printing is a field that is currently undergoing rapid development and may serve to advance tissue engineering by incorporating non-uniform characteristics that match patient anatomy and increase the ease fabrication [43,44]. The 3D printing TEVG approach enables the creation of linear or branched tubular structures using synthetic or natural biomaterials [45,46]. The main techniques used for 3D printing of biological materials are ink jet, micro extrusion, and laser assisted printing [47,48]. Within these techniques, hydrogels are the most commonly used material because of their liquid-like state and ease of chemical tunability [49,50]. However, to date, hydrogels do not have the needed initial mechanical properties required of a TEVG [51]. Therefore hydrogels are often supplemented with other biomaterials or cell seeding.

3D printed grafts can also forgo the use of hydrogels and use synthetic and/or natural materials. In fact, Hibino et al. produced an electrospun graft made out of PCL and chitosan [52]. In a sheep model, a custom mandrel was 3D printed based on preoperative image processing. Afterwards, the scaffold created by electrospinning PCL and chitosan fibers around this custom mandrel showed satisfactory remodeling 6 months post-operation.

Bioprinting is an extension of the 3D printing field and utilizes cells and/or other media to print tissue- and organ-like structures [53,54]. As individual cells are difficult to work with, they are often aggregated into "spheroids" [55]. 3D bioprinted structures rely on the self assembling nature of spheroids to fuse and create viable neotissue [56] Itoh et al. reported the use of bioprinting multicellular spheroids and transplanting the resulting scaffold into rat abdominal aortas (n = 5) [57]. The TEVGs remained patent until the five day end point of the study, but longer term evaluations are needed to further validate this paradigm.

3D bioprinting as a field has improved immensely in the last decade through the use of spheroids and the improvement of new manufacturing and bioink technologies. While this promising field will likely become more prevalent in tissue engineering applications, focus must be paid to improving ink and scaffold mechanical properties before translation to clinical studies.

3. Clinical Study in Venous Model

In 2001, Shinoka et al. reported the successful transplantation of a TEVG which replaced a 2 cm segment of a four-year-old girl's pulmonary artery [58]. The initial conduit was seeded with cells originally from an explanted peripheral vein. These cells were expanded for eight weeks in culture, then subsequently seeded onto a tubular biodegradable scaffold made of a 50:50 copolymer of ε-polycaprolactone–polylactic acid and reinforced with woven poly (glycolic acid) (PGA) fibers. The graft was fabricated in conjunction with the Japanese textile company GUNZE LTD. The PLCL sponge layer was selected because of its biodegradability and pore size which allow cell infiltration and neotissue formation. The material properties of the PLCL allow for flexibility and ease of handling, however its suture retention strength was limited. A woven layer of PLA or PGA was selected to reinforce the graft as it could be easily incorporated into the manufacturing process of the PLCL sponge layer (Figure 2a–d). The patient had no postoperative complications and displayed a patent graft upon follow-up. After the successful procedure and two additional proof of concept large animal studies, we began a pilot clinical trial investigating the use of biodegradable TEVGs in congenital heart surgery.

Between September 2001 and December 2004, 25 Japanese patients underwent extracardiac total cavopulmonary connection (TCPC) operations with a TEVG [59]. Patient demographics, diagnosis, graft type, and size at the time of implantation are presented in Table 1. The median patient age at the time of operation and mean follow-up time was 5.5 and 11.1 years, respectively [60,61]. There were no incidences of graft-rupture, aneurysmal formation, or ectopic calcification. While eight patients died within the follow-up period, none of the mortalities were due to graft-related complications. In fact, the autopsy of one patient who died 13 years after TEVG implantation revealed a structure similar to that of a native vein or pulmonary artery (Figure 3) [62]. However, seven patients presented with asymptomatic graft stenosis and underwent successful balloon angioplasty, including one that required a repeat catheterization and stent placement. Additionally, one patient's TEVG had a thrombus formation one year after implantation, but this was successfully resolved with anticoagulation drug therapy. When contacted, all surviving patients reported no functional limitations (Figure 4) [61].

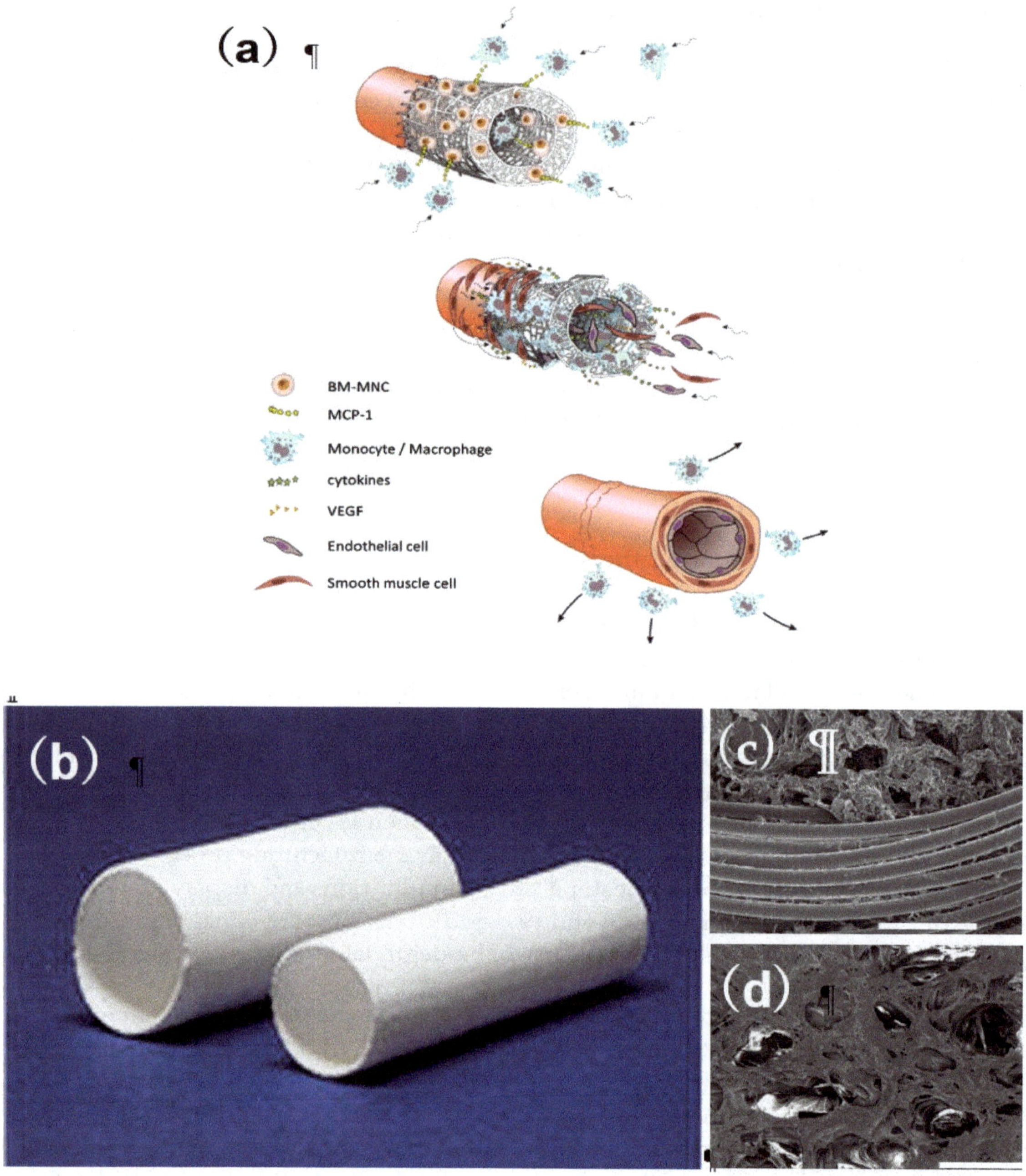

Figure 2. (**a**) Proposed mechanism of neovessel formation after implantation of a cell-seeded biodegradable scaffold. Early pulse of monocyte chemoattractant protein-1 (MCP-1) and related cytokines from seeded bone marrow-derived mononuclear cells (BM-MNCs) enhances early monocyte recruitment to the scaffold. Infiltrating monocytes release multiple angiogenic cytokines and growth factors (e.g., vascular endothelial growth factor (VEGF)), which recruit smooth muscle cells. (**b**) Appearance of tissue engineered vascular graft (TEVG). TEVG has a thickness of 1 mm, and mainly has a length of 13 cm; they are trimmed and implanted according to the anatomy of the patient. (**c**) SEM image of Woven poly (glycolic acid) (PGA). (**d**) SEM image of luminal PCLA; the bar shows 100 μm adopted with permission from Shinoka et al.

Table 1. Characteristics of the patients.

Patient	Main Diagnosis	Age	Graft Type	Graft Size
1	Asplenia, AVSD(A), small RV	2	PLA	16
2	Asplenia, SRV, TAPVC(Ib+III)	1	PLA	20
3	Concordant criss-cross heart, DORV, PAA, MS	8	PLA	18
4	TA(Ib)	22	PLA	24
5	PPA, ASD(II), sinusoidal communication	13	PLA	22
6	SRV, DORV, AVVA	4	PLA	20
7	Total sinus defect, ASD, TR(IV)	14	PLA	24
8	Asplenia, SLV, CAVVR	17	PLA	24
9	TA(Ib)	22	PLA	22
10	Polysplenia, SRV	4	PLA	12
11	HLHS, MA, IAA(A)	2	PLA	16
12	Asplenia, SRV, PAA, non-confluent PA	2	PGA	16
13	SLV, lt AVVA	2	PGA	16
14	DORV, small LV, VSD, PS, ASD(II)	2	PGA	18
15	polysplenia, cAVSD, DORV, PS	2	PGA	12
16	Asplenia, SRV, CA, TAPVC(Ib)	2	PGA	16
17	PPA, RA thrombosis, AFL, af	24	PGA	18
18	SRV, DIRV, PA, ASD(II)	1	PGA	16
19	Asplenia, SRV, PS, CA	11	PGA	18
20	polysplenia, cAVSD, PS, CAVVR	2	PGA	14
21	DORV, VSD, small RV, PLSVC, TAPVC(IIb)	3	PGA	16
22	PPA, ASD(II), PS, Sinusoidal communication	5	PGA	18
23	SLV, DILV, PA, ASD, bilateral SVC	4	PGA	18
24	Asplenia, SRV	13	PGA	16
25	TA(IIc), SAS	2	PGA	18

af, atrial fibrillation; AFL, atrial flutter; ASD, atrial septal defect; AVSD, atrio-ventricular septal defect; AVVA, atrioventricular valve atresia; CA, common atrium; cAVSD, complete atrioventricular septal defect; CAVVR, common atrioventricular valve regurgitation; CAVV, common atrioventricular valve; DILV, double-inlet left ventricle; DIRV, double-inlet right ventricle; DORV, double-outlet right ventricle; HLHS, hypoplastic left heart syndrome; IAA, interruption of aortic arch; LV, left ventricle; MA, mitral atresia; MS, mitral stenosis; PA, pulmonary artery; PAA, pulmonary artery atresia; PLA, poly (lactide acid); PLSVC, persistent left superior vena cava; PPA, pure pulmonary atresia; PS, pulmonary stenosis; RA, right atrium; RV, right ventricle; SAS, subaortic stenosis, SLV, single left ventricle; SRV, single right ventricle; SVC, superior vena cava; TA, tricuspid atresia; TAPVC, total anomalous pulmonary venous connection; TR, tricuspid regurgitation; VSD, ventricular septal defect.

In our next steps, we focused on elucidating the cellular and molecular mechanism resulting in neotissue formation and graft stenosis. Surprisingly, in a murine model, we found that that the cells seeded onto the graft all but disappeared within 24 hrs and were replaced by an abundant macrophage response [63,64]. To characterize the effect of the macrophages, we ran experiments that knocked out macrophage function, only to find that the grafts failed to remodel into neotissue. On the other hand, in unseeded grafts, too much macrophage infiltration was found to lead to stenosis [63,64]. While the original tissue engineering paradigms believed that cells seeded onto a scaffold would eventually constitute the neotissue, we found this not to be the case. We found that host-macrophage infiltration is essential for vascular neotissue formation, while excessive infiltration underlies stenosis. Our findings suggested that achieving the proper balance of macrophage infiltration and function is critical for successful neovessel formation [65].

Subsequently, we have continued to investigate the effect of seeding bone marrow-derived mononuclear cells on TEVGs in lambs, as the ovine model is preferred by the FDA due to its propensity to undergo accelerated calcification. As previously mentioned, when we began our original large animal studies in the late 1990s, we expanded cells from an explanted vein, a process that would take anywhere from 8 to 12 weeks [66]. Cell expansion is a time-consuming and costly process. Additionally, cultured cells are susceptible to infection. Being able to utilize bone marrow as a cell source cut a process that required two separate surgeries over the course of a few months to one procedure that could be completed in a day. We are developing a closed, disposable system which will allow for improved seeding efficiency and reduce the risk of infection [67].

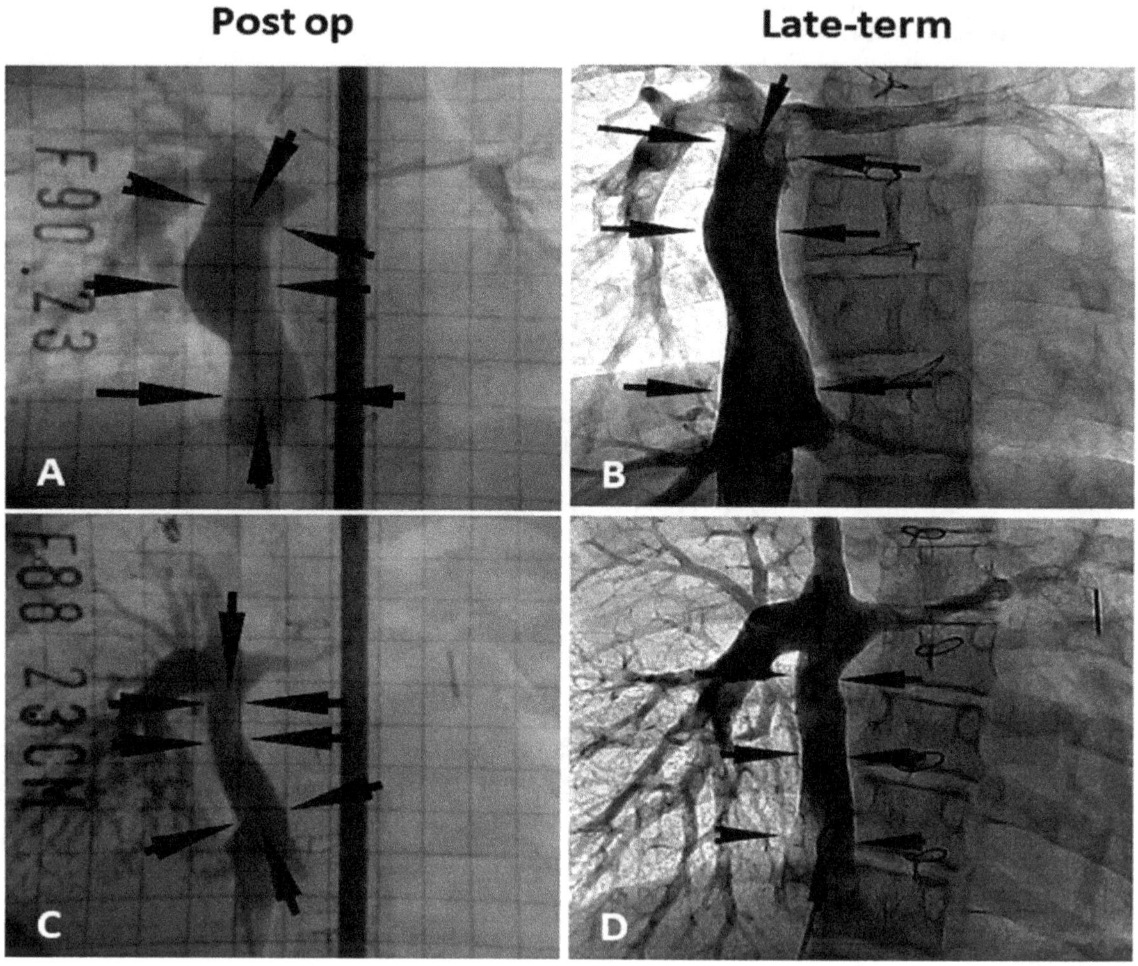

Figure 3. Postoperative and late-term TEVG angiography. (**A**) Postoperative angiography in patient 22. (**B**) Angiography 11 years after implantation in patient 22. (**C**) Postoperative angiography in patient 23. (**D**) Angiography eight years after implantation in patient 23. Arrows indicate the TEVG location. Angiography shows macroscopic growth of the TEVGs. Adopted with permission from Shinoka et al.

In regards to the development of graft stenosis, our focus is aimed at modulating the macrophage response. To date, we have shown that pharmacological treatment with a Tgfbr1 inhibitor prevents macrophage induced stenosis and future studies will look at the ability of losartan, an angiotensin II receptor blocker, to mitigate the formation of graft stenosis [68].

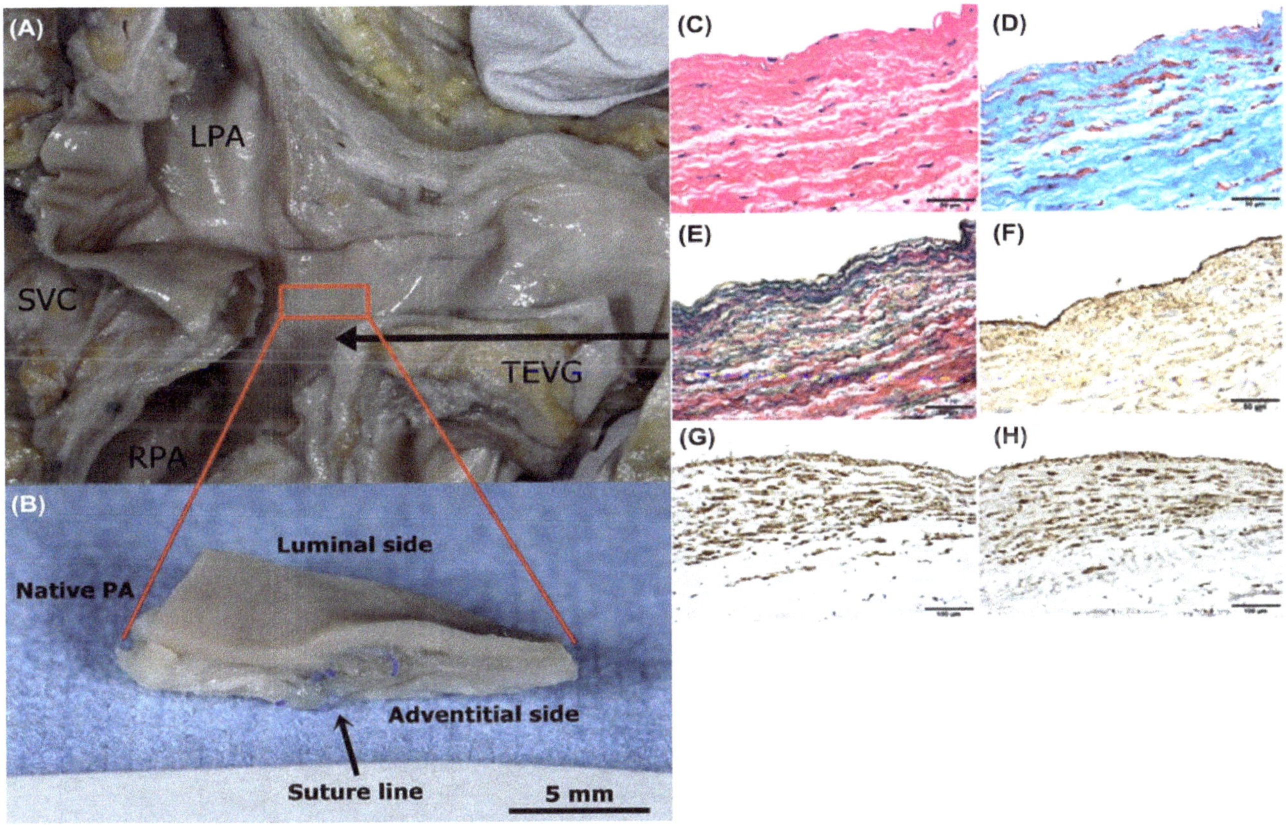

Figure 4. Macroscopic and histological images of explanted human TEVG. A female patient with a single right ventricle underwent TCPC with common atrioventricular valve plasty at age 4 years. A 12-mm-diameter biodegradable synthetic TEVG with BM-MNCs was implanted between the hepatic vein and pulmonary artery. Unfortunately, she died 12 years later and an autopsy was performed. (**A**) Macroscopic imaging of the TEVG. No difference appears between native PA and TEVG. (**B**) Cross-section view of the border between native PA and TEVG. (**C**) Hematoxylin-eosin staining. (**D**) Masson trichrome staining. (**E**) Victoria blue-van Gieson staining. (**F**) Factor VIII–positive cells (brown). (**G**) α-Smooth muscle actin–positive cells (brown). (**H**) Calponin-positive cells (brown). LPA, left pulmonary artery; PA, pulmonary artery; RPA, right pulmonary artery; SVC, superior vena cava; TCPC, total cavopulmonary connection; TEVG, tissue engineered vascular graft. Modified from Matsumura G, Shinoka T. First report of histological evaluation of human tissue-engineered vasculature. J Biotechnol Biomater 2015; 5:200 Adopted with permission from Shinoka et al.

4. Clinical Study in Arterial Model

Historically, the development of TEVGs in the arterial system has faced many difficulties as the currently available materials have been unable to withstand high arterial pressures while simultaneously allowing for graft degradation and host remodeling. The human acellular TEVG for dialysis access in patients with End-Stage Renal Disease (is a promising new technology that has been developed by Niklason et al. of [9]. In their approach organ donor-derived SMCs are seeded onto PGA scaffolds and then cultured in a pulsatile bioreactor to stimulate extracellular matrix production. The ester hydrolysis which occurs on the PGA fiber surface results in increased hydrophilicity with an increase in the adsorption of serum proteins and contributes to SMC adhesion. After the initial SMC seeding period of 30 minutes, the bioreactor was filled with medium and the SMCs were cultured for eight weeks under conditions of beating radial stress. The histological examination suggests that pulsatile stimulation is required to promote smooth muscle cell migration. [69]. After the successful creation of an ECM rich scaffold, the grafts were decellularized to remove allogeneic antigens and implanted as vascular scaffolds within baboons and canines to evaluate their in vivo function and remodeling over time.

Their first set of animal experiments evaluated a small diameter (3–4 mm) TEVG in a canine peripheral arterial and coronary bypass model. The graft was created as detailed above with the requirement that cells were sourced from a canine in order to avoid cellular rejection after implantation. It should be noted that following the decellularization process they additionally seeded the grafts with ECs over an additional two days [69]. After excluding for surgical mortality in the setting of patent grafts, they demonstrated long-term patency in five out of six grafts at one month [69].

A baboon model preclinical evaluation was undertaken to evaluate the graft as an arteriovenous shunt. Briefly, grafts 6 mm in diameter were implanted as arteriovenous shunts between an axillary artery and brachial vein. A total of eight grafts were implanted, followed by routine ultrasound to determine patency and evaluated at explant of one, three, or six months. Patency rates were 100%, 66%, and 100% at one, two, and six month explants, respectively. Only one graft showed thrombosis at three months, likely because of technical difficulties with access, which required prolonged manual pressure that led to graft clotting. Hence, the sum total patency of the arteriovenous 6 mm TEVGs in the baboon was 88% (seven of eight) [70]. Following these encouraging preclinical results, human clinical trials were conducted. Two phase two clinical trials were conducted in a total of 60 patients with the graft implanted as an arteriovenous shunt. Mean follow up was 16 months with 12 month patency rates of 28% primary patency, 38% primary assisted patency, and 89% secondary patency [9]. Secondary patency was defined as functional access patency. These cell-free transplants did not elicit an immune response and no aneurysms were reported in the study. An acellular TEVG partially biopsied at 16 weeks showed re-population of host SMC, fibroblasts, and luminal ECs. This host cell repopulation appears to progress over time, as another specimen obtained at 55 weeks showed further progressive remodeling with SMA more highly expressed throughout the vessel [9].

5. Conclusions

In recent years, we have seen the adaptation of tissue engineering techniques from the bench to the bedside to advance the field of cardiovascular biology and improve patient care. The methods of vascular tissue engineering are diverse and seek to capitalize on advances in material design and cellular biology. Clinical trials have demonstrated innovative applications of tissue engineering principles but highlight the limitations of the currently employed techniques. The ideal TEVG should be readily available, cost effective, easy to handle, and offer growth potential if required. Furthermore, the scaffold should be resistant to the development of thrombosis, stenosis, calcification, or infection as neotissue assumes physiologic vascular function.

Further research will focus on optimizing scaffolds to improve the prospects of current technologies and advance the field of cardiovascular surgery. The difficulty in scaling graft technologies from small to large animal models within the arterial circulation underscores the challenges that remain before the more widespread adoption of these innovations to patients. Despite these difficulties, the clinical translation of TEVGs is greatly anticipated based on market forces and patient needs.

Author Contributions: (I) Conception and design: All authors; (II) Administrative support: All authors; (III) Provision of study materials or patients: All authors; (IV) Collection and assembly of data: All authors; (V) Data analysis and interpretation: All authors; (VI) Manuscript writing: All authors; (VII) Final approval of manuscript: All authors.

Acknowledgments: Matsuzaki was the recipient of a Funding Award from the Uehara Memorial Foundation 2019 (Tokyo, Japan).

References

1. Van der Linde, D.; Konings, E.E.; Slager, M.A.; Witsenburg, M.; Helbing, W.A.; Takkenberg, J.J.; Roos-Hesselink, J.W. Birth prevalence of congenital heart disease worldwide: A systematic review and meta-analysis. *J. Am. Coll. Cardiol.* **2011**, *58*, 2241–2247. [CrossRef] [PubMed]
2. Simeone, R.M.; Oster, M.E.; Cassell, C.H.; Armour, B.S.; Gray, D.T.; Honein, M.A. Pediatric inpatient hospital resource use for congenital heart defects. *Birth Defects Res. A Clin. Mol. Teratol.* **2014**, *100*, 934–943. [CrossRef] [PubMed]
3. Mozaffarian, D.; Benjamin, E.J.; Go, A.S.; Arnett, D.K.; Blaha, M.J.; Cushman, M.; De Ferranti, S.; Després, J.P.; Fullerton, H.J.; Howard, V.J.; et al. Heart Disease and Stroke Statistics—2015 update: A report from the American Heart Association. *Circulation* **2015**, *131*, e29–e322. [CrossRef] [PubMed]
4. van der Slegt, J.; Steunenberg, S.L.; Donker, J.M. The current position of precuffed expanded polytetrafluoroethylene bypass grafts in peripheral vascular surgery. *J. Vasc. Surg.* **2014**, *60*, 120–128. [CrossRef] [PubMed]
5. Drews, J.D.; Miyachi, H.; Shinoka, T. Tissue-engineered vascular grafts for congenital cardiac disease: Clinicalexperience and current status. *Trends Cardiovasc. Med.* **2017**, *27*, 521–531. [CrossRef] [PubMed]
6. Langer, R.; Vacanti, J.P. Tissue engineering. *Science* **1993**, *260*, 920–926. [CrossRef] [PubMed]
7. Weinberg, C.B.; Bell, E. A blood vessel model constructed from collagen and cultured vascular cells. *Science* **1986**, *231*, 397–400. [CrossRef] [PubMed]
8. Matsumura, G.; Hibino, N.; Ikada, Y.; Kurosawa, H.; Shinoka, T. Successful application of tissue engineered vascular autografts: Clinical experience. *Biomaterials* **2003**, *24*, 2303–2308. [CrossRef]
9. Lawson, J.H.; Glickman, M.H.; Ilzecki, M.; Jakimowics, T.; Jaroszynski, A.; Peden, E.K.; Piglim, A.J.; Prichaed, H.L.; Guziewics, M.; Przywana, S.; et al. Bioengineered human acellular vessels for dialysis access in patients with end-stage renal disease: Two phase 2 single-arm trials. *Lancet* **2016**, *387*, 2026–2034. [CrossRef]
10. Rosso, F.; Marino, G.; Giordano, A.; Barbarisi, M.; Parmeggiani, D.; Barbarisi, A. Smart materials as scaffolds for tissue engineering. *J. Cell. Physiol.* **2005**, *203*, 465–470. [CrossRef] [PubMed]
11. Crapo, P.M.; Gilbert, T.W.; Badylak, S.F. An overview of tissue and whole organ decellularization processes. *Biomaterials* **2011**, *32*, 3233–3243. [CrossRef] [PubMed]
12. Hashi, C.K.; Zhu, Y.; Yang, G.Y.; Young, W.L.; Hsiao, B.S.; Wang, K.; Chu, B.; Li, S. Antithrombogenic property of bone marrow mesenchymal stem cells in nanofibrous vascular grafts. *Proc. Natl. Acad. Sci. USA* **2007**, *104*, 11915–11920. [CrossRef] [PubMed]
13. Xue, L.; Greisler, H.P. Biomaterials in the development and future of vascular grafts. *J. Vasc. Surg.* **2003**, *37*, 472–480. [CrossRef]
14. Tara, S.; Rocco, K.A.; Hibino, N.; Sugiura, T.; Kurobe, H.; Breuer, C.K.; Shinoka, T. Vessel bioengineering. *Circ. J.* **2014**, *78*, 12–19. [CrossRef]
15. Hajiali, H.; Shahgasempour, S.; Naimi-Jamal, M.R.; Peirovi, H. Electrospun PGA/gelatin nanofibrous scaffolds and their potential application in vascular tissue engineering. *J. Mater. Sci.* **2010**, *21*, 1761–1769. [CrossRef] [PubMed]
16. Treiser, M.; Abramson, S.; Langer, R.; Kohn, J. Degradable and resorbable materials. In *Biomaterials Science An Introduction to Materials in Medicine. Chapeter I.2.6. Degradable and Resorbable Biomaterials*; Elsevier: London, UK, 2013. [CrossRef]
17. Hashi, C.K.; Derugin, N.; Janairo, R.R.; Lee, R.; Schultz, D.; Lotz, J.; Li, S. Antithrombogenic modification of small-diameter microfibrous vascular grafts. *Arterioscler. Thromb. Vasc. Biol.* **2010**, *30*, 1621–1627. [CrossRef] [PubMed]
18. Sugiura, T.; Tara, S.; Nakayama, H.; Kurobe, H.; Yi, T.; Lee, A.Y.; Breuer, C.K.; Shinoka, T. Novel Bioresorbable Vascular Graft With Sponge-Type Scaffold as a Small-Diameter Arterial Graft. *Ann. Thorac. Surg.* **2016**, *102*, 720–727. [CrossRef]
19. Garg, K.; Pullen, N.A.; Oskeritzian, C.A.; Ryan, J.J.; Bowlin, G.L. Macrophage functional polarization (M1/M2) in response to varying fiber and pore dimensions of electrospun scaffolds. *Biomaterials* **2013**, *34*, 4439–4451. [CrossRef]

20. Miyamoto, S.; Shoji, T.; MIyachi, H.; Shinoka, T. Smart Biomaterials for Cardiovascular Tissue Engineering. In *Smart Materials for Tissue Engineering: Application*; Royal Society of Chemistry: London, UK, 2017; pp. 230–257.
21. Pektok, E.; Nottelet, B.; Tille, J.C. Degradation and healing characteristics of small-diameter poly(epsilon-caprolactone) vascular grafts in the rat systemic arterial circulation. *Circulation* **2008**, *118*, 2563–2570. [CrossRef]
22. de Valence, S.; Tille, J.C.; Mugnai, D. Long term performance of polycaprolactone vascular grafts in a rat abdominal aorta replacement model. *Biomaterials* **2012**, *33*, 38–47. [CrossRef] [PubMed]
23. Nottelet, B.; Pektok, E.; Mandracchia, D.; Tille, J.C.; Walpoth, B.; Gurny, R.; Moller, M. Factorial design optimization and in vivo feasibility of poly(epsilon-caprolactone)-micro- and nanofiber-based small diameter vascular grafts. *J. Biomed. Mater. Res. Part A* **2009**, *89*, 865–875. [CrossRef] [PubMed]
24. Tara, S.; Kurobe, H.; Rocco, K.A.; Maxfield, M.W.; Best, C.A.; Yi, T.; Breuer, C.K.; Shinoka, T. Well-organized neointima of large-pore poly(L-lactic acid) vascular graft coated with poly(L-lactic-*co*-ε-caprolactone) prevents calcific deposition compared to small-pore electrospun poly(L-lactic acid) graft in a mouse aortic implantation model. *Athelioscrerosis* **2014**, *237*, 684–691. [CrossRef] [PubMed]
25. Wang, Y.; Ameer, G.A.; Sheppard, B.J.; Langer, R. A tough biodegradable elastomer. *Nat. Biotechnol.* **2002**, *20*, 602–606. [CrossRef] [PubMed]
26. Allen, R.A.; Wu, W.; Yao, M.; Dutta, D.; Duan, X.; Bachman, T.N. Nerve regeneration and elastin formation within poly(glycerol sebacate)-based synthetic arterial grafts one-year post-implantation in a rat model. *Biomaterials* **2014**, *35*, 165–173. [CrossRef] [PubMed]
27. Yokota, T.; Ichikawa, H.; Matsumiya, G.; Kuratani, T.; Sakaguchi, T.; Iwai, S. In situ tissue regeneration using a novel tissue-engineered, small-caliber vascular graft without cell seeding. *J. Thorac. Cardiovasc. Surg.* **2008**, *136*, e900–e907. [CrossRef] [PubMed]
28. Pektok, E.; Nottelet, B.; Tille, J.C.; Gurny, R.; Kalangos, A.; Moeller, M. Degradation and healing characteristics of small-diameter poly(ε-capro-lactone) vascular grafts in the rat systemic arterial circulation. *Circulation* **2008**, *118*, 2563–2570. [CrossRef]
29. Taylor, M.S.; Shalaby, S.W. Sutures. In *Biomaterials Science: An Introduction to Materials in Medicine*; Elsevier: Amsterdam, The Netherlands, 2013; pp. 1010–1024.
30. Raboud, M.; Lefebvre, F.; Ducassou, D. In vitro association of type III collagen with elastin and with its solubilized peptides. *Biomaterials* **1991**, *12*, 313–319. [CrossRef]
31. Wise, S.; Byrom, M.J.; Waterhouse, A.; Bannon, P.G.; Weiss, A.S.; Ng, M.K. A multilayered synthetic human elastin/polycaprolactone hybrid vascular graft with tailored mechanical properties. *Acta Biomater.* **2011**, *7*, 295–303. [CrossRef]
32. Kim, I.Y.; Seo, S.J.; Moon, H.S.; Yoo, M.K.; Park, I.Y.; Kim, B.C.; Cho, C.S. Chitosan and its derivatives for tissue engineering applications. *Biotechnol. Adv.* **2008**, *26*, 21–32. [CrossRef]
33. Fukunishi, T.; Best, C.A.; Sugiura, T.; Shoji, T.; Yi, T.; Udelsman, B.; Ohst, D.; Ong, C.S.; Zhang, H.; Shinoka, T.; Breuer, C.K.; Johnson, J.; Hibino, N. Tissue-engineered small diameter arterial vascular grafts from cell-free nanofiber PCL/chitosan scaffolds in a sheep model. *PLoS ONE* **2016**, *11*, e0158555. [CrossRef]
34. Greisler, H.P.; Joyce, K.A.; Kim, D.U.; Pham, S.M.; Berceli, S.A.; Borovetz, H.S. Spatial and temporal changes in compliance following implantation of bio-resorbable vascular grafts. *J. Biomed. Mater. Res.* **1992**, *26*, 1449–1461. [CrossRef]
35. Greisler, H.P.; Cabusao, E.B.; Lam, T.M.; Murchan, P.M.; Ellinger, J.; Kim, D.U. Kinetics of collagen deposition within bioresorbable and nonresorbable vascular prostheses. *ASAIO Trans.* **1991**, *37*, M472–M475.
36. Wang, Z.; Cui, Y.; Wang, J.; Yang, X.; Wu, Y.; Wang, K.; Gao, X.; Li, D.; Li, Y.; Zheng, X.L.; Kong, D.; Zhao, Q. The effect of thick fibers and large pores of electrospun poly (epsilon-caprolactone) vascular grafts on macrophage polarization and arterial regeneration. *Biomaterials* **2014**, *35*, 5700–5710. [CrossRef]
37. Janairo, R.R.R.; Zhu, Y.; Chen, T.; Li, S. Mucin covalently bonded to microfibers improves the patency of vascular grafts. *Tissue Eng. Part A* **2014**, *20*, e285–e293. [CrossRef]
38. Walles, T.; Gorler, H.; Puschmann, C.; Mertsching, H. Functional neointima characterization of vascular prostheses in human. *Ann. Thorac. Surg.* **2004**, *77*, 864–868. [CrossRef] [PubMed]
39. Rosenman, J.E.; Kempczinski, R.F.; Pearce, W.H.; Edward, B.S. Kinetics of endothelial cell seeding. *J. Vasc. Surg.* **1985**, *2*, 778–784. [CrossRef]

40. L'Heureux, N.; Dusserre, N.; Konig, G.; Victor, B.; Keire, P.; Wight, T.N. Human tissue-engineered blood vessels for adult arterial revascularization. *Nat. Med.* **2006**, *12*, 361–365. [CrossRef] [PubMed]
41. McAllister, T.N.; Maruszewski, M.; Garrido, S.A.; Wystrychowski, W.; Dusserre, N.; Marini, A.; Zagaiski, K.; Fiorillo, A.; Avila, H.; Manglano, X.; et al. Effectiveness of haemodialysis access with an autologous tissue-engineered vascular graft: A multicentre cohort study. *Lancet* **2009**, *373*, 1440–1446. [CrossRef]
42. Mount, C.; Dusserre, N.; Mcallister, T.; L'Heureux, N. Tissue-engineered cardiovascular grafts and novel applications of tissue engineering by self-assembly (TESA): Biomaterials and tissue engineering. In *Cardiac Regeneration and Repair*; Li, R.-K., Weisel, R.D., Eds.; Woodhead Publishing: Sawston, UK, 2014; Volume 2, pp. 434–435.
43. Murphy, S.V.; Atala, A. 3D bioprinting of tissues and organs. *Nat. Biotechnol.* **2014**, *32*, 773–785. [CrossRef]
44. Borovjagin, A.V.; Ogle, B.M.; Berry, J.L.; Zhang, J. From Microscale Devices to 3D Printing: Advances in Fabrication of 3D Cardiovascular Tissues. *Circ. Res.* **2017**, *120*, 150–165. [CrossRef] [PubMed]
45. Mosadegh, B.; Xiong, G.; Dunham, S.; Min, J.K. Current progress in 3D printing for cardiovascular tissue engineering. *Biomed. Mater.* **2015**, *10*, 034002. [CrossRef] [PubMed]
46. Mota, C.; Puppi, D.; Chiellini, F.; Chiellini, E. Additive manufacturing techniques for the production of tissue engineering constructs: Additive manufacturing techniques for the production of tissue engineering constructs. *J. Tissue Eng. Regen. Med.* **2015**, *9*, 174–190. [CrossRef]
47. Hölzl, K.; Lin, S.; Tytgat, L.; Van Vlierberghe, S.; Gu, L.; Ovsianikov, A. Bioink properties before, during and after 3D bioprinting. *Biofabrication* **2016**, *8*, 032002. [CrossRef]
48. Gopinathan, J.; Noh, I. Recent trends in bioinks for 3D printing. *Biomater. Res.* **2018**, *22*, 11. [CrossRef] [PubMed]
49. Tabriz, A.G.; Hermida, M.A.; Leslie, N.R.; Shu, W. Three-dimensional bioprinting of complex cell laden alginate hydrogel structures. *Biofabrication* **2015**, *7*, 045012. [CrossRef]
50. Alemán, J.V.; Chadwick, A.V.; He, J.; Hess, M.; Horie, K.; Jones, R.G.; Kratochvíl, P.; Meisel, I.; Mita, I.; Moad, G. Definitions of terms relating to the structure and processing of sols, gels, networks, and inorganic-organic hybrid materials (IUPAC Recommendations 2007). *Pure Appl. Chem.* **2007**, *79*, 1801–1829. [CrossRef]
51. Hoffman, A.S. Hydrogels for biomedical applications. *Adv. Drug Deliv. Rev.* **2012**, *64*, 18–23. [CrossRef]
52. Fukunishi, T.; Best, C.A.; Sugiura, T.; Opfermann, J.; Ong, C.S.; Shinoka, T.; Breuer, C.K.; Krieger, A.; Johnson, J.; Hibino, N. Preclinical study of patient-specific cell-free nanofiber tissue-engineered vascular grafts using 3-dimensional printing in a sheep model. *J. Thorac. Cardiovasc. Surg.* **2017**, *153*, 924–932. [CrossRef] [PubMed]
53. Ji, S.; Guvendiren, M. Recent Advances in Bioink Design for 3D Bioprinting of Tissues and Organs. *Front. Bioeng. Biotechnol.* **2017**, *5*, 23. [CrossRef]
54. Gelinsky, M. Biopolymer hydrogel bioinks. In *3D Bioprinting for Reconstructive Surgery*; Thomas, D.J., Jessop, Z.M., Whitaker, I.S., Eds.; Elsevier Science & Technology: Cambridge, UK, 2018; pp. 125–136.
55. Vijayavenkataraman, S.; Yan, W.-C.; Lu, W.F.; Wang, C.-H.; Fuh, J.Y.H. 3D bioprinting of tissues and organs for regenerative medicine. *Adv. Drug Deliv. Rev.* **2018**, *13*, 296–332. [CrossRef] [PubMed]
56. Mironov, V.; Visconti, R.P.; Kasyanov, V.; Forgacs, G.; Drake, C.J.; Markwald, R.R. Organ printing: Tissue spheroids as building blocks. *Biomaterials* **2009**, *30*, 2164–2174. [CrossRef] [PubMed]
57. Itoh, M.; Nakayama, K.; Noguchi, R.; Kamohara, K.; Furukawa, K.; Uchihashi, K.; et al. Correction: Scaffold-free tubular tissues created by a Bio-3D printer undergo remodeling and endothelialization when implante in rat aortae. *PLoS ONE* **2015**, *10*, e0145971. [CrossRef]
58. Shinoka, T.; Imai, Y.; Ikada, Y. Transplantation of a tissue-engineered pulmonary artery. *N. Engl. J. Med.* **2001**, *344*, 532–533. [CrossRef] [PubMed]
59. Shinoka, T.; Matsumura, G.; Hibino, N.; Naito, Y.; Watanabe, W.; Konuma, T.; Sakamoto, T.; Nagatsu, M.; Kurosawa, H. Midterm clinical result of tissue-engineered vascular autografts seeded with autologous bone marrow cells. *J. Thorac. Cardiovasc. Surg.* **2005**, *129*, 1330–1338. [CrossRef] [PubMed]
60. Hibino, N.; McGillicuddy, E.; Matsumura, G.; Ichihara, Y.; Naito, Y.; Breuer, C.K.; Shinoka, T. Late-term results of tissue- engineered vascular grafts in humans. *J. Thorac. Cardiovasc. Surg.* **2010**, *139*, 431–436. [CrossRef] [PubMed]

61. Sugiura, T.; Matsumura, G.; Miyamoto, S.; Miyachi, H.; Breuer, C.K.; Shinoka, T. Tissue-engineered Vascular Grafts in Children With Congenital Heart Disease: Intermediate Term Follow-up. *Semin. Thoracic. Surg.* **2018**, *30*, 175–179. [CrossRef] [PubMed]
62. Shinoka, T. What is the best material for extracardiac Fontan operation? *J. Thorac. Cardiovasc. Surg.* **2017**, *153*, 1551–1552. [CrossRef]
63. Harrington, J.K.; Chahboune, H.; Criscione, J.M.; Li, A.Y.; Hibino, N.; Yi, T.; Villalona, G.A.; Kobsa, S.; Meijas, D.; Duncan, D.R.; et al. Determining the fate of seeded cells in venous tissue-engineered vascular grafts using serial MRI. *FASEB J.* **2011**, *25*, 4150–4161. [CrossRef]
64. Brennan, M.P.; Dardik, A.; Hibino, N.; Roh, J.D.; Nelson, G.N.; Papademitris, X.; SHinoka, T.; Breure, C.K. Tissue-engineered vascular grafts demonstrate evidence of growth and development when implanted in a juvenile animal model. *Ann. Surg.* **2008**, *248*, 370–377. [CrossRef]
65. Hibino, N.; Yi, T.; Duncan, D.R.; Dean, E.; Naito, Y.; Dardik, A.; Kyriakides, T.; Madri, J.; Pober, J.S.; Shinoka, T.; Breuer, C.K. A critical role for macrophages in neovessel formation and the development of stenosis in tissue-engineered vascular grafts. *FASEB J.* **2011**, *25*, 4253–4263. [CrossRef] [PubMed]
66. Watanabe, M.; Shin'oka, T.; Tohyama, S.; Hibino, N.; Konuma, T.; Matsumura, G.; Kosaka, Y.; Ishida, T.; Imai, Y.; Yamanaka, M.; et al. Tissue-engineered vascular autograft: Inferior vena cava replacement in a dog model. *Tissue Eng.* **2001**, *7*, 429–439. [CrossRef] [PubMed]
67. Best, C.; Tara, S.; Wiet, M.; Reinhardt, J.; Pepper, V.; Ball, M.; Yi, T.; Shinoka, T.; Breuer, C.K. Deconstructing the tissue engineered vascular graft; evaluating scaffold pre-wetting, conditioned media incubation, and determining the optimal mononuclear cell source. *ACS Biomater. Sci. Eng.* **2017**, *3*, 1972–1979. [CrossRef]
68. Ruiz-Rosado, J.D.; Mahler, N.; Yi, T.; Robledo, A.F.; Martinez, S.D.; Lee, A.Y.; Shoji, T.; Lee, A.Y.; Heuer, E.; Yates, A.R. Angiotensin II receptor I blockade prevents stenosis of tissue engineered vascular grafts. *FASEB J.* **2018**, *15*, fj201800458. [CrossRef] [PubMed]
69. Niklason, L.E.; Gao, J.; Abbott, W.M.; Hirschi, K.K.; Houser, S.; Marini, R.; Langer, R. Functional Arteries Grown in Vitro. *Science* **1999**, *284*, 489–493. [CrossRef]
70. Prichard, H.L.; Manson, R.J.; Di Bernardo, L.; Nikalson, L.E.; Lawson, J.H.; Dash, S.L. An early study on the mechanisms that allow tissue-engineered vascular grafts to resist intimal hyperplasia. *J. Cardiovasc. Transl. Res. J. Cardiovasc. Transl.* **2011**, *4*, 674–682. [CrossRef]

2

Finite Element Simulation and Additive Manufacturing of Stiffness-Matched NiTi Fixation Hardware for Mandibular Reconstruction Surgery

Ahmadreza Jahadakbar [1], Narges Shayesteh Moghaddam [1], Amirhesam Amerinatanzi [1], David Dean [2], Haluk E. Karaca [3] and Mohammad Elahinia [1,*]

1 Dynamic and Smart Systems Laboratory, The University of Toledo, Toledo, OH 43606, USA; ajahada@rockets.utoledo.edu (A.J.); Narges.ShayestehMoghaddam@rockets.utoledo.edu (N.S.M.); Amirhesam.Amerinatanzi@rockets.utoledo.edu (A.A.)
2 Department of Plastic Surgery, The Ohio State University, Columbus, OH 43212, USA; David.Dean@osumc.edu
3 Department of Mechanical Engineering, The University of Kentucky, Lexington, KY 40506, USA; karacahaluk@uky.edu
* Correspondence: mohammad.elahinia@utoledo.edu.

Academic Editor: Gou-Jen Wang

Abstract: Process parameters and post-processing heat treatment techniques have been developed to produce both shape memory and superelastic NiTi using Additive Manufacturing. By introducing engineered porosity, the stiffness of NiTi can be tuned to the level closely matching cortical bone. Using additively manufactured porous superelastic NiTi, we have proposed the use of patient-specific, stiffness-matched fixation hardware, for mandible skeletal reconstructive surgery. Currently, Ti-6Al-4V is the most commonly used material for skeletal fixation devices. Although this material offers more than sufficient strength for immobilization during the bone healing process, the high stiffness of Ti-6Al-4V implants can cause stress shielding. In this paper, we present a study of mandibular reconstruction that uses a dry cadaver mandible to validate our geometric and biomechanical design and fabrication (i.e., 3D printing) of NiTi skeletal fixation hardware. Based on the reference-dried mandible, we have developed a Finite Element model to evaluate the performance of the proposed fixation. Our results show a closer-to-normal stress distribution and an enhanced contact pressure at the bone graft interface than would be in the case with Ti-6Al-4V off-the-shelf fixation hardware. The porous fixation plates used in this study were fabricated by selective laser melting.

Keywords: additive manufacturing (AM); superelastic NiTi; porosity; mandibular reconstructive surgery; finite element analysis; stiffness matching

---

1. Introduction

Additive manufacturing (AM), also known as 3D printing, is useful for creating complex parts directly from Computer Aided Design (CAD) software. In general, all AM processes create physical parts directly from CAD data by adding material in successive layers. This layer-by-layer production process makes it possible to fabricate structures with engineered porosity. Current 3D printing devices used for the additive manufacturing of metals create layers by sintering or melting metal powders with a laser or an electron beam. These powder-bed technologies, such as Selective Laser Sintering (SLS), Selective Laser Melting (SLM), and direct metal laser sintering are the most common AM processes for AM fabrication of metal parts [1,2].

Figure 1 illustrates the core components of conventional SLM or SLS 3D printing. First, the shape of the part as presented in the CAD file has to be converted into horizontal slices, layers that can be individually 3D printed. Subsequently, the file that contains the information for all of the layers is transferred to the AM machine. For powder-bed SLM processes, the powder material is spread by a blade, knife, or roller on a build plate. Then the laser melts and solidifies selective areas of the powder bed and creates the first layer of the part. After the fabrication of each layer, a new layer of powder is spread on top of the previous layer, and the laser sinters or melts the new layer onto the previously formed layer. The process is repeated until the fabrication process is completed. At the end of the process, the final part is surrounded by loose powder and the part is removed from the build plate [3].

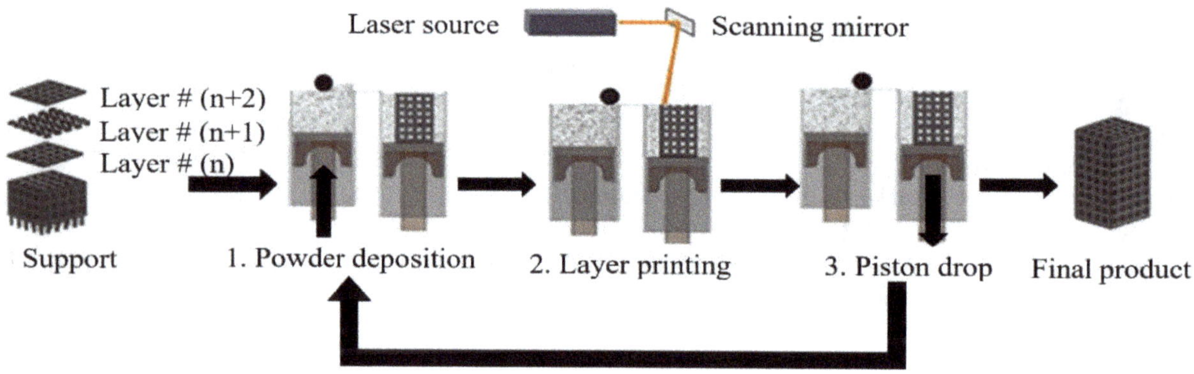

Figure 1. Additive Manufacturing (AM; 3D Printing) of metal parts.

NiTi is the most common shape memory alloy (SMA) showing unique functional properties, i.e., shape memory and superelasticity behavior [4,5]. Porous superelastic NiTi, in particular, has attracted much attention to be used in metallic implants due to their low stiffness close to that of cortical bone (i.e., 10–31.2 GPa), biocompatibility, hysteresis behaviors, and appropriate mechanical properties [1,6–8]. AM processes make it possible to fabricate implants with engineered porosity [9]. Recently, we have used SLM to create porous NiTi implants and medical devices [10–16].

Habijan et al. [17] have shown that the additively manufactured dense and porous NiTi samples are suitable carriers for human mesenchymal stem cells (hMSC) and the ion release (with the maximum concentration of 3.2 μg/L) is significantly below cytotoxic concentrations (25 mg/L). These achievements confirmed the biocompatibility and cytocompatibility of dense and porous NiTi [18]. These values are comparable to those obtained for the most common biocompatible material, i.e., Ti-6Al-4V [19].

It should be pointed out that the as-fabricated Ni-rich NiTi needs post-process heat treatments (i.e., solution annealing and aging) to acquire superelasticity behavior. In this study, we have completed a case study by using AM fabricated stiffness-matched porous NiTi skeletal fixation plates that would be useful in mandibular reconstructive surgery.

The standard of the care reconstructive surgery to repair a segmental defect of the mandible (lower jaw) involves the use of bone grafts, metallic fixation plates, and metallic screws to restore the mandible's normal appearance and function (i.e., chewing, swallowing, breathing, and speech) [20]. Surgeons often use surgical grade five titanium, Ti-6Al-4V, fixation hardware in these procedures. That material has a much higher stiffness (112 GPa) than the surrounding cortical bone of mandible (10–31.2 GPa) [21,22]. Clinical reports show a high rate of complication from 7% to 69% after the surgery [23] and a low success rate, ranging from 34% to 64% [24,25]. In all cases, failed hardware necessitates removal surgery [26,27].

The high stiffness of Ti-6Al-4V fixation plates and screws can cause abnormal stress distribution throughout the mandible. Over time, this abnormal stress distribution may result in stress concentration in the fixation hardware and screws as well as stress shielding (i.e., reduced stress) of the cortical surface of the grafted bone and the host mandible. Stress-shielded bone may resorb, which may then lead to implant failure [28]. Literature reports resorption rates of 49.5% on the surrounding bone in the case of using traditional fixation plates within the first six months after grafting [29]. In addition to stress shielding, using a very stiff fixation device reduces the contact pressure between the graft/host bone, which may degrade the revascularization of the bone graft [30,31]. Traditionally, fixation plates are shaped (i.e., bent) in the operating room to fit the patient's anatomy. This process increases the time and cost of the surgery as well as the risk to the patient [32,33]. However, 3D printed fixation plates can be bent to any degree determined in the implant CAD software prior to the surgery.

Using less stiff NiTi fixation plates may reduce stress shielding of grafted bone and elevate the compression force at the graft-host bone interfaces and subsequently enhance revascularization and healing of the grafted bone [34–36]. Furthermore, superelastic NiTi fixation plates provide the possibility of inducing tension on the mandible. To this end, the fixation plates undergo enough stress to enter the strain plateau before attaching to the host mandible. This solution is therefore expected to meet three requirements: first, to achieve a more natural stress distribution in the grafted and remaining host bone, thereby decreasing the risk of stress shielding; second, to increase the level of compressive pressure at the graft/host interfaces in order to enhance graft revascularization and defect site bone remodeling; finally, prefabricating a patient-specific fixation plate, which will fit directly on the patient's mandible, reduces the time, cost, and risk of the surgery.

2. Finite Element Model for Implant Evaluation

The design of a patient-specific skeletal fixation device starts from Computed Tomography scan data (CT scan data) of the patient. CT scans use X-ray images taken from different angles to produce tomographic images [37]. The variation of local density of bone directly affects the resolution of the images in various zones. The high-resolution CT scan images of a patient's mandible provide data about the geometric variables of the mandible and also the apparent density. The former data set provides the opportunity to create fixation plates based on a patient's geometrical variation on the exterior surface of the mandible [38–40]. The latter data set allows estimation of the material properties of the surrounding bone using a quantitative scale method [41–45]. Knowledge of the exact geometry and the required fixation device stiffness allow the level of porosity to be determined in our CAD software.

This section highlights the development, calibration, and validation of a comprehensive model-based NiTi fixation hardware design work path as summarized in Figure 2. This general methodology can also be applied to design functional implants for other areas in the skeleton. Three different finite elements models were developed. A healthy mandible (model 1) and two Mandibular Reconstructive Surgery (MRS) simulated models, one with traditional dense Ti-6Al-4V (model 2) and another with stiffness-matched porous NiTi fixation plates (model 3). The first model simulates the highest bite force expected in a healthy patient with this particular patient's anatomy. The part's stiffness is then tuned to allow the desired stress distribution in the grafted bone and adjacent host mandible during maximum occlusal force. Sixty percent of the maximum bite force on the healthy mandible was incorporated into reconstructed models (i.e., model 2 and model 3 in Figure 2) [46]. The loads in both cases include muscle forces, bite forces, pre-tension and their combinations. The results are subsequently evaluated to show the performance of the fixation hardware in reducing stress shielding, stress concentrations, and improving contact pressure and reducing micro-motion at the host-graft bone interface. These are effective measures to reduce the risk associated with the mandibular segmental defect reconstructive surgery.

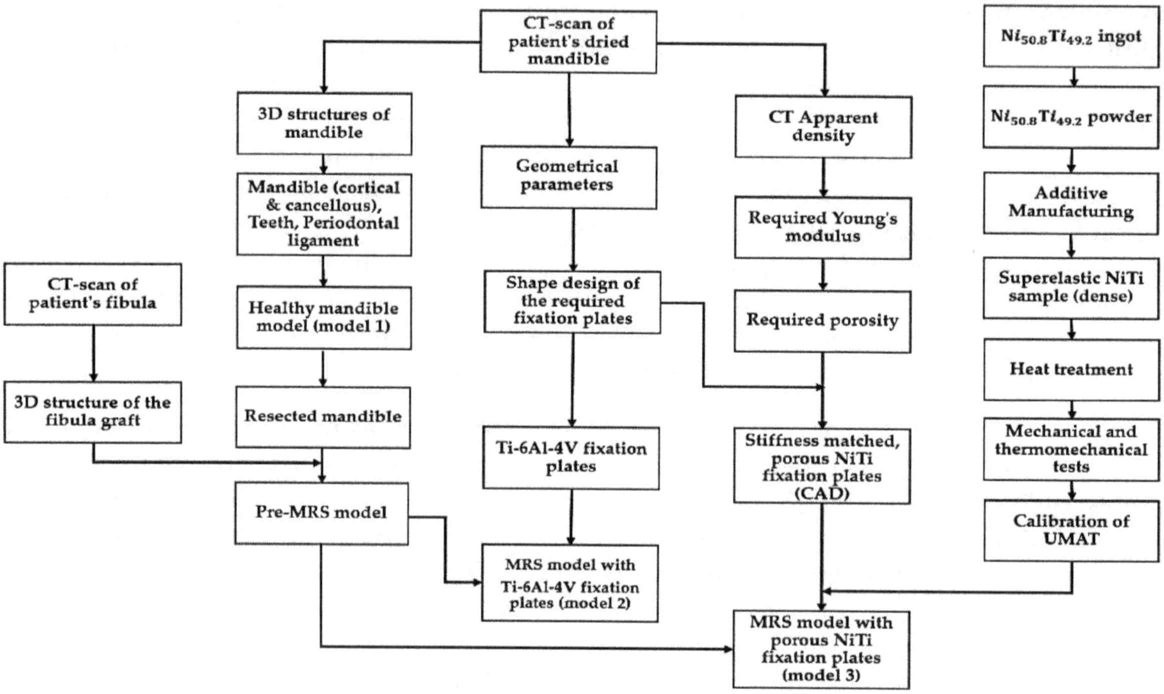

Figure 2. Flow chart for the design and fabrication of Ti-6Al-4V (standard of care) and NiTi stiffness-matched skeletal (i.e., mandible) fixation hardware. Finite Element Analysis models are used to evaluate the mandible and the fixation hardware during chewing (MRS = Mandibular Reconstructive Surgery, UMAT = User-defined Material subroutine).

A CT scan (Aquilion 64; Toshiba Medical Systems, Tokyo, Japan) of a dry cadaveric human mandible was created to produce a 3D CAD file of all mandible components including cortical bone, cancellous bone, and the teeth. This device utilizes a 64-row Quantum detector, which enables the Aquilion CT scanner to acquire 64 simultaneous slices of 0.5 mm thickness with each 400 ms gantry revolution, resulting in precise isotropic imaging of the object. The gap between the teeth and the cortical bone was graphically filled with periodontal ligament tissue in ABAQUS (CAE v6.11, Dassault Systemes, Providence, RI, USA). For this study, a segment of the left half of the mandible bearing M1-3 (i.e., molar regions) was graphically resected with a length of 40 mm. To simulate a high fidelity reconstructive surgery, a double barrel fibular graft, inferior fixation plate, superior distal fixation plate, superior mesial fixation plate and screws were modeled and implanted in the resected region using SOLIDWORKS (Dassault Systèmes, Waltham, MA, USA).

As shown in Figure 3, the double barrel fibular graft was formed by virtually cutting the fibula of a patient. The two pieces were placed together to provide a total mesiodistal length of 40 mm, a buccolingual width of 14 mm, and a height of 38 mm. The inferior fixation plate and both superior fixation plates were equipped with nine and three threaded holes, respectively (see more details in Section 3). Six bicortical screws (i.e., long screws that pierce both the buccal and lingual cortical bone) and four unicortical screws (i.e., short screws that pierce the buccal cortical bone) were included in our Finite Element Analysis (FEA) to fix the inferior fixation plate and both superior plates, respectively [47,48]. The diameter of all screws was 1.4 mm.

All of the mandible graphical components were meshed in Hypermesh (Hyperworks, Troy, MI, USA) with 4-node tetrahedral elements (C3D4), which represent 3D, Solid, Tetrahedral, Deformable element type. The optimized number of elements is reported in Table 1 based on the mesh convergence analysis of each component.

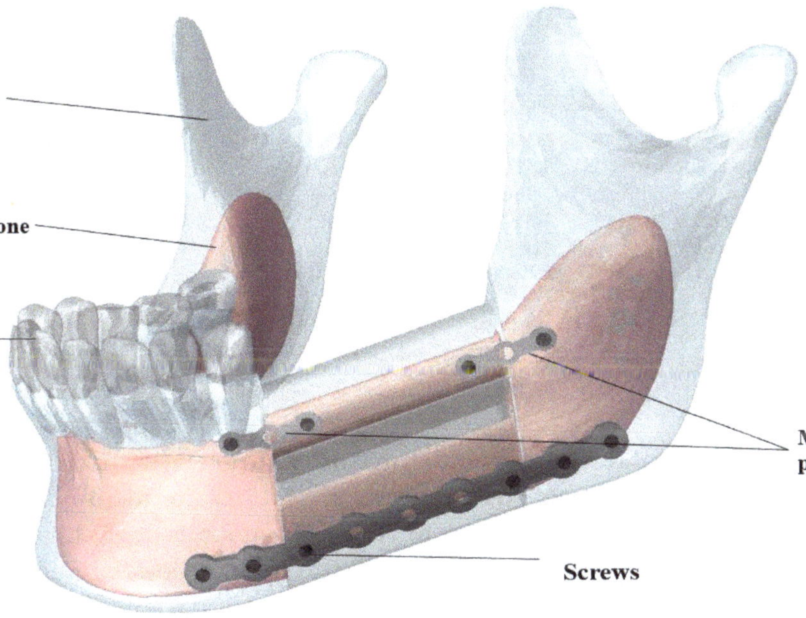

Figure 3. Components of the Reconstructed Mandible: double barrel fibular graft, one inferior fixation plate, one superior distal fixation plate, one superior mesial fixation plate, and fixation plate screws, cortical bone (**blue**) and cancellous bone (**red**).

Table 1. The number of elements for the Finite Element Analysis model components. The number of tetrahedral elements was determined by convergence analysis.

Model Component	Number of Elements
Resected mandible	218,328
Teeth (13 total)	65,179
Ligaments (13 total)	21,053
Top graft	42,065
Lower graft	45,037
Fixation hardware(s)	58,327
Screws (10 total)	67,027

All meshed parts were assembled, and constraints between screw-fixation plate, screw-host mandible, screw-fibular graft, teeth-ligaments and host mandible-ligaments were defined as tie constraints. It should be noted that the friction factors of 0 (simulation of the reconstructed mandible during the initial healing period) and 1 (simulation of the reconstructed mandible after the gaps between the grafted and host bone fragments had healed) are considered for simulation of surface to surface contact between host mandible and the fibular graft.

Table 2 summarizes the material properties of the FEA model components (i.e., fixation hardware, bone, teeth, and periodontal ligament) [1,49,50]. Cortical and cancellous bones were modeled as anisotropic material, and the other components were assumed to be linear elastic materials. It should be noted that Ti-6Al-4V material properties were assigned to the screws in all models.

The bite force created by masticatory muscles is the greatest source of stress that is usually applied to the mandible [4,51,52]. Our FEA models the peak masticatory load. Muscles are active even when the mandible is at rest. The amount of muscle forces depend on many factors including occlusion state (maximal chewing or soft food chewing) and bite loading conditions (balanced or unbalanced loading, bilateral or unilateral loading, grinding, or clenching) [53]. In this study, muscle forces related to a maximal bite force on the first right molar was considered as the loading input for the healthy mandible model (model 1) (i.e., a 526 N bite force based on Korioth et al. [46]). Three different fixation hardware scenarios (cases A, B, and C) were considered for the models 2 and 3.

Table 2. Material properties of the Finite Element Analysis mandible components [1,47,49].

Material	E_x (MPa)	E_y (MPa)	E_z (MPa)	υ_{xy}	υ_{yz}	υ_{xz}
Cortical bone-symphysis region	23,000	15,000	10,000	0.3	0.3	0.3
Cortical bone-angle region	20,000	12,000	11,000	0.3	0.3	0.3
Cortical bone-rest of mandible	17,000	8200	6900	0.315	0.325	0.31
Cancellous bone	960	390	320	0.3	0.3	0.3
Cortical-fibular graft	26,800	26,800	26,800	0.3	0.3	0.3
Cancellous-fibular graft	1650	1650	1650	0.3	0.3	0.3
Teeth	17,600	17,600	17,600	0.25	0.25	0.25
Periodontal ligament	2.7	2.7	2.7	0.45	0.45	0.45
Ti-6Al-4V	112,000	112,000	112,000	0.3	0.3	0.3
NiTi	37,000–42,000 *	37,000–42,000 *	37,000–42,000 *	0.3	0.3	0.3

* More details are discussed in Sections 4 and 5.

Case (A): The simulation of the highest bite force after surgery (without applying any pretension to the fixation hardware). Since the reconstruction surgery causes a reduction in chewing power, all the muscle force values in this study were assumed to be of 60% of Korioth et al.'s [46] values for a normal healthy mandible [47]. This is the force applied in all three FEA models; Case (B): the simulation of used NiTi fixation hardware that had received 100 N of pretension load (i.e., on both superior and the inferior plates). This value for the pretension load was obtained from the FEA model in a way that increased contact pressure of the lower section of the graft bone by 50%; Case (C): this simulation used NiTi hardware that had undergone 100 N pretension load on both superior and the inferior fixation plates; More details on the model development and boundary conditions are presented in our previous studies [10,54,55] (Figure 4).

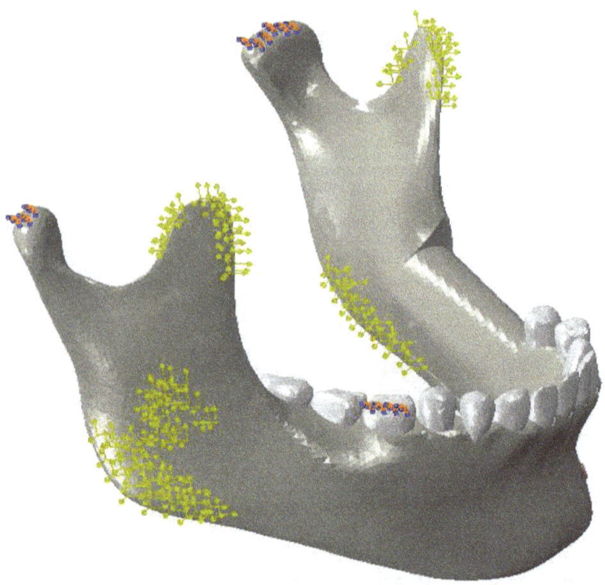

Figure 4. The finite element model of a mandible by considering the boundary conditions (**red** and **blue** points) and the muscle forces (**yellow** arrows).

3. Fixation Hardware Design

CT-scan data were used in the design of the fixation plates (i.e., patient-specific fixation plates). This eliminates the need to bend fixation plates to fit the mandible during the surgery. In this study, the local lingual side curvature of each fixation plate was designed based on the patient's mandible shape. The overall shape of the fixation plate was also designed to accommodate the insertion of screws at regular intervals and using commonly used thread geometries. The nine-hole inferior fixation plate has a buccolingual thickness of 1.5 mm, a mesiodistal length of 78 mm and a superoinferior width of 4 mm.

Each of the two three-hole superior fixation plates has the dimensions of 1 mm × 18 mm × 2.8 mm, in buccolingual, mesiodistal and superoinferior direction, respectively. Six bicortical screws (i.e., long screws that pierce both the buccal and lingual cortical bone) and four unicortical screws (i.e., short screws that pierce the buccal cortical bone) were designed to fix the inferior fixation plate and both superior plates, respectively [47], to the host and graft bone. The diameter of all screws was 1.4 mm. The developed fixation plates and screws were assembled with the pre-MRS model component to simulate the MRS with traditional Ti-6Al-4V fixation plates (model 2).

In addition to making sure that the fixation plate geometry ensures a good fit, directly on the surface of the host mandible and grafted fibular bones, this project also endeavors to ensure that the stiffness of this plate, and the screws holding it to the mandible and graft segments, have a stiffness that is matched with the stiffness of the cortical bone to which they are attached. The stiffness of cortical bone in the adult mandible varies between 10–31.2 GPa (Figure 5) [1]. The Young's modulus for different zones of the mandible can be obtained using various methods, such as using a quantitative scaling technique to analyze CT-scan data of the patient's mandible [41–45]. In our study, the estimated average Young's modulus of the dried mandible in the cut segment (i.e., Molar regions) was calculated to be 12 GPa.

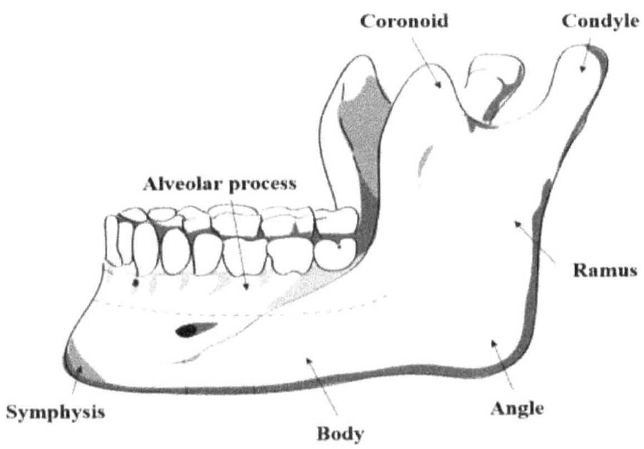

Mandible component	Cortical stiffness (MPa)
Coronoid	16,600 – 31,200
Condyle	15,900 – 26,400
Ramus	12,800 – 28,700
Angle	18,300 – 25,700
Symphysis	18,900 – 22,300

Figure 5. The stiffness in different regions of cortical bone the normal, adult mandible [1,46].

The SLM-fabricated, dense NiTi samples still had a higher stiffness (37 GPa, measured in Section 4) than the estimated Young's modulus of this mandibular cortical bone (i.e., 12 GPa). To this end, a porous NiTi part was created from a number of identical unit cells. Each unit cell was composed of three orthogonal cylinders, all with the same diameter, that intersect at their mid-point. Subsequently, a shell with the thickness of 0.2 mm was considered all around the fixation to smooth the edges. The level of porosity can be tuned by changing the diameter of the cylinders as shown in Figure 6. The level of porosity is calculated by dividing the volume of the porous unit sample to the volume of the surrounding cube. The equivalent stress on the porous part was calculated by dividing the axial force by the projected area of the unit cell on the plane normal to the loading direction. Additionally, the total displacement was used to calculate the equivalent strain. Based on the equivalent stress and strain of the porous structure, the equivalent Young's modulus can be calculated. The equivalent stress is used to evaluate the performance of the device, and the actual stress was investigated to evaluate the safety of the fixation plate [11] (i.e., will it be strong enough during the healing period). It was thus calculated that 45.7% porosity is required to achieve an equivalent Young's modulus of 12 GPa in the first fixation plate that we designed. A useful diameter in the fixation plate pore unit cells was calculated to be one millimeter. This porous structure, as Figure 7 shows, was created through imposing unit pore cells throughout the designed fixation plate. This porous hardware was assembled with the pre-MRS model component (model 3) for comparative studies.

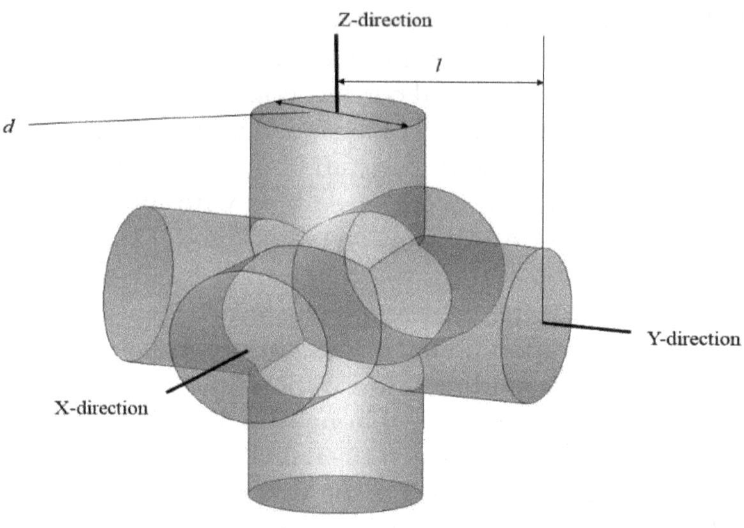

Figure 6. The unit pore cell that is used for our stiffness-matched NiTi fixation hardware. It is composed of three orthogonal hollow cylinders.

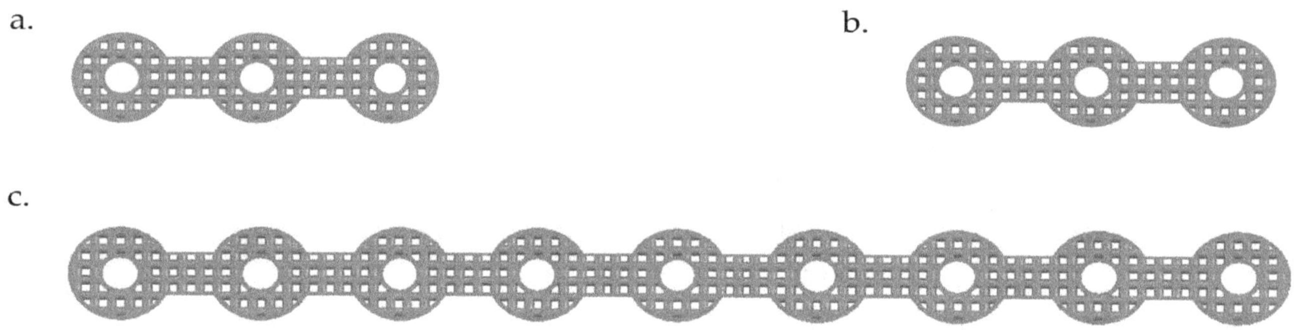

Figure 7. Porous fixation plates (i.e., superior mesial mini-plate (**a**), superior distal mini-plate (**b**), and inferior mandible bar (**c**)) with a porosity of 45.7%, created with an orthogonal cylinder geometry (see Figure 6). Note that all three plates would seat perfectly on the surface of the host and grafted bone that they will hold together.

4. Fabrication of Patient-Specific NiTi Fixation Hardware

In order to calibrate our FEA model to simulate NiTi fixation plates and screws, we fabricated dense compression specimens, performed heat treatments, and performed mechanical and Differential Scanning Calorimetry (DSC) tests to obtain the required material properties [56–59]. To this end, $Ni_{50.8}Ti_{49.2}$ (at %) ingots from NiTi Devices & Components, Inc. (Fremont, CA, USA), were atomized to powder using an Electrode Induction-melting Gas Atomization (EIGA) technique (by TLS Technique GmbH (Bitterfeld, Germany)). A PXM 3D printer (3D Systems, Rock Hill, SC, USA) equipped with a 300 W Ytterbium fiber laser for SLM was used in this study to fabricate a fully dense cylindrical shapes of 8 mm in diameter and 12 mm in length. The laser had a beam quality of $M^2 < 1.2$ and a Gaussian beam profile (TEM00). The optimized parameters of fabrication of these Ni-rich NiTi parts were from the same as in studies previously published by our group [2,13]. Those process parameters are summarized in Table 3. Finally, the designed porous superelastic NiTi fixation plates were fabricated based on the optimal parameters [10,60–65].

Table 3. Process parameters used in Selective Laser Melting (SLM) manufacturing of NiTi parts.

Effective Laser Power (W)	Layer Thickness (μm)	Scanning Velocity (m/s)	Hatch Distance (μm)	Energy Input (J/mm^3)
250	30	1.25	120	55.5

After the fabrication process, the cylindrical samples were solution annealed (1223 K, 5.5 h, H_2O), aged (623 K, 15 min), and then water quenched. To perform solution annealing, Lindberg/Blue M BF514541 Box furnace was used. To avoid oxidation of the samples, they were placed in an argon-filled quartz ampules. For determining the transformation temperatures (TTRs), a Perkin-Elmer Pyris 1 DSC with the heating/cooling rate of 10 °C/min in a nitrogen atmosphere was used. The samples were loaded up to 800 MPa (before reaching to the critical stress for plastic deformation) and unloaded using a 100 kN MTS Landmark servo-hydraulic test platform (Minneapolis, MN, USA). The strain rate of $10^{-4}\cdot s^{-1}$ was employed during loading, whereas unloading was performed under force control at a rate of 100 $N\cdot s^{-1}$. An MTS high-temperature extensometer was used to obtain strain measurements [56]. The observed mechanical properties of these SLM fabricated samples are shown in Table 4. The impurity limits for medical NiTi are prescribed in ASTM F2063-05. The impurity level for clinical applications must be below 0.05 ppm [62]. The impurity content was tested in three of the NiTi samples that we fabricated. We observed impurity levels of 0.035, 0.0500, and 0.007 ppm for carbon, oxygen, and nitrogen, respectively, for the sample with the highest level of impurity.

Table 4. Mechanical properties of fabricated parts under compression test.

Material	E (GPa)	Yield Strength (MPa)
NiTi	37	1011 [3]
Ti-6Al-4V	112	970–1030 [66]

An ABAQUS user-defined material (UMAT) subroutine based on the microplane theory [67–69] was calibrated using the experimental data of the fabricated NiTi parts. The UMAT is capable of simulation of both the superelastic and the shape memory effects of NiTi under multiaxial loading conditions regardless of the geometry of structure [70]. In order to calibrate the UMAT, the required parameters were extracted from mechanical (i.e., compression test at different temperatures) and thermomechanical experiments (i.e., DSC tests). More details on our UMAT calibration testing procedures are presented elsewhere [71].

FEA was used to determine the stiffness needed to stiffness-match the 3D printed fixation hardware. The final design of the porous NiTi fixation plates consisted of a desired level percentage of porosity, pore shape and size, and general dimension of the plate. The resulting CAD file of the designed NiTi fixation plate was used on the SLM machine for fabrication. To induce superelasticity, the same heat treatment procedures including solution annealing (1223 K, 5.5 h, H_2O) and aging (623 K, 15 min) were performed.

5. Validation and Results

The input parameters of the UMAT were found from the DSC and thermomechanical tests on dense cylindrical samples in order to calibrate, tune, and finally, validate the model. The required parameters for calibration are summarized in Table 5 [71]. Transformation temperature has been measured using DSC test (Figure 8).

Table 5. Material parameters of dense Ni-rich NiTi fabricated by SLM technique at 37 °C. (E_A and E_M are the austenitic and martensitic modulus of elasticity). Transformation temperatures have been shown by M_s, M_f, A_s and A_f.

Parameter	E_A (GPa)	E_M (GPa)	ν [72]	M_s (K)	M_f (K)	A_s (K)	A_f (K)
Value	37	42	0.33	263	243	270	280

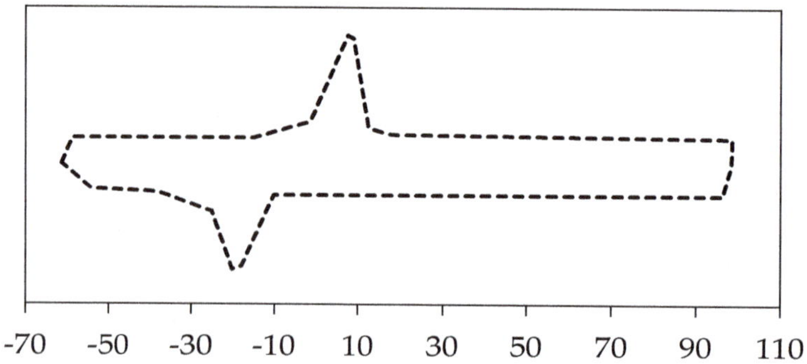

Figure 8. Differential Scanning Calorimetry (DSC) test for the 100% dense NiTi samples.

Figure 9 compares the experimental and simulation results of the compression tests of dense (98%) cylindrical specimens ($r > 0.99$, $p < 0.005$, root-mean-square error (RMSE) = 12.6 MPa and $r > 0.98$, $p < 0.005$, RMSE = 38.3 MPa for the simulation of loading and unloading responses, respectively).

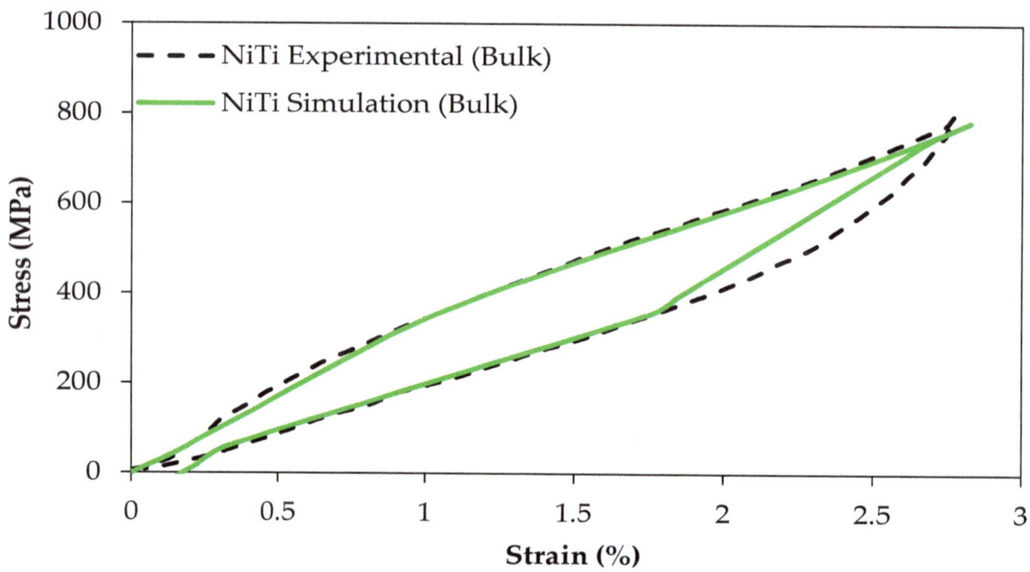

Figure 9. The simulation and experimental results of a compression test on dense NiTi.

The same UMAT was then used to simulate the behavior of porous superelastic parts. Figure 10 shows the compressive behavior of three different materials: cortical mandible bone (under compression) [73], NiTi cubes with 45.7% porosity, and Ti-6Al-V cubes [66]. We observed that the Ti-6Al-4V presents significantly higher stiffness than NiTi while the porous NiTi material shows similar stiffness to that of cortical bone (Figure 10). The results of this simulation suggest that a 45.7% porosity can be used to match the stiffness of NiTi parts to that of the cortical bone (i.e., 12 GPa) to which they are attached. This can also be done with porous Ti-6Al-4V with a very high level of porosity (see Section 6).

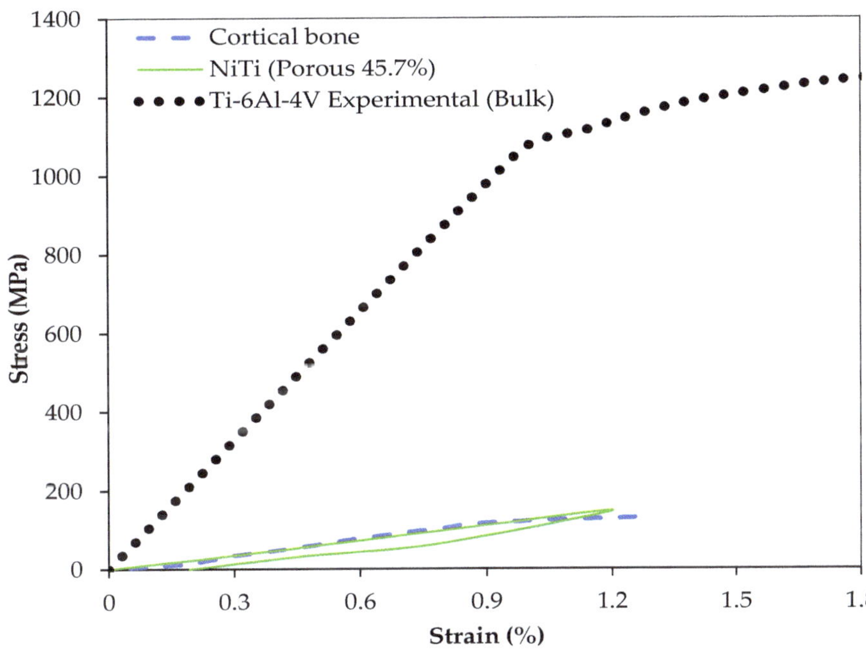

Figure 10. The equivalent stress–strain plot under compression for NiTi cubic samples with 45.7% porosity, cubes of dense Ti-6Al-4V [66] and samples of mandibular cortical bone [73].

An experimental study by Ichim et al. group [74] is comparable to our healthy mandible model (model 1). They used a dry cadaveric mandible to measure the buccal and lingual strains in mandibular cortical bone using two strain gauges. The procedure and conditions of their experiment were applied to the FEA model used in this study. Figure 11 demonstrates their experimental outcomes as well as our simulation data. The correlation between our results and theirs were statistically significant ($r > 0.99$, $p < 0.0005$, RMSE $= 2.8 \times 10^{-6}$ (%) and $r > 0.99$, $p < 0.0005$, RMSE $< 6.42 \times 10^{-6}$ (%) for the Buccal and Lingual sides of mandible cortical bone in the molar region, respectively).

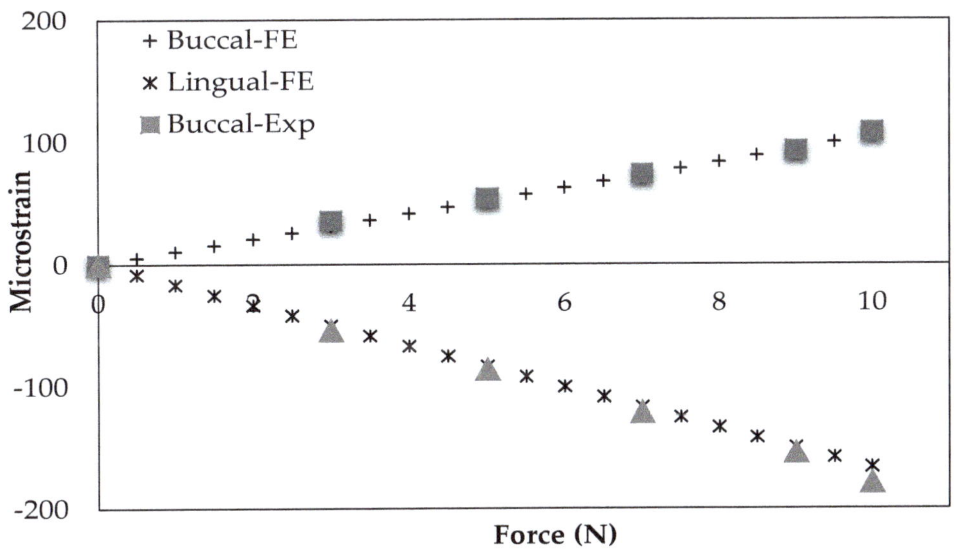

Figure 11. Model validation: a comparison between experimentally-obtained data (EXP) [74] with Finite Element Analysis (FEA)-predicted model data on the buccally and lingually placed strain gauges.

The results of our FEA models are presented at two different time points: (1) immediately following surgery, i.e., when bone fracture healing is occurring and the hardware is bearing most of the strain from chewing and other mandibular activities; and (2) post-healing where stiffness-matched fixation hardware is expected to increase the loading of the grafted bone over traditional, Ti-6Al-4V hardware, and drive the remodeling process [75,76]. One important consideration during healing period is to minimize the micromotion in the interfaces between the graft/host bone. This way, the risk of graft unvascularization caused by micromotion is minimized. Through a successful healing, the graft bone at the interfaces is integrated into the host mandible [4]. During the post healing period, the hardware should reduce the risk of stress shielding, which normally develops with the current standard of care titanium fixations.

Graft unvascularization is counted as one of the reasons for the mandibular reconstructive surgery failure. It is often caused by the relative movements, which are decreased as the contact pressure in the surfaces between the graft and the host bone increases [4]. For the loading regime during the healing and post-healing periods are studied with the current standard of care fixation hardware (Ti-6Al-4V, model 2) and the mandible reconstructed with stiffness-matched NiTi fixation hardware (model 3). It should be noted that for both cases pre-tension equal to 100 N is applied to the fixation hardware in order to increase the engagement. Two different loading scenarios are considered, at rest and under the highest occlusal load at M1. Figure 12 shows the associated average contact pressure in the interfaces between the graft and host bone.

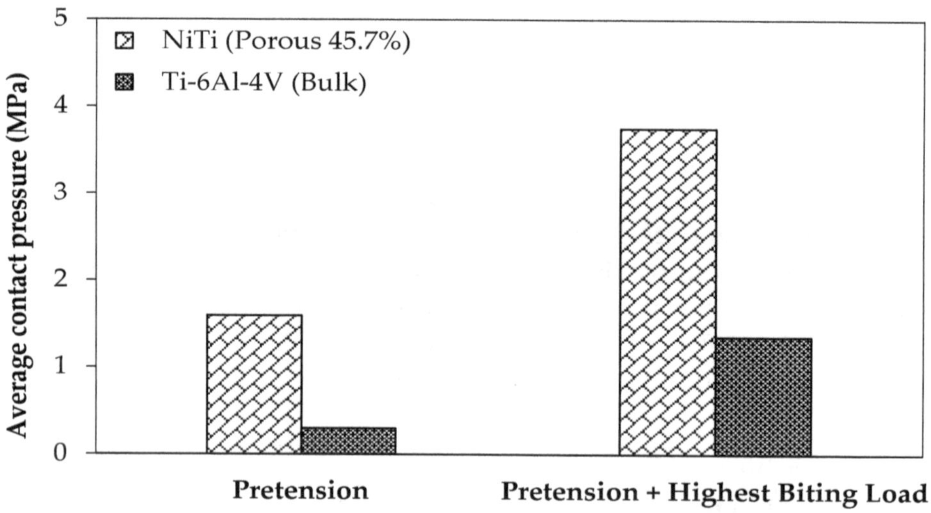

Figure 12. The effect of using NiTi and Ti-6Al-4V fixation plates on the average contact pressure at the interface between the graft and host bone (i.e., fibular bone graft and host mandible) during the healing period (i.e., in the immediate post-operative period there no strength at the graft-host bone junction).

In order to study the stress shielding effect, the von Mises stress distribution in the MRS was investigated using the current standard of care (model 2) and the mandible reconstructed with stiffness-matched NiTi (model 3). Both models were simulated in three different loading cases: case (A), applying highest biting force (i.e., 60% of the maximum bite force on the healthy mandible); case (B), applying a pure pretension (100 N) on each fixation; case (C), applying a pretension while the mandible is under highest biting force.

Figure 13 depicts the average von Mises stress for both fixations under the three loading scenarios. In a comparison with the traditional fixations, the results indicated higher average von Mises stresses on the cortical bone of the grafts in the case of using the porous NiTi fixations in all loading cases (by factors of 1.95, 1.82, and 2.14, respectively). In addition, these results were more adjusted to the average von Mises stress on the healthy mandible model (model 1), which indicates a more natural stress distribution on the grafted bone using the proposed fixations. Similarly, as shown in Figure 14, the maximum von Mises stress is higher when compared to Ti-6Al-4V fixation plates. It is worth noting that the stresses are all in a safe zone [73] (<100 MPa). It should be mentioned that the results of healthy mandible model (model 1) were attributed to the same region of the resected mandible (Figures 13 and 14). The findings show that, by taking advantage of the superelasticity and applying pretension during the procedure, the von Mises stress on the fibular grafts bone increases, which results in a better long-term outcome for the patients. This increased stress can reduce the stress shielding effects and the risk of implant failure.

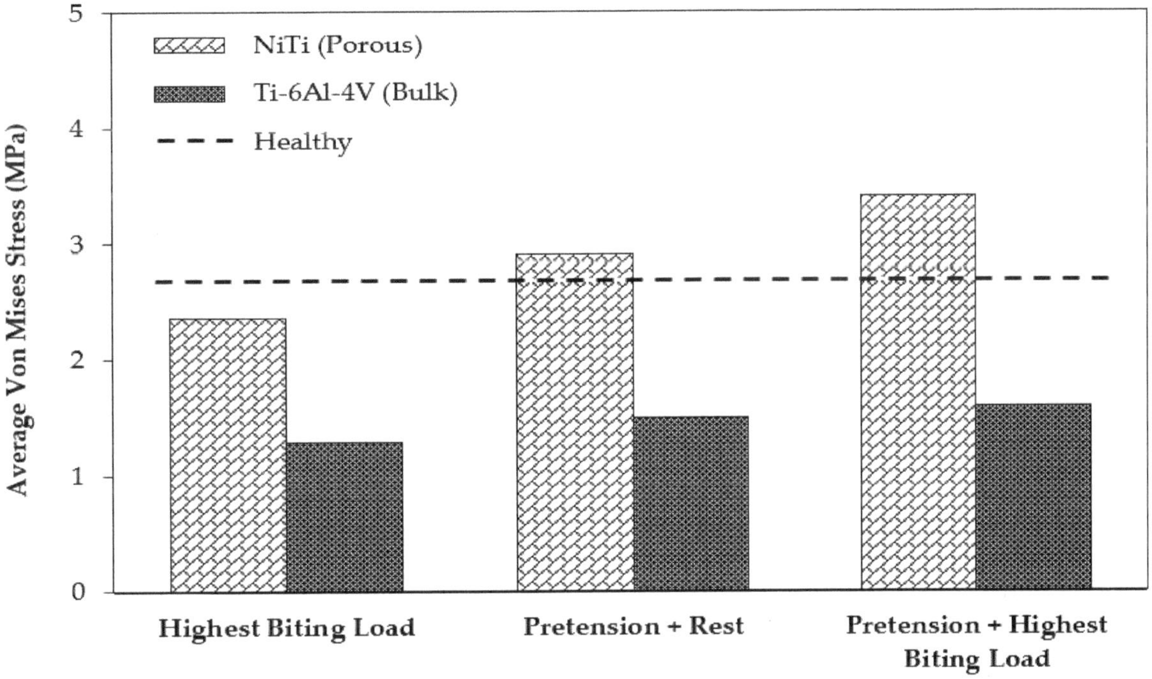

Figure 13. The average Von Mises stress on the surrounding bone in two cases of using Ti-6Al-4V and porous NiTi fixation plates, with and without applying the pretension to the fixation plates.

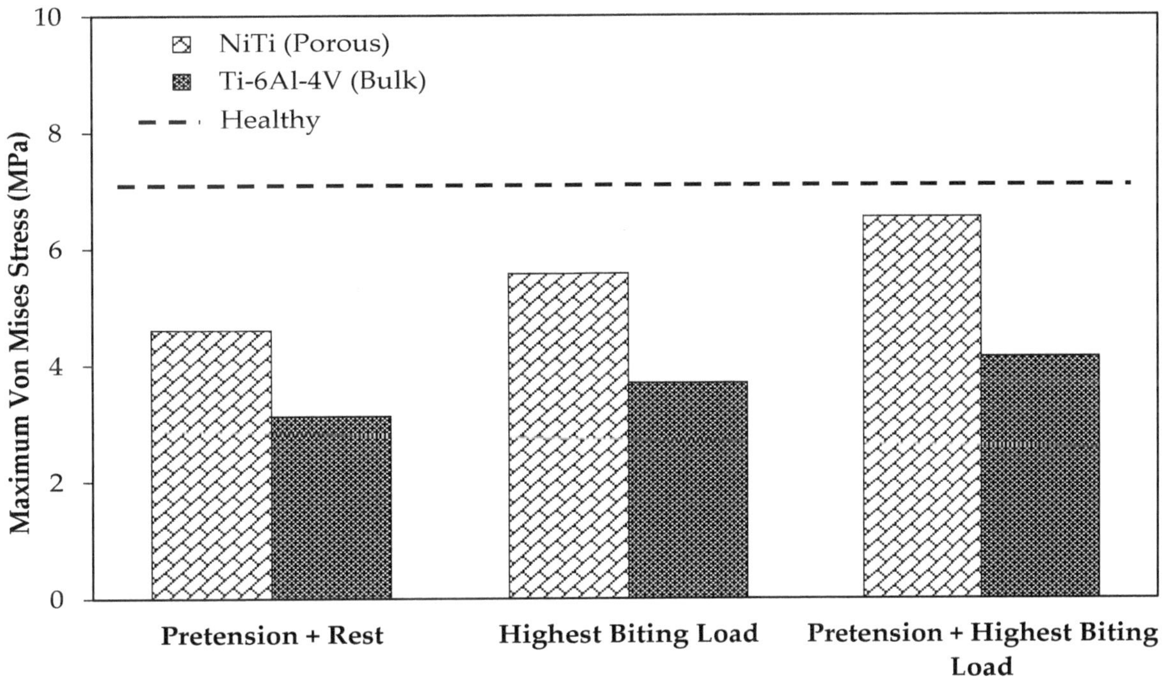

Figure 14. The maximum von Mises stress on the surrounding bone in two cases of using Ti-6Al-4V and porous NiTi fixation plates.

As Table 6 shows, the resultant maximum actual von Mises stress on the porous NiTi was higher than the dense traditional fixation plates in all loading cases. This stress for the NiTi implant at the worst cases (pretension and muscle forces) was 594 MPa, which is still in the safe region ($\sigma_y = 1011$ MPa) with the safety factor of 1.7.

Table 6. Maximum stress (MPa) on the fixation plates under different loading case.

Fixations Type	Highest Bite Loading	Pretension + REST	Pretension + Highest Biting Load
Porous NiTi fixation plate	328	485	594
Ti-6Al-4V fixation plate	98	132	299

As mentioned, a Young's modulus of 12 GPa for NiTi fixation plates can be achieved by applying a specific percentage and type of porosity (i.e., 45.7% porosity). The unit cell of the structure is made out of three perpendicular cylinders with a diameter of 1.00 mm. As a step toward the manufacturing of patient-specific fixation plates, we used a previously healthy, dried cadaver mandible. To simulate the post healing period following reconstructive surgery. Two vertical fractures were created on the left M1-3 section of the mandible. Then a set of three porous NiTi fixation plates similar to the finite element model were designed based on the geometry derived from the CT-scan image of the dried mandible. Subsequently, they were fabricated using a Phenix PXM SLM machine.

Figure 15 shows the fabricated fixation plates. Since the fixation plates were designed based on the curvature of the host mandible, they were mounted on the mandible with no need to additional bending. Figure 16 shows these patient-specific fixation plates mounted on a dried cadaver mandible in order to immobilize the resected area.

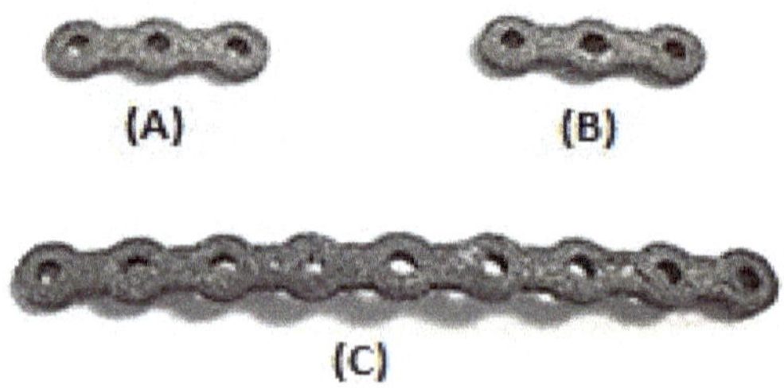

Figure 15. Additively manufactured: (**A**) superior mesial fixation plate; (**B**) superior distal fixation plate; and (**C**) inferior fixation plate (mandible bar).

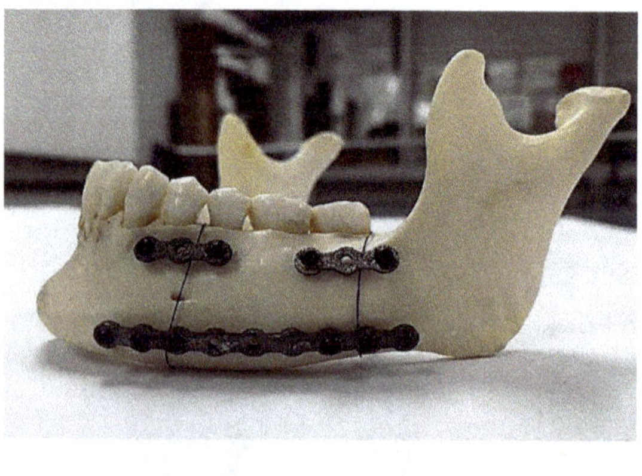

Figure 16. Reconstructed mandible using stiffness-matched, 3D printed, NiTi fixation devices.

6. Conclusions

Additive manufacturing methods have become popular for producing medical devices with high quality. The commonly used material for metallic implants, i.e., Ti-6Al-4V, presents high modulus of elasticity of 112 GPa, while the range of Young's modulus of the bone varies in the range of 10–31.2 GPa. This high stiffness may result in implant failure due to the stress shielding effect, which results in un-vascularized bone. NiTi is a good candidate for biomedical devices because of lower stiffness (37 GPa), and the superelasticity behavior similar to that of the bone. The level of stiffness of NiTi can be tuned through introducing porosity to match the desired level.

In our study, we focus on the design of a patient-specific stiffness-matched fixation hardware as a substitute for currently used fixations (Ti-6Al-4V). The purpose is to minimize the risk of implant failure (e.g., bone resorption, graft un-vascularization) and to produce the proposed fixation in a patient-specific manner. The fixation design is based on the exact shape and the required stiffness obtained by the CT-scan data of a dried mandible. Adding a 45.7% porosity to NiTi fixation hardware during 3D printing allows us to decrease the stiffness of fixation plates to stiffness of the surrounding bone (estimated from CT data). Figure 17 compares the Young's modulus of NiTi with Ti-6Al-4V when similar porosity is introduced in both alloys. The NiTi alloys offer a better solution by reaching a low stiffness at a lower percentage porosity. In general, it is desirable to keep the level of porosity low to avoid the complications during the manufacturing and to avoid the possibility of failure due to stress concentration. Figure 18 shows the superelastic simulation results for NiTi parts with different levels of porosity.

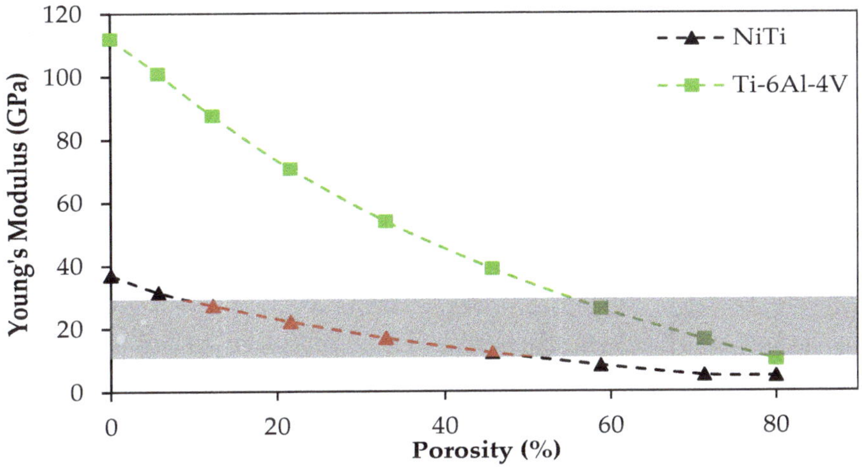

Figure 17. The effect of porosity on Young's modulus for superelastic NiTi and Ti-6Al-4V. The range of bone stiffness is shown as highlighted zone.

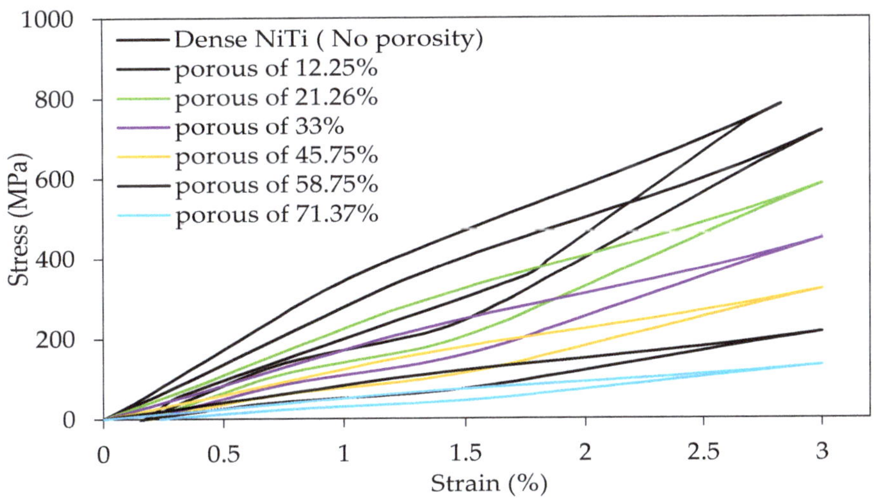

Figure 18. The effect of porosity on the compression behavior of superelastic NiTi; simulation results.

In this work, we used finite element analysis to evaluate the effect of using this reduced stiffness for the post-surgical process. Based on this, two models of MRS were simulated in different loading scenarios. Our finite element results indicate a higher level of contact pressure (177%) during initial periods of healing due to pre-tension load in the case of using porous NiTi fixation plates. Such improvements can increase the chance of vascularization during the healing period [34,35]. Also, the results show that the average von Mises stress increased on host mandible (83%) and grafted bone (126%) for MRS simulation with porous NiTi implant. Considering stress distribution on the healthy mandible as a reference, the porous NiTi can cause better results compared to Ti-6Al-4V fixations.

These porous fixation plates may be fabricated using additive manufacturing (3D printing). For showing a patient-specific design for the fixation plates, a dried cadaver mandible was used. We successfully applied the design process for a case of reconstruction surgery on a dried cadaver mandible (patient-specific study). After the design stage, using Selective Laser Melting (SLM) we could fabricate these patient-specific fixation plates and assemble them on the dried mandible. These 3D printed, porous, NiTi fixation plates not only provide the required level of stiffness (12 GPa) and minimize the stress shielding probability, they also ensure hardware well-fitting that can be quickly placed, thereby reducing operation room time.

We have compared the use of NiTi and Ti-6Al-4V as the material for a patient-specific fixation plate. To this end, we created two different porous specimens with the same equivalent Young's modulus of 12 GPa (estimated from CT scan data) using Ti-6Al-4V and Ni-rich NiTi. The required level porosity for the two specimens was different, 45.7% for the NiTi and 78.3% for the Ti-6Al-4V. Then we applied two percent equivalent strain (the recoverable strain by the cortical bone [14–16,73]) to both structures and reported the actual stress on the pore elements. The simulation results indicate that at in case of using porous Ti-6Al-4V the actual maximum stress (2981 MPa) exceeds the yield stress of the Ti-6Al-4V (970-1030 MPa) [66], and the porous structure failed (i.e., for the new and traditional porous fixation plates that have same equivalent stress-strain curve, a certain amount equivalent strain leads to much higher actual stress on the porous Ti-6Al-4V implants). Therefore, since it was not practical, we have not considered the use of a highly porous Ti-6Al-4V fixation. However, in the case of using NiTi for the porous specimen, thanks to the superelastic response of the material, this high value of equivalent strain (two percent) on the part can be completely recovered and the actual maximum stress (578 MPa) on the pore elements does not reach the yield stress $(\sigma_y = 1011 \text{ MPa})$. Regarding this fact, the superelastic response of the Ni-rich NiTi makes it the proper choice for the patient-specific fixation plates.

Acknowledgments: The authors would like to acknowledge the financial support of the ASM International through an SMST 2015 inaugural fellowship. The authors would also like to acknowledge the financial support of the Ohio Third Frontier Technology Validation and Startup Fund.

Author Contributions: Ahmadreza Jahadakbar, Narges Shayesteh Moghaddam, and Amirhesam Amerinatanzi each participated in the process of design, simulation and fabrication. They also provided the content for various parts of this article. Mohammad Elahinia provided the facilities for simulation and fabrication of the specimens. Haluk E. Karaca provided the facilities for testing the specimens. David Dean and Mohammad Elahinia have reviewed the whole document.

References

1. Andani, M.T.; Moghaddam, N.S.; Haberland, C.; Dean, D.; Miller, M.J.; Elahinia, M. Metals for bone implants. Part 1. Powder metallurgy and implant rendering. *Acta Biomater.* **2014**, *10*, 4058–4070. [CrossRef] [PubMed]
2. Elahinia, M.; Moghaddam, N.S.; Andani, M.T.; Amerinatanzi, A.; Bimber, B.A.; Hamilton, R.F. Fabrication of NiTi through additive manufacturing: A review. *Prog. Mater. Sci.* **2016**, *83*, 630–663. [CrossRef]
3. Haberland, C.; Elahinia, M.; Walker, J.; Meier, H. Visions, concepts and strategies for smart nitinol actuators and complex nitinol structures produced by additive manufacturing. In Proceedings of the ASME 2013 Conference on Smart Materials, Adaptive Structures and Intelligent Systems, Snowbird, UT, USA, 16–18 September 2013.

4. Amerinatanzi, A.; Zamanian, H.; Moghaddam, N.S.; Ibrahim, H.; Hefzy, M.S.; Elahinia, M. On the Advantages of Superelastic Niti in Ankle Foot Orthoses. In Proceedings of the ASME 2016 Conference on Smart Materials, Adaptive Structures and Intelligent Systems, Stowe, VT, USA, 28–30 September 2016.
5. Hadi, A.; Alipour, K.; Kazeminasab, S.; Amerinatanzi, A.; Elahinia, M. Design and Prototyping of a Wearable Assistive Tool for Hand Rehabilitation using Shape Memory Alloys. In Proceedings of the ASME 2016 Conference on Smart Materials, Adaptive Structures and Intelligent Systems, Stowe, VT, USA, 28–30 September 2016.
6. Mahtabi, M.; Shamsaei, N.; Mitchell, M. Fatigue of nitinol: The state-of-the-art and ongoing challenges. *J. Mech. Behav. Biomed. Mater.* **2015**, *50*, 228–254. [CrossRef] [PubMed]
7. Mahtabi, M.; Shamsaei, N.; Rutherford, B. Mean strain effects on the fatigue behavior of superelastic nitinol alloys: An experimental investigation. *Procedia Eng.* **2015**, *133*, 646–654. [CrossRef]
8. Mahtabi, M.; Shamsaei, N. Multiaxial fatigue modeling for nitinol shape memory alloys under in-phase loading. *J. Mech. Behav. Biomed. Mater.* **2015**, *55*, 236–249. [CrossRef] [PubMed]
9. Esfahani, S.N.; Andani, M.T.; Moghaddam, N.S.; Mirzaeifar, R.; Elahinia, M. Independent tuning of stiffness and toughness of additively manufactured titanium-polymer composites: Simulation, fabrication, and experimental studies. *J. Mater. Process. Technol.* **2016**, *238*, 22–29. [CrossRef]
10. Moghaddam, N.S.; Elahinia, M.; Miller, M.; Dean, D. Enhancement of bone implants by substituting nitinol for titanium (Ti-6Al-4V): A modeling comparison. In Proceedings of the ASME 2014 Conference on Smart Materials, Adaptive Structures and Intelligent Systems, Newport, RI, USA, 8–10 September 2014.
11. Rahmanian, R.; Moghaddam, N.S.; Haberland, C.; Dean, D.; Miller, M.; Elahinia, M. Load Bearing and Stiffness Tailored Niti Implants Produced by Additive Manufacturing: A Simulation Study. In *Behavior and Mechanics of Multifunctional Materials and Composites 2014*; SPIE Press: Bellingham, WA, USA, 9–13 March 2014.
12. Hadi, A.; Qasemi, M.; Elahinia, M.; Moghaddam, N. Modeling and experiment of a flexible module actuated by shape memory alloy wire. In Proceedings of the ASME 2014 Conference on Smart Materials, Adaptive Structures and Intelligent Systems, Newport, RI, USA, 8–10 September 2014.
13. Skoracki, R.; Miller, M.; Jahadakbar, A.; Taheri Andani, M.; Shayesteh Moghaddam, N.; Haberland, C.; Dean, D.; Walker, J.; Karaca, H.; Elahinia, M. *Additive Manufacturing of Nitinol Fixation Hardware for Reconstructing Mandibular Segmental Defects*; ASM International: Almere, The Netherlands, 2015.
14. Amerinatanzi, A.; Moghaddam, N.S.; Ibrahim, H.; Elahinia, M. Evaluating a Niti Implant Under Realistic Loads: A Simulation Study. In Proceedings of the ASME 2016 Conference on Smart Materials, Adaptive Structures and Intelligent Systems, Stowe, VT, USA, 28–30 September 2016.
15. Amerinatanzi, A.; Moghaddam, N.S.; Ibrahim, H.; Elahinia, M. The Effect of Porosity Type on the Mechanical Performance of Porous Niti Bone Implants. In Proceedings of the ASME 2016 Conference on Smart Materials, Adaptive Structures and Intelligent Systems, Stowe, VT, USA, 28–30 September 2016.
16. Moghaddam, N.S.; Amerinatanzi, A.; Saedi, S.; Turabi, A.S.; Karaca, H.; Elahinia, M. Stiffness Tuning of Niti Implants Through Aging. In Proceedings of the ASME 2016 Conference on Smart Materials, Adaptive Structures and Intelligent Systems, Stowe, VT, USA, 28–30 September 2016.
17. Habijan, T.; Haberland, C.; Meier, H.; Frenzel, J.; Wittsiepe, J.; Wuwer, C.; Greulich, C.; Schildhauer, T.; Köller, M. The biocompatibility of dense and porous nickel–titanium produced by selective laser melting. *Mater. Sci. Eng. C* **2013**, *33*, 419–426. [CrossRef] [PubMed]
18. Moghaddam, N.S.; Andani, M.T.; Amerinatanzi, A.; Haberland, C.; Huff, S.; Miller, M.; Elahinia, M.; Dean, D. Metals for bone implants: Safety, design, and efficacy. *Biomanuf. Rev.* **2016**, *1*, 1. [CrossRef]
19. Es-Souni, M.; Es-Souni, M.; Fischer-Brandies, H. Assessing the biocompatibility of NiTi shape memory alloys used for medical applications. *Anal. Bioanal. Chem.* **2005**, *381*, 557–567. [CrossRef] [PubMed]
20. Moghaddam, N.S.; Jahadakbar, A.; Elahinia, M.; Dean, D.; Miller, M. The effect of adding dental implants to the reconstructed mandible comparing the effect of using Ti-6Al-4V and NiTi hardware. In *Tissue Engineering Part A*; Mary Ann Liebert, Inc.: New Rochelle, NY, USA, 2015; p. S398.
21. Martola, M.; Lindqvist, C.; Hänninen, H.; Al-Sukhun, J. Fracture of titanium plates used for mandibular reconstruction following ablative tumor surgery. *J. Biomed. Mater. Res. B Appl. Biomater.* **2007**, *80*, 345–352. [CrossRef] [PubMed]
22. Spencer, K.; Sizeland, A.; Taylor, G.; Wiesenfeld, D. The use of titanium mandibular reconstruction plates in patients with oral cancer. *Int. J. Oral Maxillofac. Surg.* **1999**, *28*, 288–290. [CrossRef]

23. Wei, F.-C.; Celik, N.; Yang, W.-G.; Chen, I.-H.; Chang, Y.-M.; Chen, H.-C. Complications after reconstruction by plate and soft-tissue free flap in composite mandibular defects and secondary salvage reconstruction with osteocutaneous flap. *Plast. Reconstr. Surg.* **2003**, *112*, 37–42. [CrossRef] [PubMed]
24. Mariani, P.; Kowalski, L.; Magrin, J. Reconstruction of large defects postmandibulectomy for oral cancer using plates and myocutaneous flaps: A long-term follow-up. *Int. J. Oral Maxillofac. Surg.* **2006**, *35*, 427–432. [CrossRef] [PubMed]
25. Moghaddam, N.; Ahmadi, M.; Webb, J.; Rahmani, M.; Sadegi, H.; Musavi, M.; Ismail, R. Modeling of graphene nano-ribbon schottky diodes in the parabolic band structure limit. In Proceedings of the Sixth Global Conference on Power Control and Optimization, Las Vegas, NV, USA, 6–8 August 2012; AIP Publishing: College Park, MD, USA, 2012; pp. 268–271.
26. Yilmaz, M.; Vayvada, H.; Menderes, A.; Demirdover, C.; Kizilkaya, A. A comparison of vascularized fibular flap and iliac crest flap for mandibular reconstruction. *J. Cranio-fac. Surg.* **2008**, *19*, 227–234. [CrossRef] [PubMed]
27. Rahmani, M.; Ahmadi, M.; Kiani, M.J.; Ismail, R. Monolayer graphene nanoribbon p–n junction. *J. Nanoeng. Nanomanuf.* **2012**, *2*, 375–378. [CrossRef]
28. Nagasao, T.; Miyamoto, J.; Tamaki, T.; Kawana, H. A comparison of stresses in implantation for grafted and plate-and-screw mandible reconstruction. *Oral Surg. Oral Med. Oral Pathol. Oral Radiol. Endodontol.* **2010**, *109*, 346–356. [CrossRef] [PubMed]
29. Johansson, B.; Grepe, A.; Wannfors, K.; Hirsch, J. A clinical study of changes in the volume of bone grafts in the atrophic maxilla. *Dentomaxillofac. Radiol.* **2001**, *30*, 157–161. [CrossRef] [PubMed]
30. Goh, B.T.; Lee, S.; Tideman, H.; Stoelinga, P.J. Mandibular reconstruction in adults: A review. *Int. J. Oral Maxillofac. Surg.* **2008**, *37*, 597–605. [CrossRef] [PubMed]
31. Bagby, G.W.; Janes, J.M. The effect of compression on the rate of fracture healing using a special plate. *Am. J. Surg.* **1958**, *95*, 761–771. [CrossRef]
32. Ayache, N.; Delingette, H. Surgery simulation and soft tissue modeling. In Proceeding of the International Symposium, IS4TM 2003, Juan-Les-Pins, France, 12–13 June 2003; Springer Science & Business Media: Berlin/Heidelberg, Germany, 2003; Volume 2673.
33. Elahinia, M.; Moghaddam, N.S.; Andani, M.T.; Skoracki, R.; Valerio, I.; Miller, M.; Dean, D. Mitigating implant failure through design and manufacturing of nitinol fixation hardware. In *Tissue Engineering Part A*; Mary Ann Liebert, Inc.: New Rochelle, NY, USA, 2015; p. S10.
34. Binger, T.; Hell, B. Resorption of microsurgically vascularized bone grafts after augmentation of the mandible. *J. Cranio-Maxillofac. Surg.* **1999**, *27*, 82–85. [CrossRef]
35. Li, L.; Blake, F.; Heiland, M.; Schmelzle, R.; Pohlenz, P. Long-term evaluation after mandibular reconstruction with fibular grafts versus microsurgical fibular flaps. *J. Oral Maxillofac. Surg.* **2007**, *65*, 281–286. [CrossRef] [PubMed]
36. Bidabadi, M.; Natanzi, A.H.A.; Mostafavi, S.A. Thermophoresis effect on volatile particle concentration in micro-organic dust flame. *Powder Technol.* **2012**, *217*, 69–76. [CrossRef]
37. Amerinatanzi, A.; Summers, R.; Ahmadi, K.; Goel, V.K.; Hewett, T.E.; Nyman, E. A novel 3d approach for determination of frontal and coronal plane tibial slopes from mr imaging. *The Knee* **2016**. [CrossRef] [PubMed]
38. Kunchur, M.; Dean, C.; Moghadam, N.S.; Knight, J.; He, Q.; Liu, H.; Wang, J.; Lortz, R.; Sou, I.; Gurevich, A. Current-induced depairing in the $Bi_2Te_3/FeTe$ interfacial superconductor. *Phys. Rev. B* **2015**, *92*, 094502. [CrossRef]
39. Kunchur, M.N.; Dean, C.; Liang, M.; Moghaddam, N.S.; Guarino, A.; Nigro, A.; Grimaldi, G.; Leo, A. Depairing current density of $Nd_{2-x}Ce_xCuO_{4-\delta}$ superconducting films. *Phys. C Supercond.* **2013**, *495*, 66–68. [CrossRef]
40. Rahmani, M.; Ahmadi, M.T.; Shayesteh, N.; Amin, N.A.; Rahmani, K.; Ismail, R. Current-voltage modeling of bilayer graphene nanoribbon schottky diode. In Proceedings of the 2011 IEEE Regional Symposium on Micro and Nanoelectronics (RSM), Kota Kinabalu, Malaysia, 28–30 September 2011; pp. 256–258.
41. Schileo, E.; Dall'Ara, E.; Taddei, F.; Malandrino, A.; Schotkamp, T.; Baleani, M.; Viceconti, M. An accurate estimation of bone density improves the accuracy of subject-specific finite element models. *J. Biomech.* **2008**, *41*, 2483–2491. [CrossRef] [PubMed]

42. Schileo, E.; Taddei, F.; Cristofolini, L.; Viceconti, M. Subject-specific finite element models implementing a maximum principal strain criterion are able to estimate failure risk and fracture location on human femurs tested in vitro. *J. Biomech.* **2008**, *41*, 356–367. [CrossRef] [PubMed]
43. Zannoni, C.; Mantovani, R.; Viceconti, M. Material properties assignment to finite element models of bone structures: A new method. *Med. Eng. Phys.* **1999**, *20*, 735–740. [CrossRef]
44. Taddei, F.; Pancanti, A.; Viceconti, M. An improved method for the automatic mapping of computed tomography numbers onto finite element models. *Med. Eng. Phys.* **2004**, *26*, 61–69. [CrossRef]
45. Morgan, E.F.; Bayraktar, H.H.; Keaveny, T.M. Trabecular bone modulus–density relationships depend on anatomic site. *J. Biomech.* **2003**, *36*, 897–904. [CrossRef]
46. Korioth, T.W.; Romilly, D.P.; Hannam, A.G. Three-dimensional finite element stress analysis of the dentate human mandible. *Am. J. Phys. Anthropol.* **1992**, *88*, 69–96. [CrossRef] [PubMed]
47. Lovald, S.T.; Wagner, J.D.; Baack, B. Biomechanical optimization of bone plates used in rigid fixation of mandibular fractures. *J. Oral Maxillofac. Surg.* **2009**, *67*, 973–985. [CrossRef] [PubMed]
48. Rahmani, M.; Ahmadi, M.; Webb, J.; Shayesteh, N.; Mousavi, S.; Sadeghi, H.; Ismail, R. Trilayer graphene nanoribbon carrier statistics in degenerate and non degenerate limits. In Proceedings of the Sixth Global Conference on Power Control and Optimization, Las Vegas, NV, USA, 6–8 August 2012; AIP Publishing: College Park, MD, USA, 2012; pp. 272–275.
49. Nagasao, T.; Miyamoto, J.; Kawana, H. Biomechanical evaluation of implant placement in the reconstructed mandible. *Int. J. Oral Maxillofac. Implant.* **2008**, *24*, 999–1005.
50. Shetty, P.P.; Meshramkar, R.; Patil, K.N.; Nadiger, R.K. A finite element analysis for a comparative evaluation of stress with two commonly used esthetic posts. *Eur. J. Dent.* **2013**, *7*, 419–422. [CrossRef] [PubMed]
51. Moghaddam, N.S. Toward Patient Specific Long Lasting Metallic Implants for Mandibular Segmental Defects. Ph.D. Thesis, The University of Toledo, Toledo, OH, USA, August 2015.
52. Moghaddam, N.S.; Jahadakbar, A.; Amerinatanzi, A.; Elahinia, M.; Miller, M.; Dean, D. Metallic fixation of mandibular segmental defects: Graft immobilization and orofacial functional maintenance. *Plast. Reconstr. Surg. Glob. Open* **2016**, *4*, e858. [CrossRef] [PubMed]
53. Tanaka, E.; Koolstra, J. Biomechanics of the temporomandibular joint. *J. Dent. Res.* **2008**, *87*, 989–991. [CrossRef] [PubMed]
54. Amerinatanzi, A.; Moghaddam, N.S.; Jahadakbar, A.; Dean, D.; Elahinia, M. On the effect of screw preload on the stress distribution of mandibles during segmental defect treatment using an additively manufactured hardware. In Proceedings of the ASME 2016 11th International Manufacturing Science and Engineering Conference, Blacksburg, VA, USA, 27 June–1 July 2016.
55. Raad, B.; Moghaddam, N.S.; Elahinia, M. A numerical simulation of the effect of using porous superelastic nitinol and stiff titanium fixation hardware on the bone remodeling. In *Nanosensors, Biosensors, and Info-Tech Sensors and Systems 2016*; SPIE Press: Bellingham, WA, USA, 2016.
56. Saedi, S.; Turabi, A.; Taheri Andani, M.; Elahinia, M.; Karaca, H. Thermo-mechanical characterization of NiTi alloys manufactured by selective laser melting. In Proceedings of the ASME Conference on Smart Materials, Adaptive Structures and Intelligent Systems (SMASIS), Colorado Springs, CO, USA, 21–23 September 2015; ASME: Colorado Springs, CO, USA, 2015.
57. Saedi, S.; Turabi, A.S.; Andani, M.T.; Haberland, C.; Karaca, H.; Elahinia, M. The influence of heat treatment on the thermomechanical response of Ni-rich NiTi alloys manufactured by selective laser melting. *J. Alloy. Compd.* **2016**, *677*, 204–210. [CrossRef]
58. Ahmadi, A.; Mirzaeifar, R.; Moghaddam, N.S.; Turabi, A.S.; Karaca, H.E.; Elahinia, M. Effect of manufacturing parameters on mechanical properties of 316l stainless steel parts fabricated by selective laser melting: A computational framework. *Mater. Des.* **2016**, *112*, 328–338. [CrossRef]
59. Ahmadi, A.; Moghaddam, N.S.; Elahinia, M.; Karaca, H.E.; Mirzaeifar, R. Finite element modeling of selective laser melting 316l stainless steel parts for evaluating the mechanical properties. In Proceedings of the ASME 2016 11th International Manufacturing Science and Engineering Conference, Blacksburg, VA, USA, 27 June–1 July 2016.
60. Shayesteh Moghaddam, N.; Dean, D.; Miller, M.; Elahinia, M. Improving bone implant success by using nitinol as a substitute for titanium: A modeling comparison. In Proceedings of the ASME 2014 Smart Materials, Adaptive Structures and Intelligent Systems, Newport, RI, USA, 8–10 September 2014.

61. Elahinia, M.H.; Hashemi, M.; Tabesh, M.; Bhaduri, S.B. Manufacturing and processing of NiTi implants: A review. *Prog. Mater. Sci.* **2012**, *57*, 911–946. [CrossRef]
62. Haberland, C.; Elahinia, M.; Walker, J.M.; Meier, H.; Frenzel, J. On the development of high quality NiTi shape memory and pseudoelastic parts by additive manufacturing. *Smart Mater. Struct.* **2014**, *23*, 104002. [CrossRef]
63. Dadbakhsh, S.; Speirs, M.; Kruth, J.-P.; Van Humbeeck, J. Influence of SLM on shape memory and compression behaviour of NiTi scaffolds. *CIRP Ann. Manuf. Technol.* **2015**, *64*, 209–212. [CrossRef]
64. Dadbakhsh, S.; Speirs, M.; Kruth, J.P.; Schrooten, J.; Luyten, J.; Van Humbeeck, J. Effect of SLM parameters on transformation temperatures of shape memory nickel titanium parts. *Adv. Eng. Mater.* **2014**, *16*, 1140–1146. [CrossRef]
65. Dadbakhsh, S.; Vrancken, B.; Kruth, J.-P.; Luyten, J.; van Humbeeck, J. Texture and anisotropy in selective laser melting of NiTi alloy. *Mater. Sci. Eng. A* **2016**, *650*, 225–232. [CrossRef]
66. Lee, W.-S.; Lin, C.-F. Plastic deformation and fracture behaviour of Ti-6Al-4V alloy loaded with high strain rate under various temperatures. *Mater. Sci. Eng. A* **1998**, *241*, 48–59. [CrossRef]
67. Mehrabi, R.; Kadkhodaei, M.; Ghaei, A. Numerical implementation of a thermomechanical constitutive model for shape memory alloys using return mapping algorithm and microplane theory. *Adv. Mater. Res.* **2012**, *516*, 351–354. [CrossRef]
68. Mehrabi, R.; Kadkhodaei, M.; Andani, M.T.; Elahinia, M. Microplane modeling of shape memory alloy tubes under tension, torsion, and proportional tension–torsion loading. *J. Intell. Mater. Syst. Struct.* **2014**, *26*, 144–155. [CrossRef]
69. Mehrabi, R.; Kadkhodaei, M. 3D phenomenological constitutive modeling of shape memory alloys based on microplane theory. *Smart Mater. Struct.* **2013**, *22*, 025017. [CrossRef]
70. Andani, M.T.; Haberland, C.; Walker, J.M.; Karamooz, M.; Turabi, A.S.; Saedi, S.; Rahmanian, R.; Karaca, H.; Dean, D.; Kadkhodaei, M. Achieving biocompatible stiffness in NiTi through additive manufacturing. *J. Intell. Mater. Syst. Struct.* **2016**, *4*, 2661–2671. [CrossRef]
71. Andani, M.T.; Alipour, A.; Eshghinejad, A.; Elahinia, M. Modifying the torque–angle behavior of rotary shape memory alloy actuators through axial loading: A semi-analytical study of combined tension–torsion behavior. *J. Intell. Mater. Syst. Struct.* **2013**, *24*, 1524–1535. [CrossRef]
72. Taheri, A.M. Modeling, simulation, additive manufacturing, and experimental evaluation of solid and porous NiTi. Ph.D. Thesis, The University of Toledo, Toledo, OH, USA, August 2015.
73. Van Eijden, T. Biomechanics of the mandible. *Crit. Rev. Oral Boil. Med.* **2000**, *11*, 123–136. [CrossRef]
74. Ichim, I.; Kieser, J.; Swain, M. Functional significance of strain distribution in the human mandible under masticatory load: Numerical predictions. *Arch. Oral Biol.* **2007**, *52*, 465–473. [CrossRef] [PubMed]
75. Raad, B.; Moghaddam, N.S.; Elahinia, M. A comparison between porous NiTi and Ti-6Al-4V fixation hardware on bone remodeling after a reconstruction surgery. In Proceedings of the ASME 2016 11th International Manufacturing Science and Engineering Conference, Blacksburg, VA, USA, 27 June–1 July 2016.
76. Elahinia, M.; Moghaddam, N.S.; Andani, M.T.; Rahmanian, R.; Walker, J.; Miller, M.J.; Dean, D. Site-Specific Material Properties and the Additive Manufacturing of Nitinol Musculoskeletal Implants. In *Tissue Engineering Part A*; Mary Ann Liebert, Inc.: New Rochelle, NY, USA, 2014; Volume 20, pp. S120–S121.

3

Patient-Specific Surgical Implant using Cavity-Filled Approach for Precise and Functional Mandible Reconstruction

Khaja Moiduddin [1,*], Syed Hammad Mian [1], Wadea Ameen [1], Mohammed Alkindi [2], Sundar Ramalingam [2] and Osama Alghamdi [2]

1 Advanced Manufacturing Institute, King Saud University, Riyadh 11421, Saudi Arabia; smien@ksu.edu.sa (S.H.M.); wqaid@ksu.edu.sa (W.A.)

2 Department of Oral and Maxillofacial Surgery, College of Dentistry, King Saud University, Riyadh 11545, Saudi Arabia; malkindi@ksu.edu.sa (M.A.); smunusamy@ksu.edu.sa (S.R.); oghamdi@ksu.edu.sa (O.A.)

* Correspondence: khussain1@ksu.edu.sa.

Abstract: Mandibular reconstruction is a complicated task because of the complex nature of the regional anatomy. Computer-assisted tools are a promising means of improving the precision and safety of such complex surgeries. The digital techniques utilized in the reconstruction of mandibular defects based on medical data, computer-aided-design approaches, and three-dimensional (3D) printing are widely used to improve the patient's aesthetic appearance and function, as well as the accuracy and quality of diagnosis, and surgical outcomes. Nevertheless, to ensure an acceptable aesthetical appearance and functional outcomes, the design must be based on proper anatomical reconstruction, mostly done in a virtual environment by skilled design engineers. Mirroring is one of the widely used techniques in the surgical navigation and reconstruction of mandibular defects. However, there are some discrepancies and mismatches in the mirrored anatomical models. Hence, in order to overcome these limitations in the mirroring technique, a novel approach called the cavity-filled technique was introduced. The objective of this study was to compare the accuracy of the newly recommended cavity-filled technique with the widely used mirror reconstruction technique in restoring mandibular defects. A prominent 3D comparison technique was employed in this work, where the resected and the reconstructed mandibles were superimposed to quantify the accuracy of the two techniques. From the analysis, it can be inferred that the cavity-filled technique with a root-mean-square value of 1.1019 mm produced better accuracy in contrast to the mirroring approach, which resulted in an error of 1.2683 mm. Consequently, by using the proposed cavity-filled design, the discrepancy between the reconstruction plate and the bone contour was mitigated. This method, owing to its high precision, can decrease the number of adjustments and the time of surgery, as well as ensure a quick recovery time with better implant tissue in-growth.

Keywords: 3D printing; custom-specific implant; mirror reconstruction; 3D comparison; cavity-filled approach

---

1. Introduction

Functional and aesthetic defects in the maxillofacial region occur primarily due to various ailments, such as tumor excision, trauma, malformation, jaw atrophy, and benign or malignant neoplasm [1,2]. Immediate reconstruction is the most effective way to achieve improved and long-term functional outcomes [3]. Recent advances in technology and innovations in the patient-specific implants and their treatment led to the minimization of surgical time and cost. Precise design and production of patient-specific implants are essential in the surgical outcome. One of the biggest challenges, even for experienced surgeons, is to precisely fit the implant onto the bone contours and eliminate postoperative revisions. The success rate of any reconstructive implant surgery depends on several factors, such as medical evaluation, implant design, and the surgeon's skill [4]. The majority of conventionally manufactured reconstructive implants are of standard size and form. Such implants must be adjusted by manual bending or twisting according to the bone contour of the patient, resulting in poor adaptation and prolonged operating time [5]. Most patients undergo secondary surgical reconstruction to refine the cosmetic and functional outcomes that result in psychological stress and social implications [6,7]. The pre-operative preparation and three-dimensional (3D) printed patient-specific implant assessment are crucial to mitigate these instances. In addition, accurate patient-specific implants and their evaluation will result in reduced operating time, predictability of surgical outcome, and increased implant accuracy [8,9]. Virtual pre-operative planning and 3D-printed polymer models help minimize revision, as well as errors, eventually providing better aesthetic and functional results [10].

The technique of 3D printing developed in the mid-1980s laid the foundation for the efficient manufacturing of complex anatomical models, whereby anatomical defects can be measured and pre-planned by surgeons, and surgeries can be simulated [11]. The anatomical curvature of the skull and its facial bone is extremely complex, and it is often a demanding process for skilled surgeons to accurately align and rebuild the implant [12]. In the past, several computer-assisted design (CAD) and 3D planning strategies were proposed for the reconstruction of mandibular and dental implants [13,14]. These concepts utilized a preoperative virtual simulation of the proposed mandibular defect, and they could easily modify the 3D file multiple times, rather than relying heavily on the traditional intraoperative manual assessment [15]. In addition, 3D reconstruction planning improved the surgical precision, reduced the operating time, and ultimately enhanced the structural and functional outcomes [16]. Bartier et al. [17] demonstrated that a 3D reconstruction technique maintained the symmetrical accuracy, as well as improved the functional and aesthetic outcomes, in mandibular reconstruction when compared to traditional freehand technique. Mascha et al. [18] and Yang et al. [19] also developed a patient-specific mandibular reconstruction plate using a CAD procedure and proved that it was more effective and satisfying for accurate mandibular reconstruction. According to Davies et al. [20], the segmental mirroring technique could be exploited satisfactorily for creating reasonably accurate 3D models to enable mandibular reconstruction in instances where preoperative adjustment of a reconstruction plate was constrained by the complexity of the mandibular defect. This strategy was rather less effective when the complicated mandibular condyle anatomy was involved. Similarly, Mahendru et al. [21] advocated the application of CAD/computer-aided manufacturing (CAM) technology and 3D-printed cutting guides to accomplish realistic and cosmetic performance in patients seeking mandibular reconstruction with a free fibula flap. However, the higher costs coupled with CAD/CAM technology can be easily compensated for by reducing the operating time and adequate rehabilitation. Darwich et al. [22] also documented a report of sizeable mandibular tumor removal and reconstruction of the deformity using a personalized 3D-printed titanium implant. The analysis provided impressive functional and aesthetic postoperative outcomes without serious side effects. As per the researcher, titanium implants represented an optimal alloplastic material for mandibular reconstruction since they were versatile, bioinert, impervious, and easily workable, particularly with the aid of 3D digital planning tools. An integrated two-phase strategy was developed by Linares et al. [23] for the segmentation of cone-beam computed tomography (CBCT). They firstly executed an automatic segmentation of bone geometries with super-voxels, permitting a reasonable graph estimate of the 3D data. A user-placed seed operation, then directed a graph partitioning algorithm, which divided the extracted bones into mandible and cranium. The exploration of the algorithm led to a precise segmentation and was resilient to parameter variations. The segmentation of the mandible in computer tomography (CT) scans is greatly affected by metal objects such as dental filling materials and by substantial variations in shape and size between patients. To resolve these challenges, Qiu et al. [24] implemented an automated mandibular segmentation approach in CT scans that identified the spectrum of anatomical forms across multiple planes. The mechanism relied on the architecture of the convolution neural network and then merged the resultant two-dimensional (2D) segmentations from three orthogonal planes into a 3D segmentation.

Restoration of maxillary defects following tumor removal is a complex process owing to anatomical and functional complications, and autografts along with fixation plates are amongst the most frequently used methods. The disadvantage of this standard approach is the fairly prolonged time required in manipulating the plate during the process, which not only increases the surgical time but also induces metal fatigue in the plate. The vulnerability of the conventional fixation plates was resolved by Abbai et al. [25], who fused stereolithography with mirror reconstruction through the projection of the unaffected side onto the affected side. Mirroring is one of the most widely used reconstruction techniques, and several research studies proved that the mirror technique successfully restored the facial symmetry [26,27]. Hatamleh et al. [28] also consolidated the mirror restoration method with selective laser sintering for bimaxillary surgery and mandibular reconstruction. The concerned patient reported the capabilities of 3D CAD/CAM technologies in improving surgical results for cranio-maxillofacial reconstruction. Mirror restoration is among the extensively used procedures of 3D reconstruction in medical applications where the impaired section is substituted by a healthy symmetrical region [29]. However, the technique of cavity-filled reconstruction is a new or perhaps uncommon approach where the bone cavity is filled with mass to create a solid bone portion. Since, implant fitting has always depended on the reconstructed area, the accuracy assessment of the restored region is mandatory. This implies that, with better accuracy or placement of the implant, the overall aesthetics of the facial anatomy would improve. The primary goal of this work was to assess the effectiveness of the cavity-filled approach in terms of implant fitting accuracy. It also aimed to compare the performance of the cavity-filled technique with respect to the mirror reconstruction method. For statistical inference, two hypotheses were tested in this work: the null hypothesis of no effect and the alternative hypothesis of an effect [30,31]. The null hypothesis included that there was no difference in the accuracy of the two reconstruction techniques. The alternative hypothesis was that the accuracy of the implant using the cavity-filled approach was significantly different than the mirror reconstruction technique.

In this research, the two techniques (i.e., mirror and cavity-filled reconstruction techniques) were firstly employed in 3D model design and recreation of the implants. The two reconstructed design models were subsequently fabricated in a fused deposition technology (FDM)-based 3D-printing machine (Stratasys, Eden Prairie, MN, USA). These implant models were then evaluated and compared using a 3D comparison technique. The 3D comparison is one of the most thorough and useful techniques for quantifying the error deviations between the two models [32]. The accuracy analysis using a 3D comparison was performed in Geomagics Control® software, employing the Faro arm scanner. The two hypotheses were also tested depending on the acquired results. Finally, the implant acquired with the cavity-filled reconstruction approach was fabricated utilizing an electron beam melting (EBM) machine in case the null hypothesis was rejected.

2. Proposed Methodology

The proposed research methodology adopted for the reconstructive design consisted of six stages as shown in Figure 1.

2.1. Tumor Diagnosis

A patient with a progressive expanding mass on his left cheek was subjected to an incisional biopsy procedure, which showed a plexiform ameloblastoma. A GE (General Electric) light speed VCT XTe 64-row spiral CT scan was used, and the scanned images were then saved as a DICOM (digital imaging and communication in medicine) file. DICOM is a de facto international standard for sharing, exchanging, and storing digital medical images. The DICOM file contained 2D images of the anatomical structure.

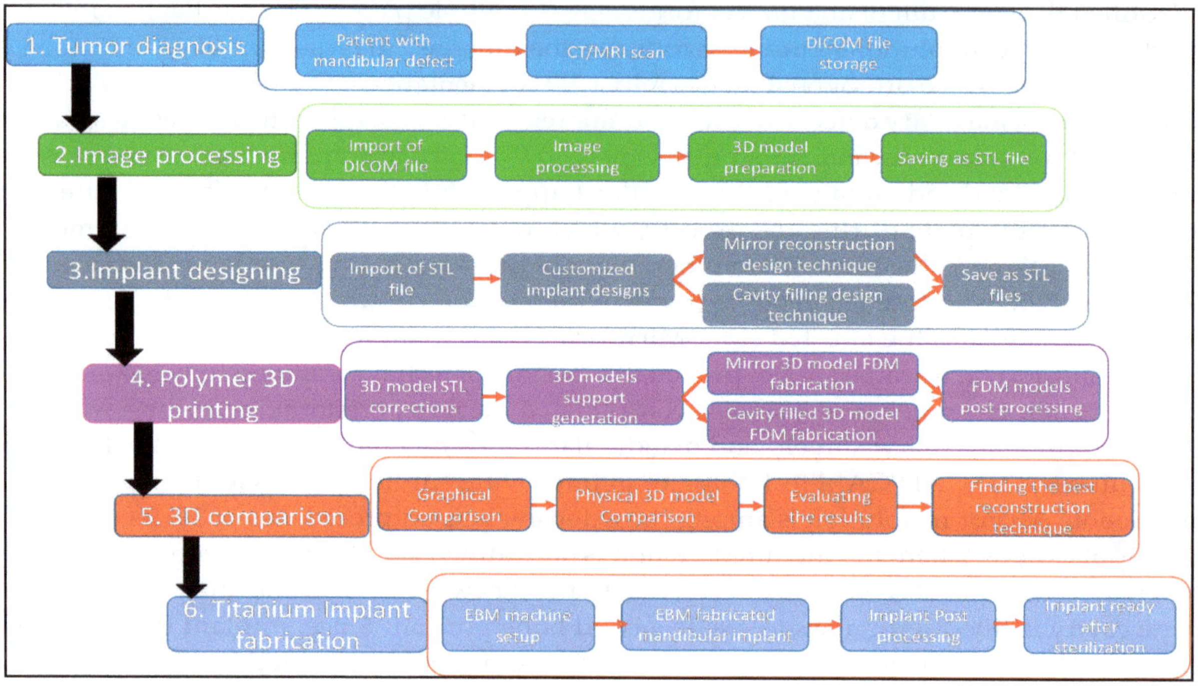

Figure 1. Flowchart illustrating the steps in the selection of implant reconstruction technique.

2.2. Image Acquisition and Processing

The DICOM file consists of a series of 2D images that do not provide enough information for clinical diagnosis. There are many image visualizations and surgical planning software available in the market such as 3D Slicer, Scan IP, etc. In this study, MIMICS® 17.0 (Materialise NV, Leuven, Belgium, 2014), a powerful image processing software for 3D design and modeling, was utilized in the conversion of medical DICOM data into a 3D surface model. In MIMICS®, the 2D DICOM images were stacked upon each other to create a perfect 3D surface model, as shown in Figure 2. The 3D model showed a cystic cavity with a cortical bone defect in the left mandibular body region.

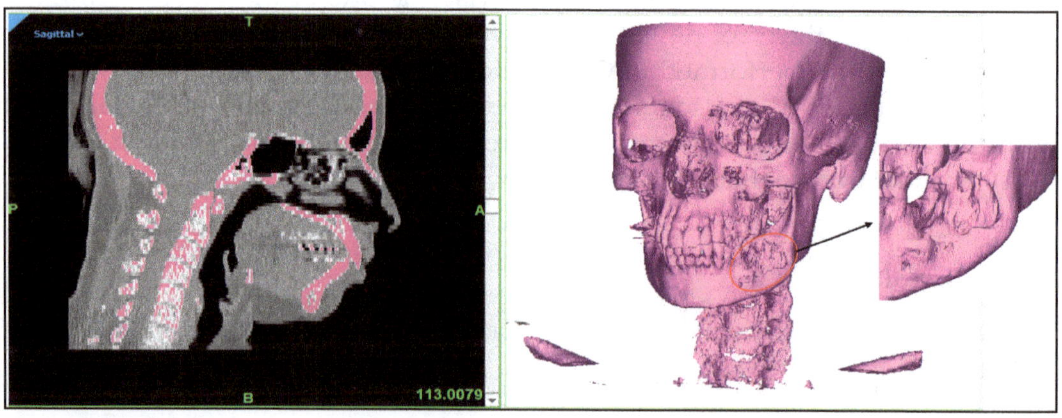

Figure 2. Patient anatomical model revealing the tumor mass and the resultant bone destruction on the left side of the mandible.

A custom Hounsfield unit (HU) of upper threshold value 3012 and a lower threshold value of 260 was used for the bone identification and to separate the hard and soft tissues. The next step was to segment the full mask into a series of smaller elements using a region-growing technique, until the region of interest (mandible) was obtained (Figure 3). The surface irregularities were smoothened with a compensating shrinkage factor and the obtained mandible was then saved as an STL (Standard Triangle Language) file.

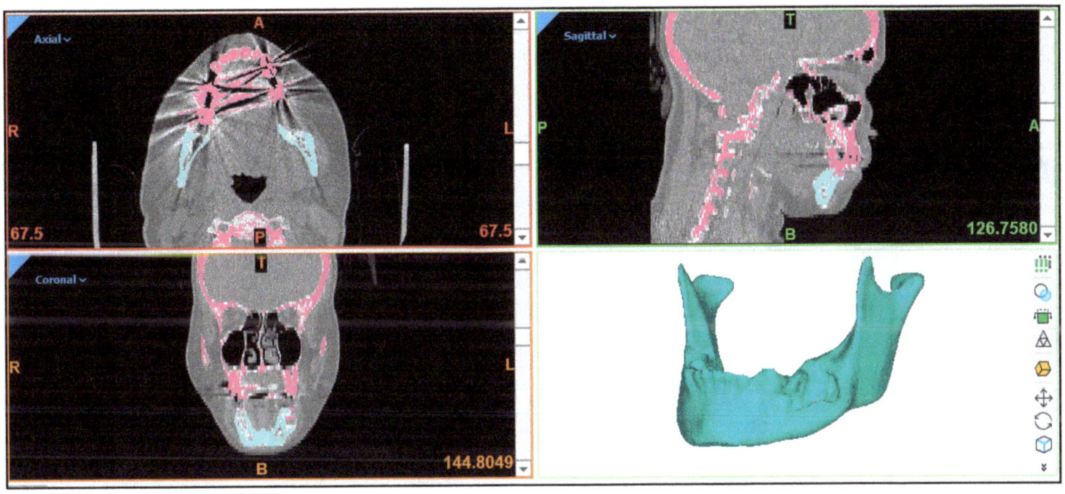

Figure 3. Segmentation of the region of interest (mandible) from the skull region.

2.3. Custom Implant Design

The mandible model from MIMICS® was imported in 3-Matic® 13.0 (Materialise NV, Leuven, Belgium, 2018) software to model and custom-design the reconstruction plate. The steps involved in mirror reconstruction are explained in Figure 4. The mandibular STL file obtained from MIMICS® was imported in 3-Matic® (Figure 4a), where the left tumor region was cut down by a cut-and-punch operation (Figure 4b). The mandibular model was then split into two regions (Figure 4c), where the tumor region was removed (Figure 4d) for mirror operation. Mirroring was performed (Figure 4e) where the symmetrical healthy right mandibular region was mirrored to the left side. The two symmetrical right and left mandibular regions were then merged (Figure 4f) and wrapped to remove the voids and gaps (Figure 4g). The final obtained mirror model was then aligned with the mandibular tumor model (Figure 4h) to evaluate the anatomical positions. Upon closer examination of the aligned models, a small upper portion of the condyle regions mismatched the original tumor mandible. Several attempts at re-mirroring and re-adjustment failed to match the orientation to the original mandible.

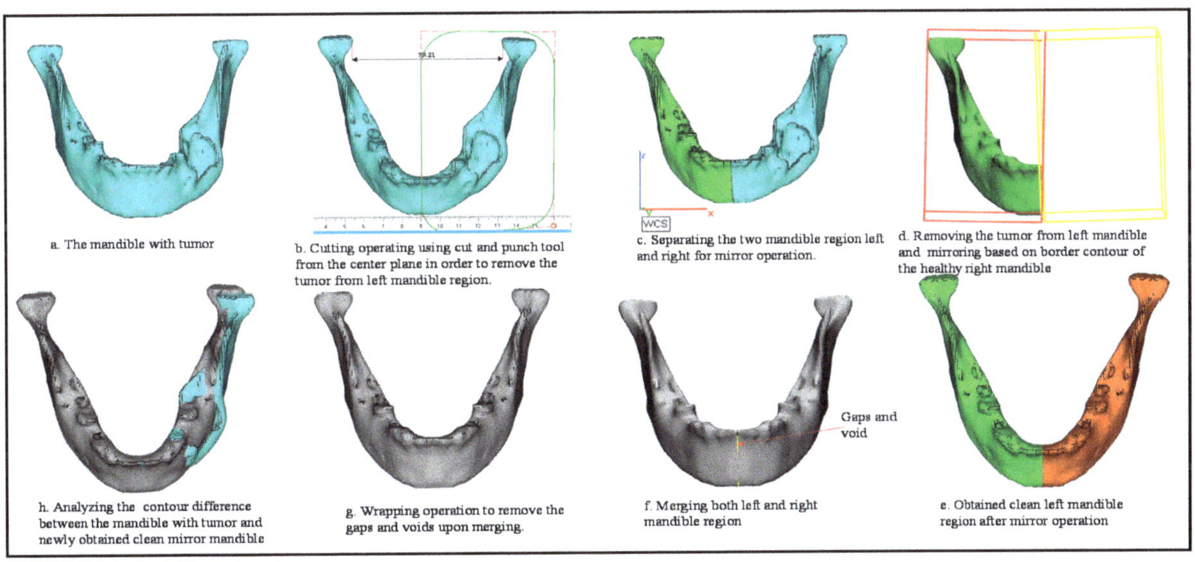

Figure 4. Steps involved in the three-dimensional reconstruction of the clean, healthy mandible using the mirroring technique.

To overcome the misalignment between the mirroring and original tumor mandible, a newly design reconstruction technique was proposed. In this technique, the tumor model (Figure 5a) was cavity-filled to create a solid bone portion matching the original contours (Figure 5b). The benefit of such an approach was that it maintained the shape and anatomical geometry of the mandible. The additional bone portion of the tumor area was trimmed (Figure 5c), and the obtained cavity-filled mandible model was then aligned with the tumor mandible for evaluation (Figure 5d).

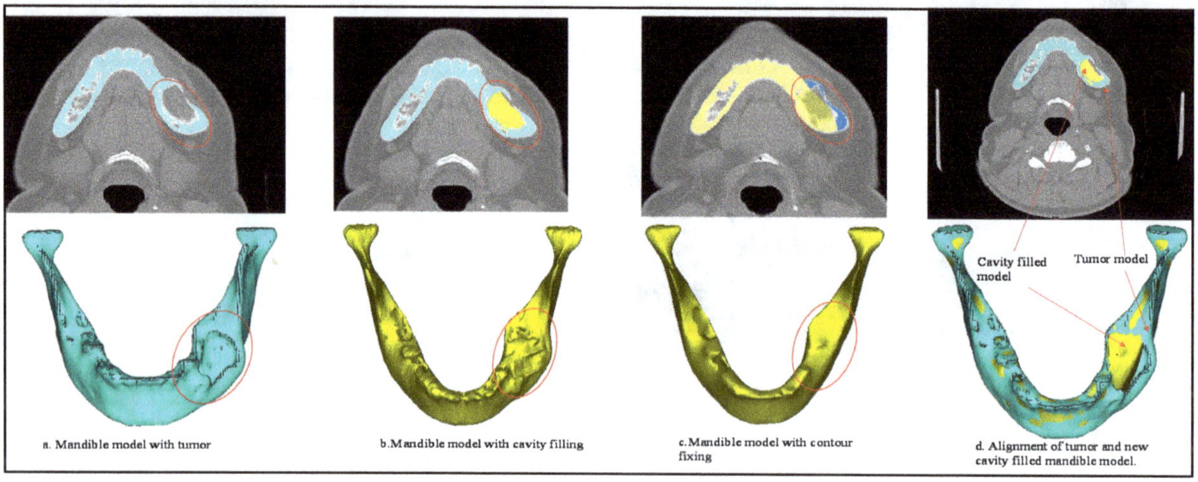

Figure 5. Sequential steps involved in the reconstruction of the mandible using cavity-filled technique.

Figure 6 explains the design steps involved in the resection of the mandible model, where the tumor part (Figure 6a) was resected using a cut-and-punch operation (Figure 6b,c). The resected model was the patient's mandible bony region on which the surgeons operated the implant after tumor removal. The resected tumor mandible (Figure 6d) was used for the 3D comparison and the fitting of the customized implant design in this study.

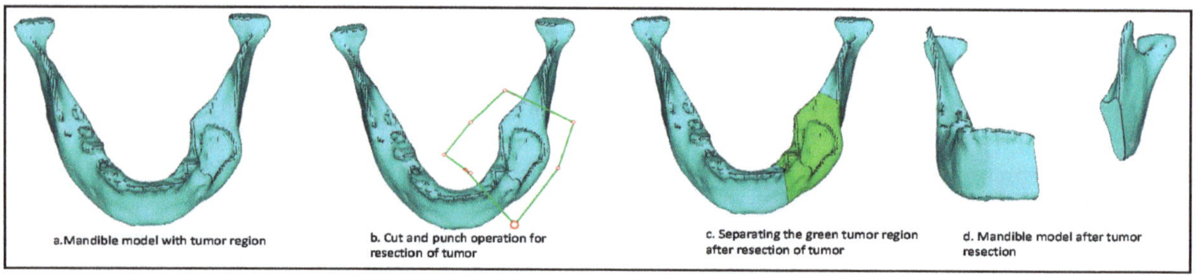

Figure 6. Design steps in the creation of resected mandible.

Figure 7 explains the steps involved in the reconstruction of the customized implant design from the cavity-filled model. The obtained cavity-filled mandible model was loaded into 3-Matic® as an STL file (Figure 7a). The model outer part was selected using the brush mark technique (Figure 7b,c) and extracted for custom implant design (Figure 7d). Trimming and splitting operations were performed (Figure 7e,f) on the extracted bone mask to get an implant template (Figure 7g). An offset thickness of 2 mm was added (Figure 7h), and screw holes were incorporated for fitting (Figure 7i). The final obtained prefabricated custom-designed mandibular implant was aligned with the resected mandible for assembly and fitting evaluation (Figure 7j). The prefabricated implant designed from the cavity-filled model fitted precisely onto the tumor-resected mandible model as it was created from the bone itself. Similarly, a second prefabricated implant was also designed following a similar approach to that above from the mirror reconstruction model. These steps are presented to illustrate how the custom-designed implant was created from the healthy mandible after tumor removal through a mirroring or cavity-filled approach. Hence, reconstructing a healthy mandible model is important whether through mirroring or cavity-filled approaches. The modeling and designing of the customized implant from the healthy mandible is the same for both models.

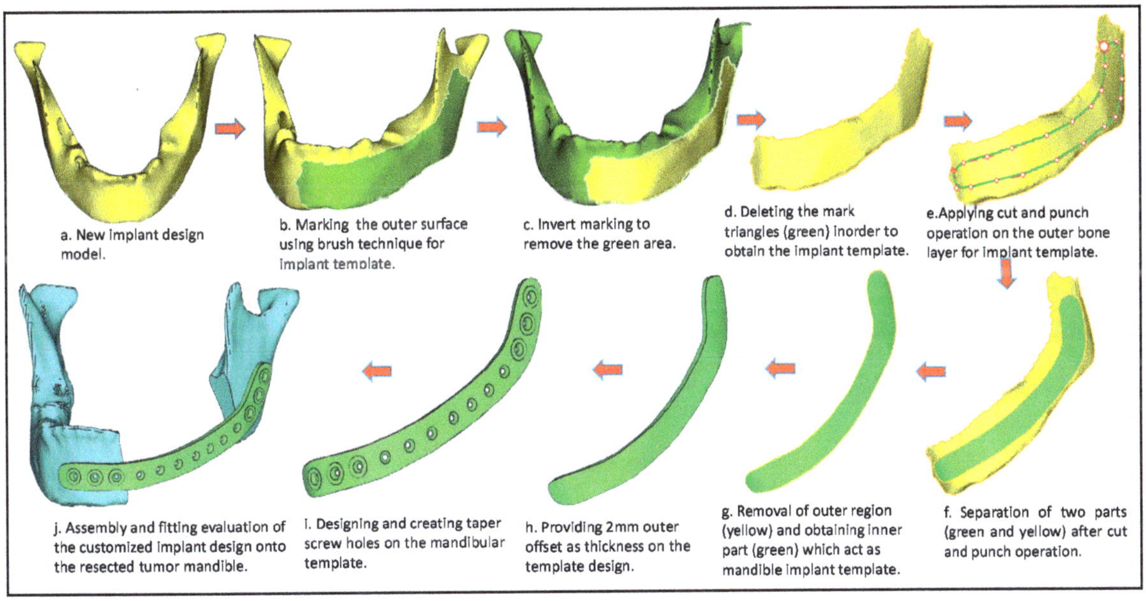

Figure 7. Steps involved in the design of a customized mandibular implant from a healthy design model.

3. 3D Printing

The technique of 3D printing was used in this study for the fabrication of the mandibles and the subsequent 3D comparison of the reconstructed design models. The polymer-based Stratasys FDM machine was used for the 3D printing of models. The FDM machine used ABS (acrylonitrile butadiene styrene) material, which is a common thermoplastic resin allowing functional testing of medical products, and which is relatively safe to handle [33]. The ABS material contributes a good balance of chemical and heat resistance, along with tensile strength and a good glossy finish on the finished surface [34]. The FDM process started by importing the model STL file into a pre-processing software where the model was sliced into a series of horizontal 2D layers. Support structures were created where needed as per the model geometry. The built and support filaments were unwound from a coil and fed through the printer extrusion nozzle. The nozzle melted the filament and extruded it on top of the previous extrusion layer, thus creating parts layer by layer.

3.1. STL Corrections and Support Generations

The mirror and cavity-filled reconstructed models were firstly subjected to Magics® 18.0 (Materialise NV, Leuven, Belgium, 2013) to repair the STL file and to generate support. Repairing the STL file before 3D printing was a mandatory operation, because any faulty STL file could lead to geometric inaccuracies and a defective build [35]. Support structures were used to dissipate the heat and to assist in overhanging structures [36]. Moreover, Magics® was also used for the orientation and best possible position during the build process to minimize the build time for the support structure.

3.2. FDM Fabrication

The error-free STL files of the reconstruction models were imported into the FDM machine for the fabrication of polymer mandibular models. Figure 8 illustrates the FDM machine and its fabricated original resected mandible with support structures.

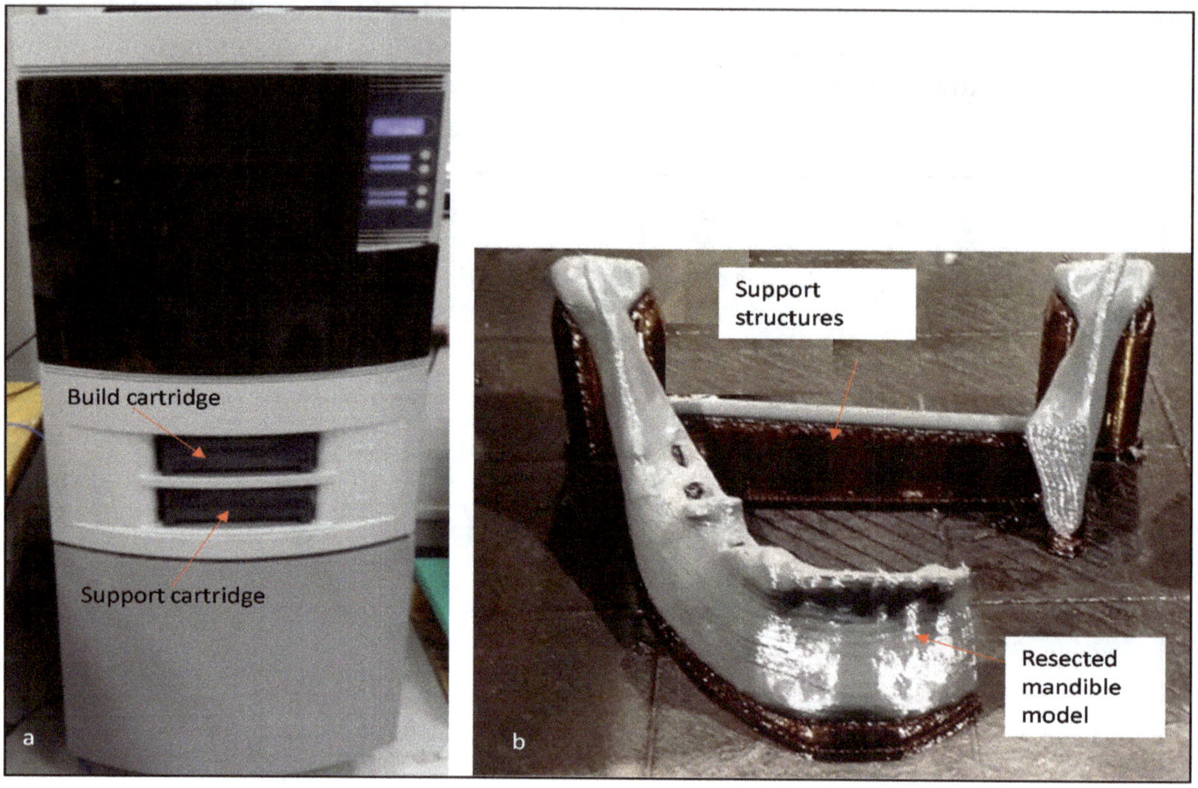

Figure 8. Fused deposition modeling (FDM) machine (**a**) with built resected mandible model, and (**b**) with support structures.

The supports were removed by releasing the fabricated parts into a heated water-based soluble solution where the support structure was dissolved. Figure 9 illustrates the final obtained FDM fabricated models after support removal.

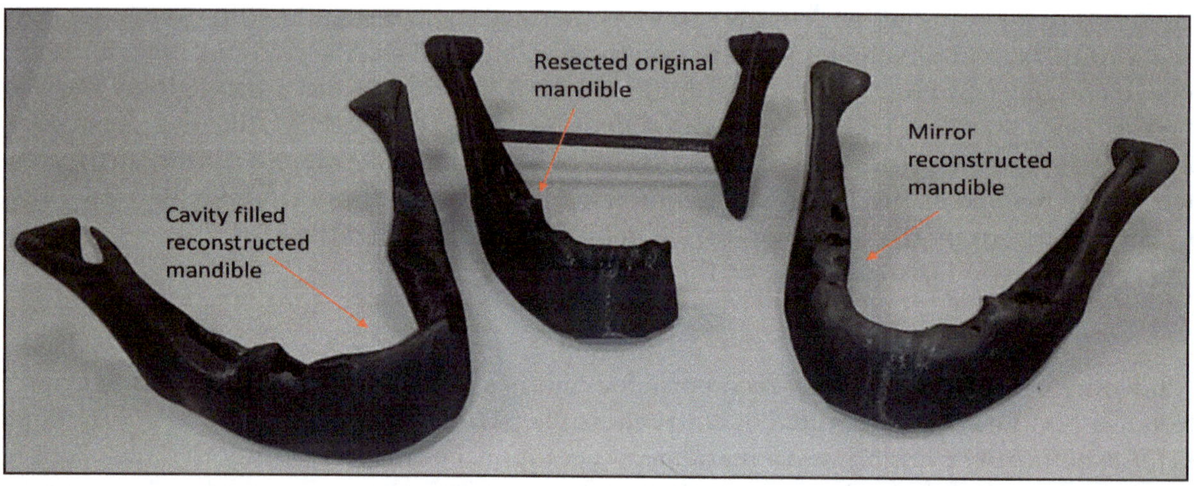

Figure 9. FDM-fabricated polymer models: cavity-filled reconstructed model (**right**), resected original model (**center**), and mirror reconstructed model (**left**) after support removal.

4. Accuracy Assessment

Convenient and precise fitting of the implant is necessary for an aesthetic and functional mandibular restoration. The accuracy of the implant fitting is invaluable, especially when a defect is present on facial features, such as the mandible. The implant fitting is indeed dependent on the reconstructed area obtained via mirroring and cavity-filled techniques. The restoration of the defective area for implant design requires several phases from data acquisition to eventual fabrication. Certainly, errors can occur at each step, and the final accuracy is the sum of all errors at each stage. Therefore, accuracy assessment is mandatory to enhance the placement of the implant and the overall aesthetics of the facial anatomy.

The accuracy evaluation in this investigation was based on a comparison between the resected and the reconstructed mandible models. This analysis was conducted in two steps, to validate and corroborate the findings. Firstly, the STL files of the resected and recovered mandibles were compared, and the polymer-based prototypes were examined in a subsequent stage to achieve a precise fitting of the implants. The goal of this step was, therefore, to estimate the accuracy or precision of the defect reconstruction methods in partially edentulous patients by superimposing 3D digital (STL) files, as well as physical prototypes. The overall workflow for accuracy evaluation is shown in Figure 10.

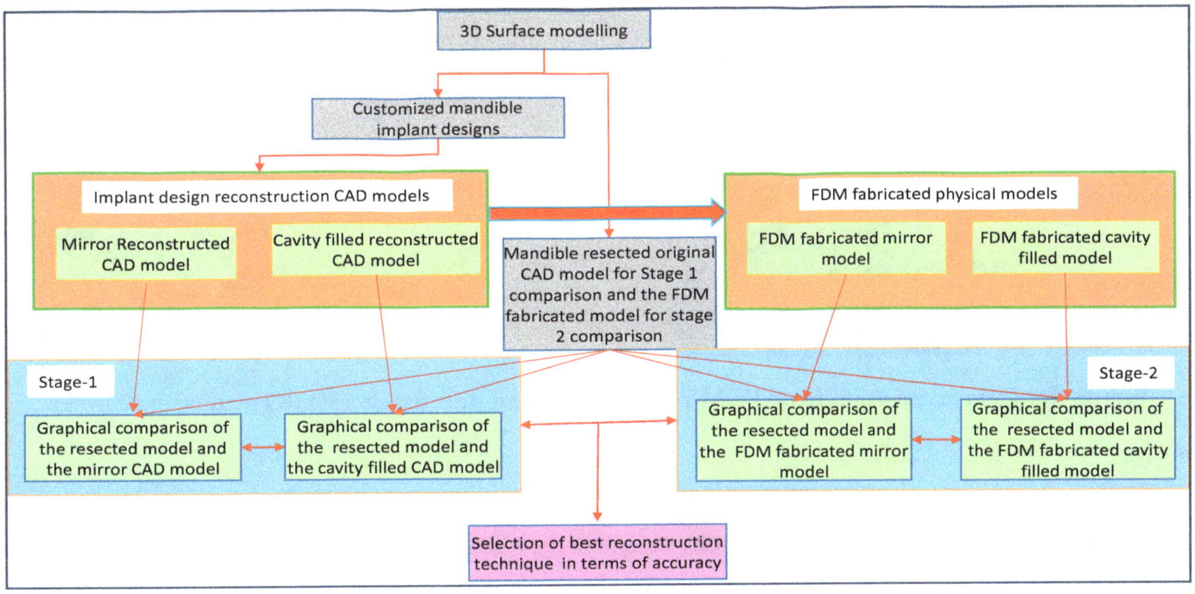

Figure 10. Evaluation of an implant design reconstruction technique using a comparison approach.

For assessment based on physical prototypes, the FDM-produced mirroring and cavity-filled models, as well as the resected model, were scanned using the FARO arm laser scanner (Faro, Lake Mary, FL, USA), as shown in Figure 11. The obtained files were imported into the Geomagics Control 2014 software (3D Systems, Rock Hill, SC, USA) for analysis. For STL-based analysis, the STL files of mirroring, cavity-filled, and resected models were directly imported into the Geomagics Control software from MIMICS. To analyze the deviation (or accuracy), the STL files of the resected mandible were superimposed one by one on both mirror and cavity-filled mandibles via perfect matching using the best-fit algorithm. The resected model was set as a reference, while the mirrored and cavity-filled models were set as test models to facilitate the accuracy assessment.

The following 3D deviations were measured for accuracy analysis using Geomagics Control: root-mean square (RMS) and average deviation (AD). The AD required estimating the variations in the inside and outward directions between the test and the reference files. The RMS (Equation (1)) determined the average error magnitude between both datasets or models. It also quantified the overall accuracy of the models. The two statistics were considered to ascertain and substantiate the results.

$$\mathrm{RMS} = \frac{1}{\sqrt{n}}\sqrt{\sum\nolimits_{i=1}^{n}(X_{1,i} - X_{2,i})^2}, \quad (1)$$

where $X_{1,i}$ is the i-th digitized point in the reference dataset, $X_{2,i}$ is the i-th digitized point in the test dataset, and n represents the number of digitized points. The units of measurement considered for the RMS and AD were mm.

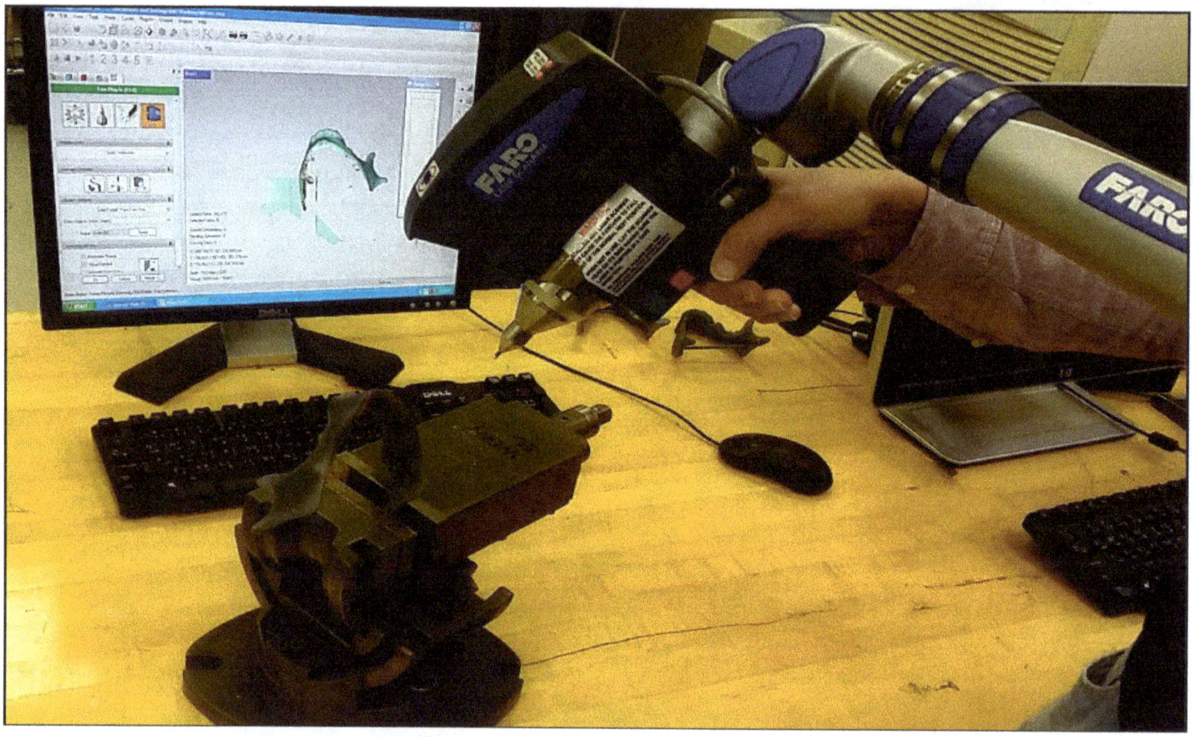

Figure 11. Data acquisition from FDM-reconstructed models using a FARO arm laser scanner.

5. Results

The 3D inspection results shown in Figure 12 illustrated that the majority of the surface was mapped green in the cavity-filled approach, suggesting a high degree of precision between reference (R) and test (T) models.

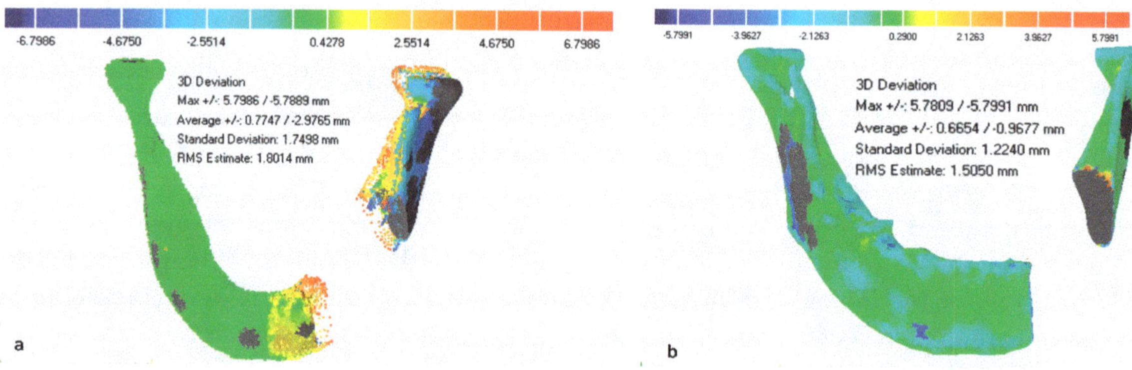

Figure 12. Three-dimensional (3D) inspection results of the resected original mandible model with (**a**) mirror reconstruction model and (**b**) cavity-filled reconstruction model.

A 2D analysis was also conducted to determine the variance around a specific cross-section. A 2D comparison is useful for matching the cross-section of the test object to the cross-section of the reference component. The section plane, shown in Figure 13, was taken across the middle of the mandible to divide the part into top and bottom halves. Figure 13a implies that the top half of the mandible in the test portion was not precisely aligned with the reference artifact. This could be due to either inaccurate symmetrical measurement of the plane or differences on both sides of the mandible of the patient. Indeed, the 2D analysis in Figure 13b demonstrated the higher precision of the cavity-filled approach as compared to the mirror-reconstructed mandible.

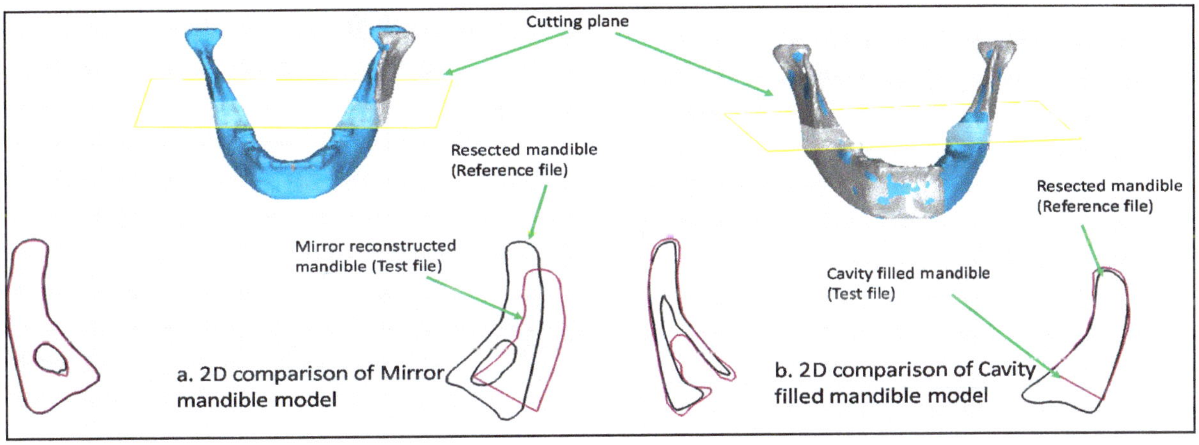

Figure 13. Two-dimensional (2D) comparison results of the cross-sectional plane of resected mandible with (**a**) mirror mandible model and (**b**) cavity-filled model.

The findings of the STL file comparison were further assisted by examining the FDM-produced physical prototype scans using the Faro arm laser scanner. The 3D color map, shown in Figure 14a, further determined that the cavity-filled reconstruction technique resulted in higher accuracy.

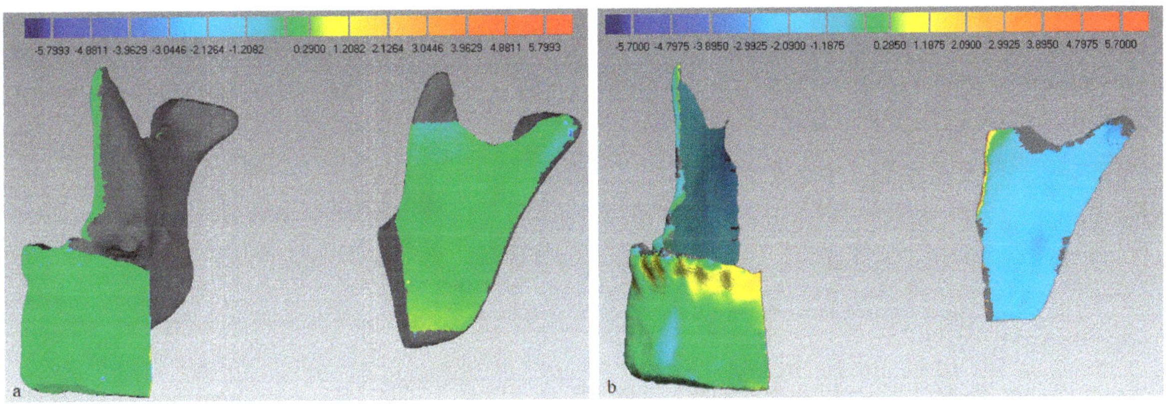

Figure 14. The 3D comparison results for physical prototypes with (**a**) Cavity-filled with resected comparison (**b**) Mirror with resected comparison.

The Geomagics program produced the statistical information, including the RMS and AD (positive and negative sides), upon alignment of the two models. There was a positive deviation when the test model was outside the reference model and conversely for a negative deviation. A series of five measurements was conducted for each mode under study to validate the consistency of the method, as shown in Table 1. The placement and positioning of the specimen or mandible was altered at each measurement run. A comparative analysis of the mirror and cavity-filled techniques with respect to their accuracy (RMS and AD) was made using the two sample t-test. As the p-value was less than the significance level (α) of 0.05, the null hypothesis was discarded, and it could be inferred that the two reconstruction techniques differed significantly.

Furthermore, the one-way ANOVA test also verified that the p-values for the RMS and AD between mirror and cavity-filled groups were less than 0.05. This finding substantiated yet again that both techniques (mirror and cavity-filled) varied considerably. The outcomes of both the sample t-test and the one-way ANOVA led to the rejection of the null hypothesis and concluded that the population means from two reconstruction techniques were not equal.

The mean RMS values observed for mirroring and cavity-filled techniques in the physical prototype evaluation were 1.2683 and 1.1019 mm, respectively. This implied an error decline of nearly 13% in 3D-printed mandibles restored using a cavity-filled approach, as depicted in Figure 15. Similarly, when the STL files from the mirror and the cavity-filled rehabilitated virtual variants were assessed, the RMS error value decreased from 1.8018 to 1.5048 mm, resulting in an approximately 16% drop. The significant decrease in AD (both positive and negative in Table 1) can also be noted in the cavity-filled procedure relative to the mirror reconstruction solutions. This provided mean values of 0.5194/−0.5392 mm (AD) for the cavity-filled approach as compared to the mirroring technique, which resulted in corresponding higher values of 0.7441/−0.8682 mm (see Table 1). This reduction in error is very competitive, given the simplicity and ease of use of the cavity-filled method. The preceded analysis underlines that the cavity-filled method would lead to a more reliable implant that should meet the aesthetic requirements. However, in mirror reconstruction, the approximation of the midsagittal plane is done using manual landmark points, which leads to deviation and causes implant placement issues, as well as concerns in post-surgical rehabilitation and movement. In contrast, cavity-filled reconstruction is a rather more straightforward and robust technique without any landmarks.

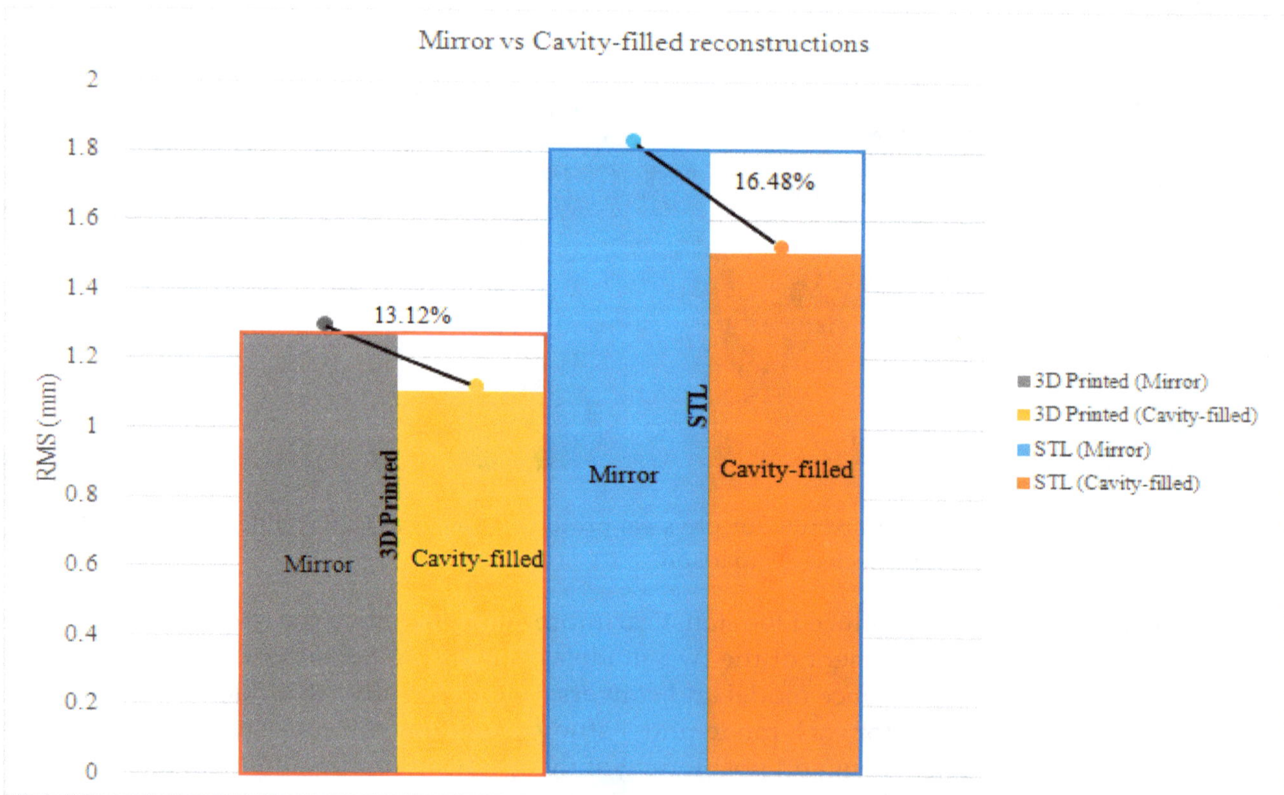

Figure 15. Graphical depiction of error reduction with cavity-filled approach.

Table 1. The 3D comparison results of the mirror and the cavity-filled reconstruction techniques.

Sample Number	Mode (R-T)											
	Scanned (Resected)- Scanned (Mirror)			STL (Resected)- STL (Mirror)			Scanned (Resected)- Scanned (Cavity-Filled)			STL (Resected)- STL (Cavity-Filled)		
	RMS	Average		RMS	Average		RMS	Average		RMS	Average	
		Negative	Positive		Negative	Positive		Negative	Positive		Negative	Positive
1	1.2695	−0.8676	0.7432	1.8014	−2.9765	0.7747	1.1021	−0.5386	0.5192	1.5050	−0.9677	0.6654
2	1.2690	−0.8672	0.7434	1.8017	−2.9760	0.7753	1.1011	−0.5390	0.5193	1.5047	−0.9680	0.6650
3	1.2672	−0.8693	0.7432	1.8031	−2.9762	0.7730	1.1014	−0.5397	0.5195	1.5054	−0.9671	0.6655
4	1.2664	−0.8690	0.7424	1.8025	−2.9769	0.7742	1.1023	−0.5389	0.5193	1.5046	−0.9670	0.6652
5	1.2692	−0.8678	0.7483	1.8004	−2.9779	0.7758	1.1028	−0.5399	0.5190	1.5044	−0.9679	0.6649
Mean	1.2683	−0.8682	0.7441	1.8018	−2.9767	0.7746	1.1019	−0.5392	0.5194	1.5048	−0.9675	0.6652

6. EBM Fabrication

The finally obtained cavity-filled implant was produced through EBM technology. EBM is one of the latest rapid manufacturing techniques, which produces a fully dense part using a computer-controlled gun in a vacuum environment. EBM was first commercialized in 1997 by the Arcam AB Corporation now under General Electric [37]. The general principle of EBM is the selective melting of metal powder (Ti6Al4V) in a layer-by-layer fashion using the electron beam of an electron emitted from the tungsten filament. The beam of electrons, as illustrated in Figure 16a, is controlled by three magnetic lenses, namely, the astigmatism lens, the focus lens, and the deflection lens. The astigmatism lens helps to generate a circular electron beam with a Gaussian energy distribution. The focus lens focuses and sharpens the beam into the smallest desired (0.1 mm) diameter. The deflection lens deflects the electron beam onto a specific target of the powder bed as per the CAD file. When the high-energy beam of electrons hits the metal powder, the kinetic energy is transformed into heat and melts the powder completely. After each melt cycle, the powder hopper holding the metal powder of 45 to 100 microns in size (Figure 16b) is lowered by one layer (50 microns), and the next layer of powder is fed onto the build platform using raking blades. This process is repeated until the completion of the build.

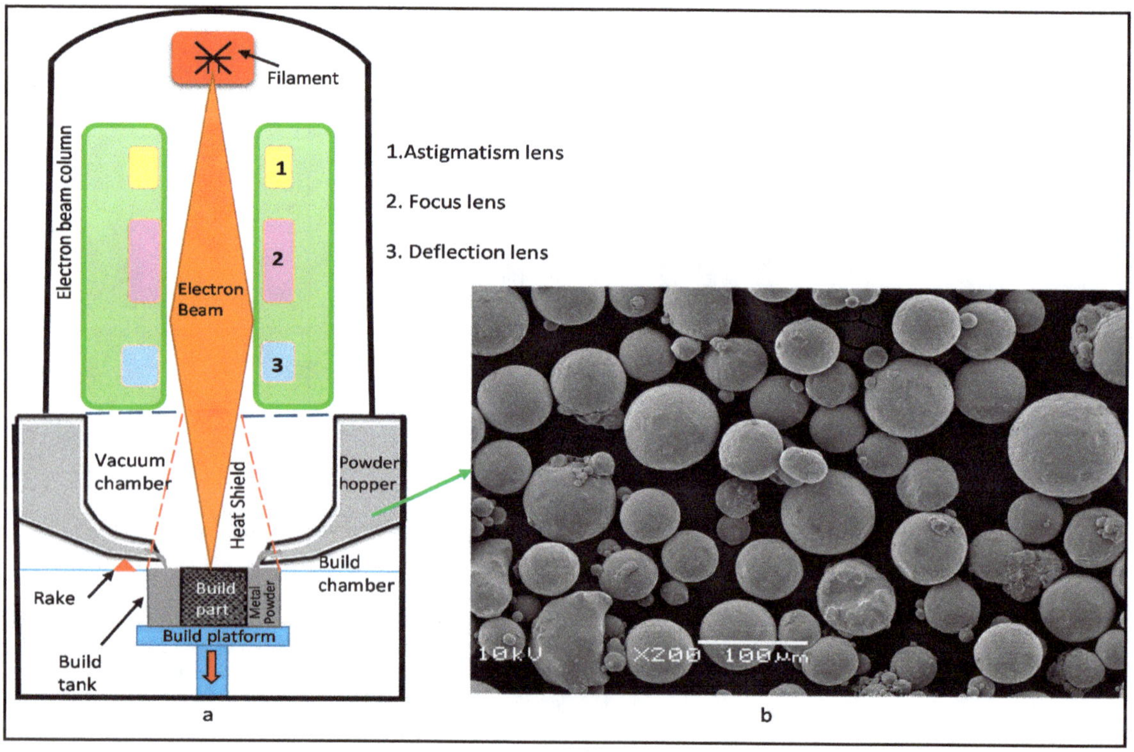

Figure 16. (**a**) Schematic diagram of the electron beam melting (EBM) A2 machine and (**b**) scanning electron microscopic image of Ti6Al4V powder.

When the build was completed, the build chamber was allowed to cool to 100 °C at 400 mbar through helium, followed by air. The cooled EBM build parts were then fed into a powder recovery system (PRS) (Figure 17) to blast away the semi-sintered titanium powder attached to the building part. All the blasted powder was recycled to minimize material loss. A filter screen and explosion-protected vacuum cleaner was also used to separate the coarse powder particles from the clean powder.

Figure 18a illustrates the EBM-fabricated cavity-filled mandibular implant with attached support structures. The support structures provided gravity support for overhanging surfaces in order to dissipate the process heat and to minimize the geometrical distortions caused by the internal stresses [38]. However, the support structures had to be removed during post-processing. The support structures were attached to the building part by the teeth (Figure 18b) which could be easily removed manually through plyers. The finally obtained titanium implant after support removal was precisely fitted onto the mandible model using bi-cortical medical screws, as shown in Figure 18c,d. This precise adaptation of the implant and bone counterpart helps in the reduction of surgical time and revision, in addition to providing better cosmesis [39].

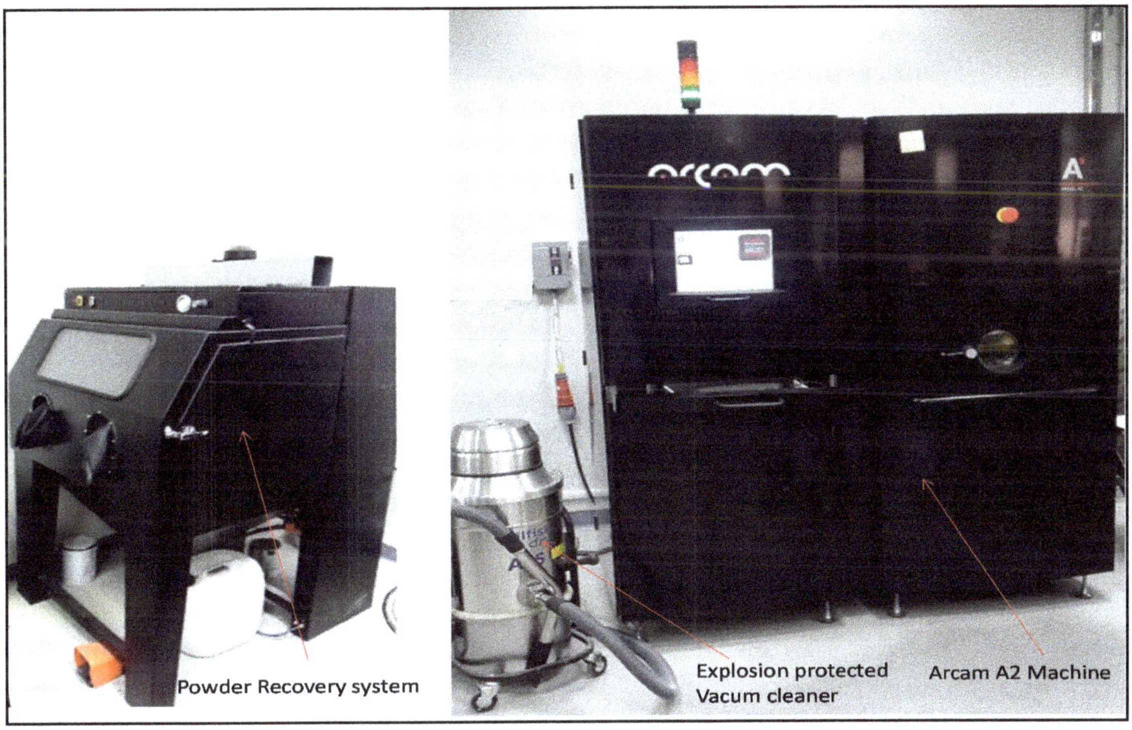

Figure 17. An Arcam EBM A2 machine (ARCAM AB, Molndal, Sweden) with accessories such as a powder recovery system and explosion-protected vacuum cleaner.

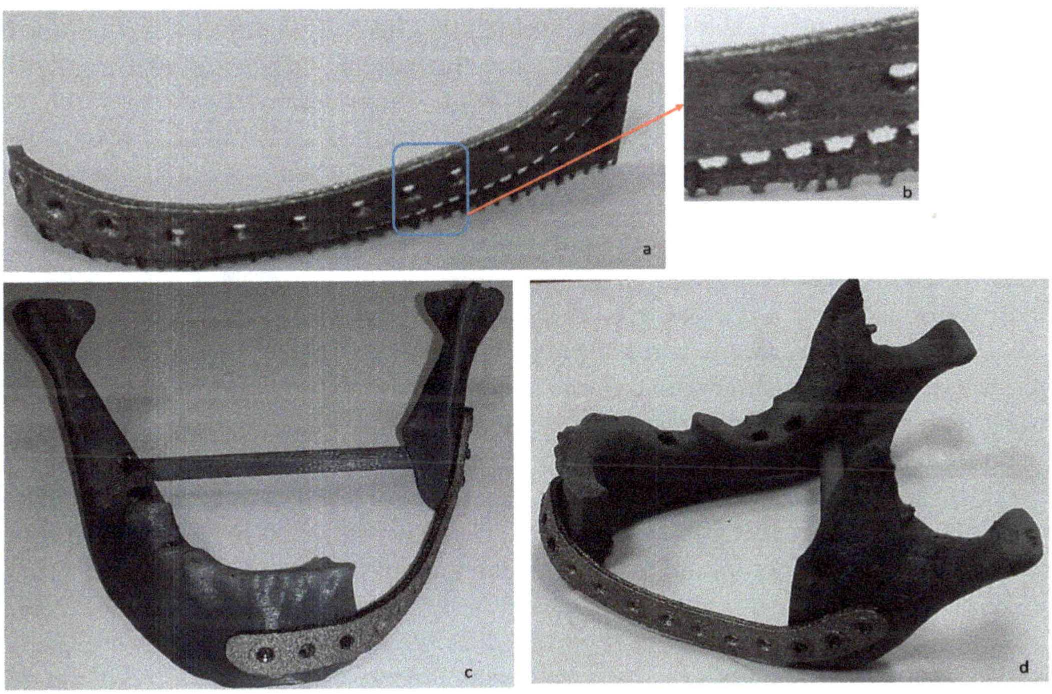

Figure 18. EBM-produced cavity-filled reconstructed titanium implant (**a**) with support structures attached to the teeth (**b**) for easy removal. Front view (**c**) and side view (**d**) of precisely fitted titanium implant onto the FDM model with bi-cortical screws after support removal.

7. Discussion

This work illustrated the significance of effective and accurate reconstruction techniques for accomplishing enhanced aesthetic and functional needs of a mandible. This is because the mandible and maxilla plays an important role in mastication, articulation, and cosmetic functions. They are both amenable to composite bone reconstruction. The WHO (World Health Organization) classifies mandibular lesions as benign and malignant, and the updated classification scheme is accessible in the ninth volume of the fourth-edition WHO series [40,41]. Benign tumors represent a broad spectrum of lesions and can be classified as odontogenic, e.g., ameloblastoma, odotoma, and myxoma, and non-odontogenic, e.g., fibro-osseous lesions and giant cell tumors [42]. Benign tumors can grow larger, but do not spread to surrounding tissues, whereas malignant tumors invade, destroy, and spread. The most common malignant tumors include squamous cell carcinomas, osteosarcomas, and giant cell tumors [42]. Tumors represents a major challenge in clinical practice as they lead to facial deformation and functional impairment. The factors influencing the choice of initial tumor treatment are primarily the size (T stage), location (anterior vs. posterior), bone proximity (mandible or maxilla), and histology, including the grade, type, and depth of invasion [43]. Certainly, adequate assessment of the tumor invasion is crucial in diagnosis and optimal surgical treatment planning.

It must be highlighted that, although the mirror image reconstruction technique is an effective tool for implant design, it is not without its drawbacks. A new approach known as cavity-filled reconstruction was, therefore, implemented to address its limitations. The two custom-design reconstruction techniques were compared and evaluated based on their virtual (STL file) and physical (3D-printed) prototypes. The accuracy assessment confirmed that the cavity-filled reconstruction technique provided higher accuracy. In the cavity-filled method, the RMS error was decreased by almost 13–16% compared to the mirror reconstruction technique. The mean RMS values recorded for mirroring and cavity-filled techniques in the physical prototype analysis were 1.2683 and 1.1019 mm, respectively. Similarly, when the STL files from the mirror and the cavity-filled reconstituted virtual equivalents were reviewed, the RMS error value was reduced from 1.8018 (mirror) to 1.5048 mm (cavity-filled). The study also established average values of 0.5194/−0.5392 mm (AD) for the cavity-filled approach as compared to the mirroring that resulted in the higher values of 0.7441/−0.8682 mm. Similar trends for AD were observed when STL data were investigated. The AD for the cavity-filled approach was −0.9675/0.6652 mm, and it was quite lower compared to the −2.9767/0.7746 mm in mirror reconstruction. It was, therefore, noted, based on the results of the 3D and 2D analysis, that the cavity-filled methodology exactly matched the bone contours. It is noteworthy that, in the cavity-filled approach, the bilateral condyle and chin were exactly in the same position unlike in the mirroring technique.

Various techniques are used in the reconstruction of mandibular and maxillary defects, and the most important is mirror reconstruction. Several researchers and surgeons illustrated how the mirror technique can be used successfully in mandibular reconstruction [20,44]. It is also widely used in the reconstruction of custom cranial implants, which replace defective parts of the skull [27,45]. Human skulls are extremely complex and irregular in shape [46]. They are never symmetrically ideal and, thus, the construction of an anatomical frame based on their reference is extremely ambiguous [47]. Throughout clinical practice, the symmetrical plane of the skull is approximated to the mid-sagittal plane and manually calculated using known landmarks [48]. The recognition of the anatomical midpoint used in the mirroring tool is not as simple as one might presume. The slightest deviation of the selected plane would result in discrepancies from the real anatomy. Although this method is simple and uses the patient's actual data as a template, it involves a high degree of user interaction and relies heavily on symmetrical plane computation. On the other hand, the cavity-filled approach is more automated, requiring minimal user intervention. It is faster, easier to use, more straightforward, and more accurate as it requires fewer repetitive tasks. This results in greater control and reliability of the implant performance, thus making it a more efficient reconstruction technique. The current research also demonstrates that the cavity-filled approach would give rise to a more robust implant that would satisfy aesthetic requirements. Contrary to this, the approximation of the midsagittal plane using manual landmark points is done in mirror reconstruction, which contributes to deviation and causes implant placement problems. It also reinforces issues in subsequent post-operative recovery and movement of the mandible.

The outcomes of the sample *t*-comparison, as well as one-way ANOVA analysis, of the two reconstruction techniques rejected the null hypothesis of the study. This underlined that the two methods, i.e., mirror and cavity-filled, varied substantially in terms of implant accuracy. It was also noted that the RMS error and AD estimates for the mirror reconstruction technique were greater than for the cavity-filled process. The current study, therefore, compared two reconstruction techniques for accurate mandible restoration, following tumor resection. It also focused on a procedure for estimating the accuracy of the reconstructed mandible models.

8. Conclusions

The success of any reconstructive operation depends on the reconstruction technique used in the reenactment of custom-design implants. The mirroring technique is the most commonly used method to recover mandibular defects, but it does have some anomalies and inaccuracies. In this research, a new technique known as the cavity-filled approach was explored as opposed to mirroring reconstruction. To estimate their performance, a 3D comparison was carried out between the reconstructed models of the two modeling techniques, analyzing the deviation. The statistical analysis utilizing hypothesis testing displayed statistically meaningful differences in the two reconstruction techniques. It was discovered on the basis of the 3D deviation study that the new or rather infrequently used cavity-filled technique provided a superior fitting as compared to the mirroring technique. The mirror reconstruction method in 3D-printed models led to a relatively higher RMS error of 1.2683 mm compared to 1.1019 mm in the cavity-filled technique due to increased user involvement and often inconsistent symmetrical plane approximation. By using the cavity-filled method, the RMS error decreased by 16.48% when the STL comparison was implemented. Moreover, the evaluation of 3D-printed models disclosed a notable 13.12% drop in RMS error with the cavity-filled in contrast to the mirror reconstruction technique. This new design approach demonstrated an integrated framework for the reconstruction of personalized mandibular implants, which provides greater facial symmetry and reduces operating time by minimizing revisions. However, the cavity-filled technique is a great and promising technique which might be limited to expanding lesions that have intact or minimal cortical wall destruction. Conversely, in the case of severe destructive lesions with distorted anatomy and loss of cortical plates or in the case of pathological mandibular fractures with loss of pre-tumor dimensions, applying such a technique might be challenging.

Author Contributions: K.M., conceptualization and experiments; K.M., methodology and draft preparation; S.H.M., analysis and investigation; K.M. and S.H.M., data curation, resources, and investigation; M.A., project administration and funding acquisition; S.R., validation; W.A. and O.A., visualization and supervision; K.M., writing; M.A. and S.R., review and editing. All authors read and agreed to the published version of the manuscript.

Acknowledgments: The authors extend their appreciation to the Deanship of Scientific Research at King Saud University for funding this work through Research Group no. RG-1440-075.

References

1. Torroni, A.; Marianetti, T.; Romandini, M.; Gasparini, G.; Cervelli, D.; Pelo, S. Mandibular Reconstruction with Different Techniques. *J. Craniofacial Surg.* **2015**, *26*, 885–890. [CrossRef] [PubMed]
2. Kumar, B.P.; Venkatesh, V.; Kumar, K.A.J.; Yadav, B.Y.; Mohan, S.R. Mandibular Reconstruction: Overview. *J. Maxillofac. Oral Surg.* **2016**, *15*, 425–441. [CrossRef] [PubMed]

3. Zeller, A.; Neuhaus, M.T.; Weissbach, L.V.M.; Rana, M.; Dhawan, A.; Eckstein, F.M.; Gellrich, N.C.; Zimmerer, R.M. Patient-Specific Mandibular Reconstruction Plates Increase Accuracy and Long-Term Stability in Immediate Alloplastic Reconstruction of Segmental Mandibular Defects. *J. Maxillofac. Oral Surg.* **2020**. [CrossRef]
4. Parthasarathy, J. 3D modeling, custom implants and its future perspectives in craniofacial surgery. *Ann. Maxillofac. Surg.* **2013**, *4*, 9–18. [CrossRef]
5. Bowers, C.A.; McMullin, J.H.; Brimley, C.; Etherington, L.; Siddiqi, F.A.; Riva-Cambrin, J. Minimizing bone gaps when using custom pediatric cranial implants is associated with implant success. *J. Neurosurg. Pediatrics* **2015**, *16*, 439–444. [CrossRef]
6. Cassoni, A.; Brauner, E.; Pucci, R.; Terenzi, V.; Mangini, N.; Battisti, A.; Monaca, M.D.; Ciolfi, A.; Laudoni, F.; Di Carlo, S.; et al. Head and Neck Osteosarcoma—The Ongoing Challenge about Reconstruction and Dental Rehabilitation. *Cancers* **2020**, *12*, 1948. [CrossRef]
7. Meyer-Marcotty, P.; Alpers, G.W.; Gerdes, A.B.M.; Stellzig-Eisenhauer, A. Impact of facial asymmetry in visual perception: A 3-dimensional data analysis. *Am. J. Orthod. Dentofac. Orthop.* **2010**, *137*, 168.e1–168.e8. [CrossRef]
8. Metzler, P.; Geiger, E.J.; Alcon, A.; Ma, X.; Steinbacher, D.M. Three-dimensional virtual surgery accuracy for free fibula mandibular reconstruction: Planned versus actual results. *J. Oral Maxillofac. Surg.* **2014**, *72*, 2601–2612. [CrossRef]
9. Alasseri, N.; Alasraj, A. Patient-specific implants for maxillofacial defects: Challenges and solutions. *Maxillofac. Plast. Reconstr. Surg.* **2020**, *42*, 15. [CrossRef]
10. Huotilainen, E.; Jaanimets, R.; Valášek, J.; Marcián, P.; Salmi, M.; Tuomi, J.; Mäkitie, A.; Wolff, J. Inaccuracies in additive manufactured medical skull models caused by the DICOM to STL conversion process. *J. Craniomaxillofac. Surg.* **2014**, *42*, e259–e265. [CrossRef]
11. Davim, J.P. *Additive and Subtractive Manufacturing: Emergent Technologies*; Walter de Gruyter GmbH & Co KG: Berlin, Germany, 2020.
12. Boyette, J.R.; Pemberton, J.D.; Bonilla-Velez, J. Management of orbital fractures: Challenges and solutions. *Clin. Ophthalmol.* **2015**, *9*, 2127–2137. [CrossRef] [PubMed]
13. Goormans, F.; Sun, Y.; Bila, M.; Schoenaers, J.; Geusens, J.; Lübbers, h.-t.; Coucke, W.; Politis, C. Accuracy of computer-assisted mandibular reconstructions with free fibula flap: Results of a single-center series. *Oral Oncol.* **2019**, *97*, 69–75. [CrossRef] [PubMed]
14. Lancellotta, V.; Pagano, S.; Tagliaferri, L.; Piergentini, M.; Ricci, A.; Montecchiani, S.; Saldi, S.; Chierchini, S.; Chierchini, S.; Cianetti, S.; et al. Individual 3-dimensional printed mold for treating hard palate carcinoma with brachytherapy: A clinical report. *J. Prosthet. Dent.* **2019**, *121*, 690–693. [CrossRef] [PubMed]
15. Pagano, S.; Moretti, M.; Marsili, R.; Ricci, A.; Barraco, G.; Cianetti, S. Evaluation of the Accuracy of Four Digital Methods by Linear and Volumetric Analysis of Dental Impressions. *Materials* **2019**, *12*, 1958. [CrossRef]
16. Kirke, D.N.; Owen, R.P.; Carrao, V.; Miles, B.A.; Kass, J.I. Using 3D computer planning for complex reconstruction of mandibular defects. *Cancers Head Neck* **2016**, *1*, 17. [CrossRef]
17. Bartier, S.; Mazzaschi, O.; Benichou, L.; Sauvaget, E. Computer-assisted versus traditional technique in fibular free-flap mandibular reconstruction: A CT symmetry study. *Eur. Ann. Otorhinolaryngol. Head Neck Dis.* **2020**. [CrossRef]
18. Mascha, F.; Winter, K.; Pietzka, S.; Heufelder, M.; Schramm, A.; Wilde, F. Accuracy of computer-assisted mandibular reconstructions using patient-specific implants in combination with CAD/CAM fabricated transfer keys. *J. Cranio-Maxillofac. Surg.* **2017**, *45*, 1884–1897. [CrossRef]
19. Yang, W.-F.; Zang, C.-Y.; Choi, W.S.; Zhu, W.-Y.; Li, D.T.S.; Chen, X.-S.; Du, R.; Su, Y.-X. A novel 'surgeon-dominated' approach to the design of 3D-printed patient-specific surgical plates in mandibular reconstruction: A proof-of-concept study. *Int. J. Oral Maxillofac. Surg.* **2020**, *49*, 13–21. [CrossRef]
20. Davies, J.C.; Chan, H.H.L.; Jozaghi, Y.; Goldstein, D.P.; Irish, J.C. Analysis of simulated mandibular reconstruction using a segmental mirroring technique. *J. Craniomaxillofac. Surg.* **2019**, *47*, 468–472. [CrossRef]
21. Mahendru, S.; Jain, R.; Aggarwal, A.; Aulakh, H.S.; Jain, A.; Khazanchi, R.K.; Sarin, D. CAD-CAM vs. conventional technique for mandibular reconstruction with free fibula flap: A comparison of outcomes. *Surg. Oncol.* **2020**, *34*, 284–291. [CrossRef]

22. Darwich, K.; Ismail, M.B.; Al-Mozaiek, M.Y.A.-S.; Alhelwani, A. Reconstruction of mandible using a computer-designed 3D-printed patient-specific titanium implant: A case report. *Oral Maxillofac. Surg.* **2020**. [CrossRef] [PubMed]
23. Linares, O.C.; Bianchi, J.; Raveli, D.; Neto, J.B.; Hamann, B. Mandible and skull segmentation in cone beam computed tomography using super-voxels and graph clustering. *Vis. Comput.* **2019**, *35*, 1461–1474. [CrossRef]
24. Qiu, B.; Guo, J.; Kraeima, J.; Glas, H.H.; Borra, R.J.H.; Witjes, M.J.H.; van Ooijen, P.M.A. Automatic segmentation of the mandible from computed tomography scans for 3D virtual surgical planning using the convolutional neural network. *Phys. Med. Biol.* **2019**, *64*, 175020. [CrossRef] [PubMed]
25. Abbasi, A.J.; Parvin, M.; Bashiri, S. Innovative use of a stereolithographic model together with the mirror image technique to reconstruct a defect in mandibular continuity. *Br. J. Oral Maxillofac. Surg.* **2018**, *56*, 887–889. [CrossRef]
26. Lin, H.; Zhu, P.; Lin, Q.; Huang, X.; Xu, Y.; Yang, X. Comprehensive Analysis of Mandibular Residual Asymmetry after Bilateral Sagittal Split Ramus Osteotomy Correction of Menton Point Deviation. *PLoS ONE* **2016**, *11*, e0161601. [CrossRef]
27. Moiduddin, K.; Darwish, S.; Al-Ahmari, A.; ElWatidy, S.; Mohammad, A.; Ameen, W. Structural and mechanical characterization of custom design cranial implant created using additive manufacturing. *Electron. J. Biotechnol.* **2017**, *29*, 22–31. [CrossRef]
28. Hatamleh, M.M.; Bhamrah, G.; Ryba, F.; Mack, G.; Huppa, C. Simultaneous Computer-Aided Design/Computer-Aided Manufacture Bimaxillary Orthognathic Surgery and Mandibular Reconstruction Using Selective-Laser Sintered Titanium Implant. *J. Craniofacial Surg.* **2016**, *27*, 1810–1814. [CrossRef]
29. Scolozzi, P. Maxillofacial reconstruction using polyetheretherketone patient-specific implants by 'mirroring' computational planning. *Aesthetic Plast. Surg.* **2012**, *36*, 660–665. [CrossRef]
30. Neyman, J.; Pearson, E.S.; Pearson, K. On the problem of the most efficient tests of statistical hypotheses. *Philos. Trans. Royal Soc. Lond. Ser. A* **1933**, *231*, 289–337. [CrossRef]
31. Giudice, A.L.; Ronsivalle, V.; Grippaudo, C.; Lucchese, A.; Muraglie, S.; Lagraere, M.O.; Isola, G. One Step before 3D Printing—Evaluation of Imaging Software Accuracy for 3-Dimensional Analysis of the Mandible: A Comparative Study Using a Surface-to-Surface Matching Technique. *Materials* **2020**, *13*, 2798. [CrossRef]
32. Mian, S.H.; Mannan, M.A.; Al-Ahmari, A.M. The influence of surface topology on the quality of the point cloud data acquired with laser line scanning probe. *Sens. Rev.* **2014**, *34*, 255–265. [CrossRef]
33. Hague, R.J.M.; Reeves, P.E. *Rapid Prototyping, Tooling and Manufacturing*; iSmithers Rapra Publishing: Shropshire, UK, 2000.
34. Material Properties of ABS-Acrylonitrile-Butadlene-Styrene. Dielectric Manufacturing. Available online: https://dielectricmfg.com/knowledge-base/abs/ (accessed on 31 January 2020).
35. Oropallo, W.; Piegl, L.A. Ten challenges in 3D printing. *Eng. Comput.* **2016**, *32*, 135–148. [CrossRef]
36. Umer, U.; Ameen, W.; Abidi, M.H.; Moiduddin, K.; Alkhalefah, H.; Alkahtani, M.; Al-Ahmari, A. Modeling the Effect of Different Support Structures in Electron Beam Melting of Titanium Alloy Using Finite Element Models. *Metals* **2019**, *9*, 806. [CrossRef]
37. About Arcam. GE Additive. Available online: https://www.ge.com/additive/who-we-are/about-arcam (accessed on 4 March 2020).
38. Calignano, F. Design optimization of supports for overhanging structures in aluminum and titanium alloys by selective laser melting. *Mater. Des.* **2014**, *64*, 203–213. [CrossRef]
39. Martinez-Marquez, D.; Mirnajafizadeh, A.; Carty, C.P.; Stewart, R.A. Application of quality by design for 3D printed bone prostheses and scaffolds. *PLoS ONE* **2018**, *13*. [CrossRef]
40. Adel, E.-N.K.; John, C.K.C.; Jennifer, G.; Takashi, T.; Pieter, J.S. *WHO Classification of Head and Neck Tumours*, 4th ed.; International Agency for Research on Cancer (IACR): Lyon, France, 2017; Volume 9.
41. Tekkeşin, M.S.; Wright, J. The World Health Organization Classification of Odontogenic Lesions: A Summary of the Changes of the 2017 (4th) Edition. *Turk. J. Pathol.* **2013**, *34*. [CrossRef]
42. Dunfee, B.L.; Sakai, O.; Pistey, R.; Gohel, A. Radiologic and Pathologic Characteristics of Benign and Malignant Lesions of the Mandible. *RadioGraphics* **2006**, *26*, 1751–1768. [CrossRef]
43. Shah, J. Cancer of the Head and Neck, Mandible Reconstruction. *Cancer Head Neck* **2013**, *19*, 355–375.

44. Essig, H.; Rana, M.; Kokemueller, H.; von See, C.; Ruecker, M.; Tavassol, F.; Gellrich, N.-C. Pre-operative planning for mandibular reconstruction—A full digital planning workflow resulting in a patient specific reconstruction. *Head Neck Oncol.* **2011**, *3*, 45. [CrossRef]
45. Jardini, A.L.; Larosa, M.A.; Filho, R.M.; de Carvalho Zavaglia, C.A.; Bernardes, L.F.; Lambert, C.S.; Calderoni, D.R.; Kharmandayan, P. Cranial reconstruction: 3D biomodel and custom-built implant created using additive manufacturing. *J. Cranio-Maxillofac. Surg.* **2014**, *42*, 1877–1884. [CrossRef]
46. White, T.D.; Folkens, P.A. Chapter 7-SKULL. In *The Human Bone Manual*; White, T.D., Folkens, P.A., Eds.; Academic Press: San Diego, CA, USA, 2005; pp. 75–126.
47. Ferrario, V.F.; Sforza, C.; Ciusa, V.; Dellavia, C.; Tartaglia, G.M. The effect of sex and age on facial asymmetry in healthy subjects: A cross-sectional study from adolescence to mid-adulthood. *J. Oral Maxillofac. Surg.* **2001**, *59*, 382–388. [CrossRef] [PubMed]
48. Yáñez-Vico, R.M.; Iglesias-Linares, A.; Torres-Lagares, D.; Gutiérrez-Pérez, J.L.; Solano-Reina, E. Three-dimensional evaluation of craniofacial asymmetry: An analysis using computed tomography. *Clin. Oral Investig.* **2011**, *15*, 729–736. [CrossRef] [PubMed]

4

"In Vivo" Validation of 3D-Printed Innovative Surgical Template for Lumbar Spinal Arthrodesis

Francesco Naddeo [1], Emilio Cataldo [2], Nicola Narciso [3], Alessandro Naddeo [1,*] and Nicola Cappetti [1]

1 Department of Industrial Engineering, University of Salerno, Via Giovanni Paolo II, 132, 84084 Fisciano, SA, Italy; frnaddeo@unisa.it (F.N.); ncappetti@unisa.it (N.C.)
2 Techno DESIGN S.r.l., via Rosa Jemma, 2, 84091 Battipaglia, SA, Italy; e.cataldo@technodesign.it
3 "San Giovanni di Dio e Ruggi d'Aragona" University Hospital, Largo Città di Ippocrate, 84131 Salerno, Italy; narcisonicola@virgilio.it
* Correspondence: anaddeo@unisa.it.

Abstract: The most common type of spine instrumentation is the pedicle screw fixation. The recent literature shows how customized drilling templates help surgeons to perform the surgery better. This work aims to validate the design of a customized template for inserting lumbar pedicle screw via a procedure based on rapid prototyping and reverse engineering techniques and to show the benefits. The novelties of this template are its low-invasive sizes, its design based on a patented algorithm, which calculates the sizes of the screws and the optimal insertion direction, the engage/disengage system, and the adaptability to every kind of surgeon's kit. Accuracy of pedicle screw location, surgery duration, and X-ray exposition have been used to evaluate the performances of the template. Mono-centric in vivo trial was performed. Twenty patients (8 women and 12 men) were enrolled randomly corresponding to sixty vertebrae treated with spinal arthrodesis (30 with and 30 without templates). Accuracy of the screw positioning and reduction in both surgery duration and patients' exposure to X-rays achieved excellent results because the time spent on the insertion of pedicle screws via the surgical template was cut down by about 63%, while the number of X-ray shots was reduced by about 92%. The proposed template performed better than the standard approach and could be helpful both for skilled and novice surgeons.

Keywords: spine surgery; surgical template; lumbar spinal arthrodesis; screw location optimisation; X-ray minimisation

---

1. Introduction

1.1. State of the Art

Increasingly, computer-aided-design and computer-aided-surgery (CAD/CAS) systems are being integrated into surgery procedures, especially in pre-operative planning and guided surgery template design. This work describes the validation of a surgical device utilized in the stabilization of the spine.

Spinal arthrodesis, consisting of the fusion of the spine's segments by implanting titanium rods anchored to transpedicular screws that are inserted into the vertebra passing by the pedicle bone structure, is the most often utilized spinal stabilization procedure [1]. Nerve roots and main blood vessels surrounding close to vertebras are critical to consider because the impairment of these structures can be fatal to the patient or can cause severe permanent injuries.

Generally, the standard procedure that uses pedicle screws involves: identifying the entry point for the screw; choosing the trajectory based on X-rays and cannulating the pedicle along it; probing with the appropriate device to detect breaches; and tapping and screw introduction.

This procedure is usually performed "hand-based" with all the related aspects that affect confidence in implantology. Even the experienced surgeons sometimes have to correct the trajectory of the screws during surgery. The correct introduction in the vertebra is normally monitored with many harmful radiographic shots [1].

New navigation systems are normally utilized to allow viewing on a screen, in real time, the anatomical structures to be treated, avoiding dangerous X-ray shots. These systems present three technical issues: positioning accuracy, calibration, and high costs [1].

For these reasons, patient-specific surgical templates produced in three-dimensional biocompatible material via rapid prototyping technology represent a valid alternative.

Ma [2] demonstrated that the surgical template improves screw placement precision by comparing the accuracy with and without templates. Kashani [3] proposed a particular surgical template that could accommodate drill having different diameters.

Normally, during the pre-operative step the identification of the screw direction is performed. The surgical template is designed based on the results of the previous step. A multilevel surgical template was designed, via CAD software, by Merc et al. [4]. Even though several aspects were automated in this way, multilevel templates did not always guarantee excellent positioning. In [5], the authors tried to find the smallest diameter of the pedicles. They calculated the optimal orientation and the maximum size of the screws via least squares method. In this case, problems raised for highly deformed spines. A method that finds the isthmus of the pedicles intended as the smallest section and from its centre projects a perpendicular straight line i.e., the optimum direction for the screws was presented in [6]. In [7], the authors have shown a computer-aided method for calculating the best path for pedicle screw insertion (sufficiently equidistant from the barycentric points of the pre-set coronal sections of the pedicle), with appropriate dimensioning of the screw based on the smallest cross section of the pedicle. Recently, other researchers [8,9] have worked on writing algorithms to find the best trajectories, diameters, and maximum length for screws. In [10], a new hook-shaped rapid-prototyped template has been tested on a single patient and a comparison with twelve similar techniques presented in previous articles has been performed, demonstrating the accuracy in surgery and the usability of the proposed template. Nevertheless, a real clinical trial has not been conducted on a sufficiently wide sample of cases.

1.2. Aims and Scopes

This paper is focused on the validation of the design of a surgical device, that is opportunely customized for the patient to optimize the lumbar pedicle screws insertion via the CAD-CAS approach and its manufacturing via rapid prototyping techniques. The optimal insertion trajectories, the length, and the diameter of the screws are designed starting from CAD model of the area of interest (insertion area). This model comes from reverse engineering (RE) techniques.

The design of the device starts from the knowledge of the screw entry point that will be chosen by the surgeon based on his experience.

Subsequently, the optimal screw insertion trajectories are determined via a patented algorithm [8,11,12]. The matching and disengage system presents several innovations. The first consists of the possibility of being able to apply not only pointers and perforators, but also to directly apply pedicle screws that can be used with any surgical instruments. In fact, the guide cylinders are designed to be able to implant different screws with different instruments thanks to a notch that allows the controlled fracture of a portion of the cylinders themselves, facilitating the last phase of screw implantology and the mask removal. An innovative contact surface between mask and vertebra has also been designed with several holes, with a diameter of about half a millimetre, that are arranged randomly on the surface of the mask to increase the probability that any presence of small tissue produced during the skeletonization will be channelled into these holes, thereby avoiding creating interference in the coupling between the mask and the vertebra with possible mismatching.

This template also allows preserving a good portion of the supraspinous longitudinal ligament (when there is no laminectomy) because the anchor points of the template on the vertebra are traceable to four portions of vertebral lamina. Finally, thanks to a semi-automatic trajectory identification algorithm that allows the surgeon to choose the first access point, it is also possible to think about designing the whole template in a semi-automatic way.

The proposed device is used only as a guide that integrates perfectly with the standard freehand surgical procedure without altering it but allowing a guided screw implantology.

In the classical freehand procedure, the radiation doses, surgery time, and risk of error are generally acceptable but high. Moreover, wrong positioning could induce to surgery failure resulting in re-intervention and, normally, an increase in surgery duration that means an increase of noxious real-time X-rays. The proposed surgical device drives surgeon throughout the best insertion direction of the screws, keeping down the risk of damaging the nervous system. Moreover, this procedure cuts down the surgery duration (resulting in an increase in surgery comfort), the blood loss, and radiation doses.

2. Materials and Methods

2.1. Patient Sample

To validate the use of the lumbar drilling template, a clinical trial was performed at San Giovanni di Dio e Ruggi D'Aragona public hospital (Salerno, Campania, Italy). Twenty patients (8 women and 12 men) were enrolled randomly. The patient inclusion criterion was people who were waiting for vertebral stabilisation surgery for degenerative disease of the lumbar spine, including *de novo scoliosis*, with a maximum age of 70 years and a minimum of 50 years, without home pharmacological therapy.

During the trial, thirty vertebrae were surgically treated by the traditional procedure, and thirty vertebrae were treated using the custom-made template. All vertebrae were in the lumbar spine except for a single patient whose vertebrae T10 and T11 were operated on, respectively, without and with the template.

The segments on which to intervene using the template and on which to proceed in a traditional way were chosen randomly. The comparison between the two approaches took place in the same operative conditions (health status of the patient, presence of staff in the operating room, side effects, etc.).

2.2. Collected Data and Statistics

During the trial, data were collected before, during, and after surgery. An example of the data sheet is included in Online Resource 1. The complete datasheet is presented in Online Resource 2.

Online Resource 1 (OR1) TEMPLATE OF THE PATIENT DATA SHEET

Online Resource 2 (OR2) PATIENT DATA SHEETS

Both objective and subjective data were collected to perform the comparison with and without the use of the template and to validate the template itself.

Data collected were:

1. Surgery times:
    a. starting from the vertebra's exposure to titanium rods implantology; and
    b. starting from screws implantology to end of screws implantology;
2. X-ray shots during single-vertebra surgery;
3. Kirshner wire positioning error; and
4. Screw positioning error (requiring a screw repositioning).

Qualitative data were organised in a synoptic table including:

1. The post-surgery evaluation of the final trajectories with scores from 1 to 5 depending on the correctness of the trajectory obtained [13];
2. Qualitative evaluation of the whole operation to evaluate the mental load and the physical effort of the surgeon.

2.3. *Patient's Spine 3D Modelling*

The 3D CAD models of the vertebral bodies were obtained starting with a CT scan that gave a DICOM output. This output was imported in Materialize Mimics software (Materialize NV—Leuven, Belgium) for human structures segmentation, which allows for reconstructions of the lumbar regions with both automatic and manual thresholding techniques, based on the Hounsfield Grayscale.

Segmentation generates 3D Standard-Triangulation-Language (STL) models of the vertebrae that were imported into Geomagic software (3D Systems— Rock Hill (SC), USA) for conversions in poli-surfaces format (IGES). This step is particularly useful because the IGES model is composed by closed surfaces that are suitable for processing with CAD modelling software. After the conversion into IGES format, the vertebral model was imported using the Rhinoceros Software (Robert McNeel & Associates—Seattle, WA, USA). Figure 1 shows a 3D reconstruction.

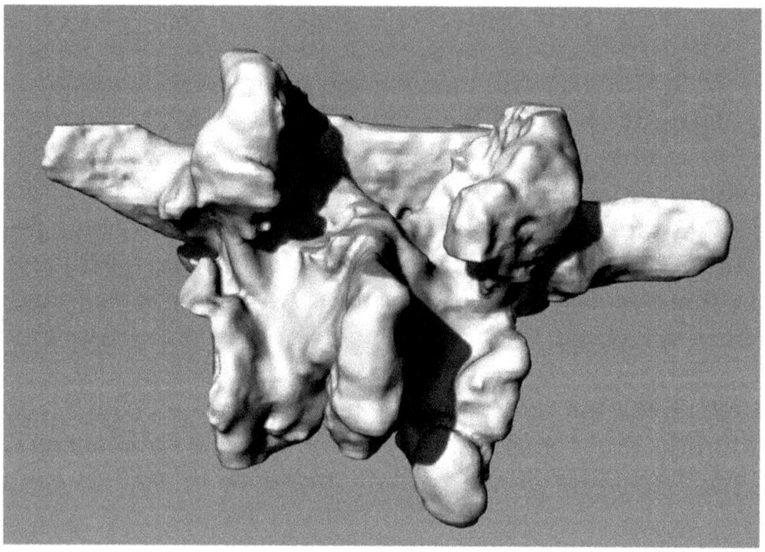

Figure 1. Computer-aided-design (CAD) reconstruction of a lumbar vertebra.

2.4. *Computer Aided Surgery Planning: Screws' Optimal Length, Diameter and Insertion Direction*

The target of the arthrodesis surgery is to locate the screws. The standard procedure expects a barycentric insertion of the screw with respect to the cross sections of the pedicle and tendentially parallel to the vertebral plate (that is the transverse plane) [14]. The standard procedure is a freehand empirical method where anatomical landmarks suggest the ideal insertion direction. The target is to find an optimized insertion of the screw from a structural and patient safety point of view, avoiding the "pull out" phenomenon. The trajectories are chosen in order to be properly convergent.

These specifications reduce the probability of damage to spinal, nerve and circulatory structures (especially in the upper part of the vertebral column).

In the proposed procedure, the search for optimal directions is carried out, as previously mentioned, through an algorithm based on a rigorous mathematical method that avoids to define a minimal section of the isthmus, unlike other research works mentioned in the introduction. In this case, in fact, the algorithm defines a free 3D space (whose volume can be safely crossed by a screw without touching the outer pedicle's surfaces) whose visibility is guaranteed because it coincides with the entry point (visible) chosen by the surgeon. The previous sections describe the innovativeness of this procedure, which includes the innovative trajectory of insertion design in [8,12,15].

The algorithm identifies the available bone space building a solid angle from the entry point located on the surface of the bone. From this point, the algorithm estimates the barycentric trajectories and the acceptable maximum screws' diameter. Moreover, it calculates the length of the screws based on the distance between the screws' tip, the vertebra external surface, and the sagittal plane, considering an opportune safety factor (for further details, see [8,11,12]).

2.5. 3D CAD Modelling of the Customized Template

The 3D modelling of the customized template is the crucial step of the methodology; it has to fit perfectly with the vertebra to direct the surgeon correctly during screw insertion.

The spine segment has to be imported into the Rhinoceros® software to check potential interferences between vertebra and the template (during the surgery) while also neglecting the vertebral natural distraction due to excision of the supraspinous ligament (which usually is foreseen in this kind of surgery or is needed in decompressive laminectomy surgery and usually is performed for vertebral distraction) that usually helps avoid interferences.

The template interfacing shape is obtained by creating a negative solid from the lamina of the vertebra through a Boolean difference operation between a sufficiently big prism and the vertebra itself. While doing that, the modelling procedure takes into consideration the spinous process to prevent under-cuts that could negatively affect the template positioning.

Therefore, it is appropriate to cut the 3D model of the template in its internal surfaces so as not to generate interference and under-cuts with the surfaces of the spinous process. On the solid, tubes and holes have to be created along the already verified trajectories for creating the guides for the screws. Figure 2 shows the final shape of the solid.

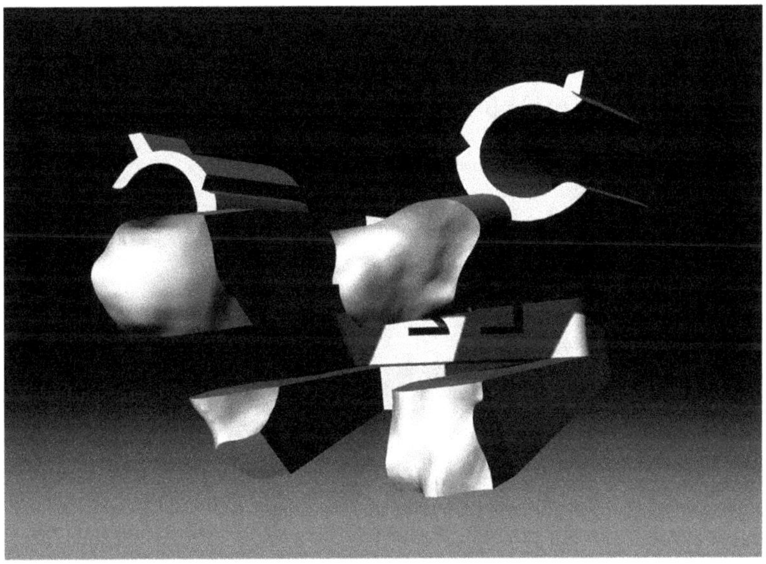

Figure 2. 3D model of template.

2.6. Innovative Engaging and Disengaging Device

The surgical operation of "skeletonization" (removing all the soft tissue attached to the bone structure of the vertebra) may generate small scraps of tissue or bone due to an imperfect cut during the skeletonization. To avoid matching problems between the vertebra and the template and to simplify the engagement and positioning of the template itself on the exposed surfaces of the vertebra, some tube structures have been generated on the interface surface of the template (see Figure 3). It has been verified that very small residual tissues or bone are about half a millimetre in diameter for two reasons: the precision capacity of the prototyping machine, and the hypothesis that any pieces of "waste" tissue larger than this size can be easily identified and removed by hand.

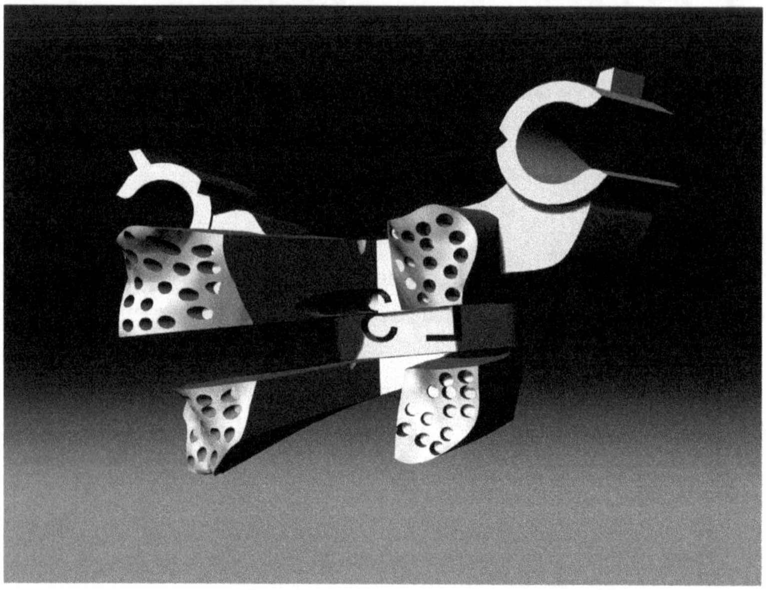

Figure 3. 3D model of template with innovative engage system.

The holes are through-holes where the geometry of the mask allows it and are arranged randomly on the surface (it would have been impossible to define a systematic criterion given that the surfaces are all extremely different from each other) to fit in the free space among the tubes and avoid generating interference in the coupling between the surfaces of the template and those of the vertebral lamina.

In in vivo testing, a pre-notched tube (see Figure 4) used as Kirschner/screw guide on the template has been designed for simplifying the template disengagement once a screw is inserted. After the insertion of the screw, the surgeon can easily break the pre-notched tube without creating plastic scraps, using the small flat spline on the tube [16].

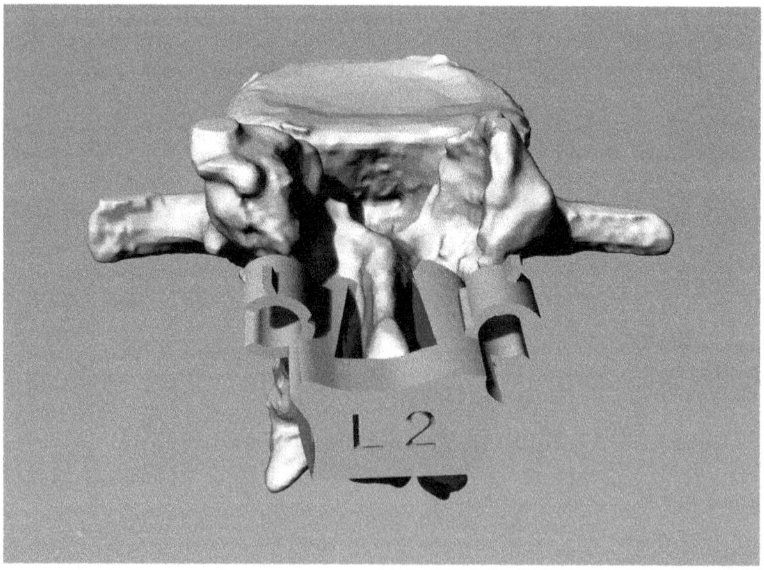

Figure 4. Customized template positioned on the L2 vertebra surface with notched tubes and tongues.

2.7. 3D Printing of the Physical Models

Physical models of templates were produced by rapid prototyping (RP) techniques using stereolithography technology (SLA) (Form 2 by Formlabs, Formlabs Inc. 35 Medford St., Suite 201, Somerville, MA 02143, USA).

All the templates used for the trial were manufactured utilizing a biocompatible resin (Dental SG, Class 1 biocompatible resin (EN-ISO 10993-1:2009/AC: 2010, USP Class VI)) that was designed to produce drill guides directly. The templates showed directional pipes having holes properly sized for the insertion of Kirschner wires. Templates' design and prototyping took about three hours. This value is the mean of the 30 treated cases. The production of 20 different templates on the same printing plate requires 3.5 h thanks to the easily scalability of the rapid manufacturing process.

2.8. Procedure for Using the Template

The target of the template is to improve and optimize the standard vertebral arthrodesis procedure by guiding the screws in the optimal directions.

This is obtained by positioning the template on the vertebral surface. The template must be positioned appropriately on the surface of the vertebra to be treated and, consequently, the template design is aimed at the appropriate choice of the contact surfaces in such a way as to make the positioning univocal and avoid errors.

An accurate skeletonization has to be performed on the vertebral lamina before the positioning of the template. This way a stable match can be obtained making a few and small movements in finding the right position on the vertebra surface (thanks also to the innovative engage system).

To simplify the positioning of the surgical template, a minor distraction will be required of the vertebral bodies via, for example, the supraspinatus ligament excision or the positioning of the patient in a hyperkyphotic position. The anchorage to the vertebra is insured by the perfectly fitting shape of the template.

Once verified the template/vertebra coupling, a first X-ray shot has to be done to evaluate the trajectories goodness and theoretical tracing via the Kirschner wires, which are introduced into the vertebral body via the guide tubes and adaptors. Positive X-ray feedback allows the surgeon to directly insert the screw using the direction tubes along the planned direction [17]. Finally, the surgeon can extract the template by breaking the tongues and disengaging the template.

This procedure has been approved by the Ethical Committee of the Italian Health Ministry.

3. In Vitro Tests

Several in vitro tests were performed to check the feasibility of the templates and the effectiveness of the procedure before beginning the in vivo tests. Several vertebrae belonging to thoracic and lumbar spine segments were acquired by CT (Computerized Tomography) exams and were 3D-modelled and rapidly prototyped in Acrylonitrile-Butadiene-Styrene (ABS) using a fused-deposition-moulding (FDM) technology (Shareboat Dual Extrusor, with a 0.8 mm of thickness and 30 mm/s of print speed) that allows physical models of the vertebrae to be created in a few hours at low cost and with a geometric error lower than 0.3 mm. The procedure was used to build templates to create a physical demonstrator of the surgery. Finally, real screws were inserted in the vertebra utilizing the templates, and the obtained trajectories investigated by simply cutting the vertebra along planned trajectories planes. The results showed the perfect match between planned surgeries and in vitro realised ones.

Clinical Trial: In Vivo Tests

Sixty vertebrae (30 with template and 30 without template), for which a spinal arthrodesis was required, were treated to test the proposed template.

For each pair of screws inserted, an intra-operative X-ray has been taken for evaluating the position of the Kirschner wire and, thereafter, the position of implanted pedicle screws.

Qualitative evaluation parameters: the evaluation of the correctness of the trajectories was expressed by the surgeon based on the good standards present in the medical literature. The X-ray shots were used to provide a good surgery rating.

Quantitative and qualitative evaluation parameters: each screw insertion was evaluated through the following parameters:

1. accuracy of screw insertion based on three geometrical parameters: centring in the pedicle cross-section, alignment with vertebral plate, screws convergence (the evaluation criterion was class 5 (no violation): the screw is placed along the planned trajectory; class 4 (precise): the screw axis deviates by <2 mm away the planned trajectory; class 3 (normal accuracy): the screw axis deviates by >2 mm but <4 mm away; class 2 (deviated): the screw axis deviates by >4 mm; and class 1 (not conform): the screw axis presents critical deviation);
2. surgery duration for each vertebra (in minutes);
3. number of X-ray shots per vertebra (n);
4. Kirshner wires repositioning times (n); and
5. pedicle screw repositioning times (n).

All procedures and criteria for the clinical trial were in line with the 1964 Helsinki Declaration, performed in accordance with the ethical standards of current Italian law and approved by the Ethical Review Board of the San Giovanni di Dio e Ruggi d'Aragona University Hospital in Salerno, where the trial/tests were conducted. The trial itself and the proposed procedure have been approved by the Ethical Committee of the Italian Health Ministry (Campania regional district). All participants were informed about the experiment protocol, the nature of the medical implements used, and risks and benefits linked to the new surgical device. Informed consent was signed by the patients.

4. Results

Quantitative comparative analysis with freehand surgery and custom-made template-assisted surgery are synthetically shown in the following tables. Data reported in the tables are mean values among the surgeries. The detailed information about each case treated is reported in Online Resource 2.

The comparative analysis of the values in Table 1 shows an improvement of the analysed parameters that is not dependent on the vertebra on which the surgery is done. The improvement is highlighted both in the mean values and in variance. The independence of the results towards the operated-upon vertebra is a strong point of the procedure.

Table 1. Quantitative parameter results.

	Number of Samples	X-Ray Shots	Time (min)	Kirshner Repositioning	Screws Repositioning
Freehand					
1.1	2	10.0	57.5	3.5	0.0
1.2	4	9.0	66.8	5.5	0.3
1.3	10	22.4	60.6	5.5	0.4
1.4	5	17.0	47.4	5.8	0.0
1.5	8	12.4	69.6	6.6	0.1
Total	*Mean*	15.8	60.9	5.7	0.2
30	*St. Dev.*	16.1	30.7	3.8	0.5
Guided hand					
1.1	5	2.6	12.6	0.4	0.0
1.2	5	2.6	12.8	0.4	0.0
1.3	4	2.3	13.8	0.5	0.0
1.4	12	3.1	15.5	0.3	0.0
1.5	3	3.7	16.7	1.3	0.0
Total	*Mean*	2.8	14.3	0.5	0.0
30	*St. Dev.*	0.9	3.9	0.7	0.0

The mean value of X-ray shots, that is, as shown in the table, about equal to 3, is perfectly matching what is required in the procedure: one X-ray shot for template positioning before the vertebra drilling, one X-ray shot for verification of the trajectories during the screw implanting, and the final X-ray shot for verifying the final screw positioning.

Rarely were the Kirschner wires repositioned during the surgery, while the screws were never repositioned (nor for freehand and for guided insertion, probably thanks to the high number of X-ray shots in the freehand cases and to the use of template in the guided cases).

Table 2 shows the comparison of the qualitative data acquired during the surgeries. The surgeon, just after the surgery, was asked to express a motivated judgement on a 5-point scale (1 = very poor, 5 = very good) about the qualitative parameters, just analysing the post-operative X-ray or CT.

Table 2. Qualitative parameter results.

	Number of Samples	Pedicle Centring	Alignment	Screws Convergence
Freehand				
1.1	2	3.5	4.0	4.0
1.2	4	4.0	4.0	3.3
1.3	10	3.6	4.3	3.7
1.4	5	4.0	3.8	3.4
1.5	8	3.9	4.0	4.1
Total	*Mean*	3.8	4.0	3.7
30	*St. Dev.*	0.6	0.7	0.6
Guided hand				
1.1	5	3.4	4.6	4.2
1.2	5	4.4	4.4	4.2
1.3	4	4.3	4.3	4.3
1.4	12	4.3	4.5	4.0
1.5	3	4.0	4.0	4.0
Total	*Mean*	4.1	4.4	4.1
30	*St. Dev.*	0.7	0.6	0.5

The comparison shows a mean value of improvement of the judgements equal to 10%. The reference value is the best judgement the surgeon expressed on the manual insertion.

To check the significance of results of qualitative comparison, a Wilcoxon signed-rank test was performed on the qualitative data: pedicle centring, alignment, and screw convergence. The Wilcoxon test is appropriate because it is a nonparametric test designed to evaluate the difference between two treatments or conditions when the samples are correlated.

The data considered for the two test cases were the case "with template" and the case "without template".

Table 3 shows the comparison results for two non-null hypotheses: p-value < 0.01 and p-value < 0.05.

Table 3. Wilcoxon tests results.

	p-Value	$p < 0.01$	$p < 0.05$
centring	0.09296	NO	NO
alignment	0.05744	NO	NO
convergence	*0.02510*	NO	YES

No significant differences were found among those data except for the case of screw convergence that was checked as significantly better (p-value < 0.05) in the case "with template".

Table 4 synthetises the percentage of improvement of each acquired data point (quantitative and qualitative) without considering the type and level of the vertebra.

Figure 5 also synthetically shows how the use of the surgical template allows improvement of every analysed parameter.

Table 4. Results on quantitative/qualitative parameters.

	Free Hand	Using Template	Improve (%)
X-ray shots reduction	15.8	2.8	82%
Time reduction	60.9	14.3	77%
Kirshner wire repositioning reduction	5.7	0.5	92%
Pedicle screw repositioning reduction	0.2	0.0	100%
Quality of screw passage via the pedicle centre	3.8	4.1	8%
Quality of the alignment to the vertebra's plane line	*4.0*	4.4	9%
Quality of pedicle screws convergence	*3.7*	4.1	11%

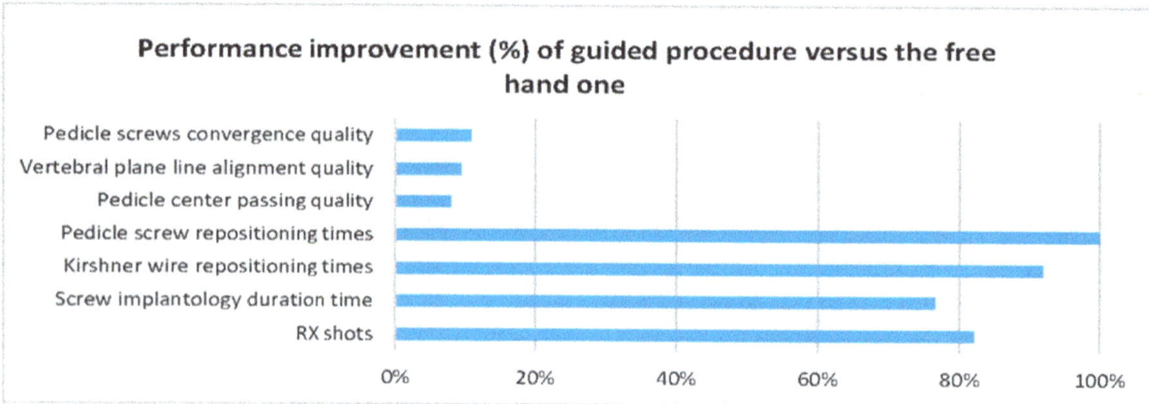

Figure 5. Performance improvement (%) of guided procedure versus the free hand one.

Figures 6–9 show examples of pre- and post-operative X-ray shots.

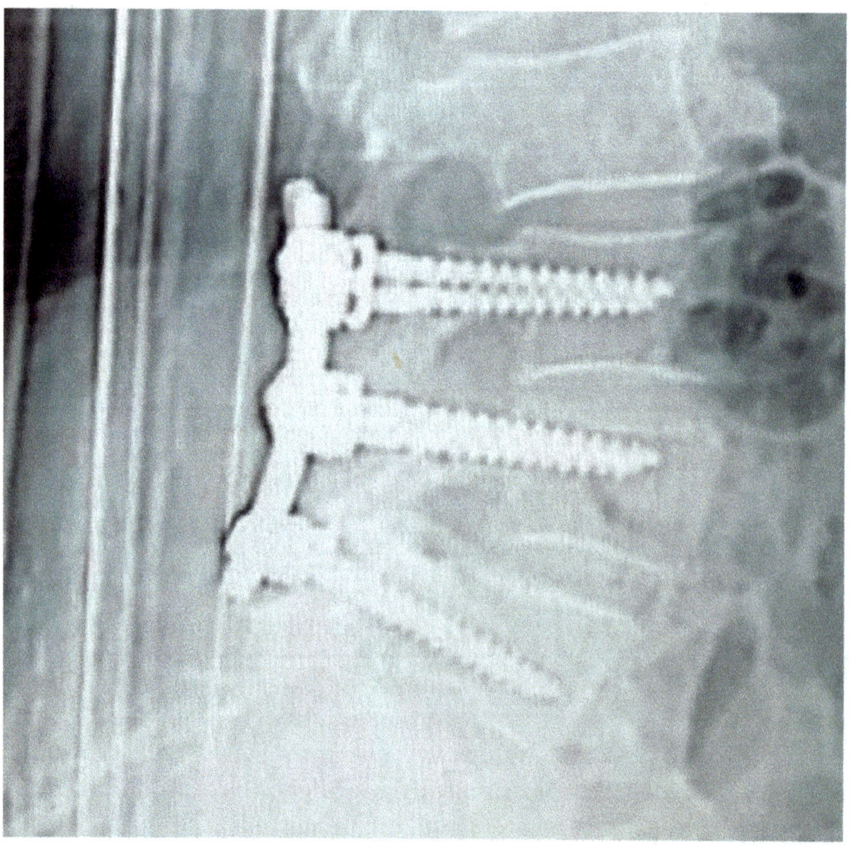

Figure 6. Post-operative sagittal X-ray check—patient code: 2ATL3L4L5110.

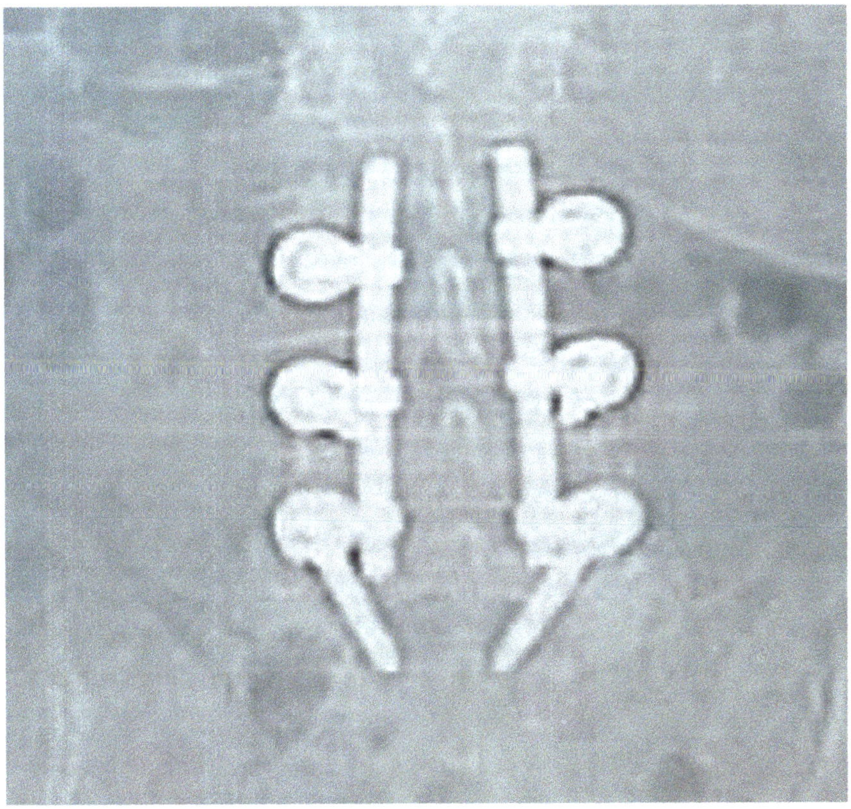

Figure 7. Post-operative coronal X-ray check—patient code: 2ATL3L4L5110.

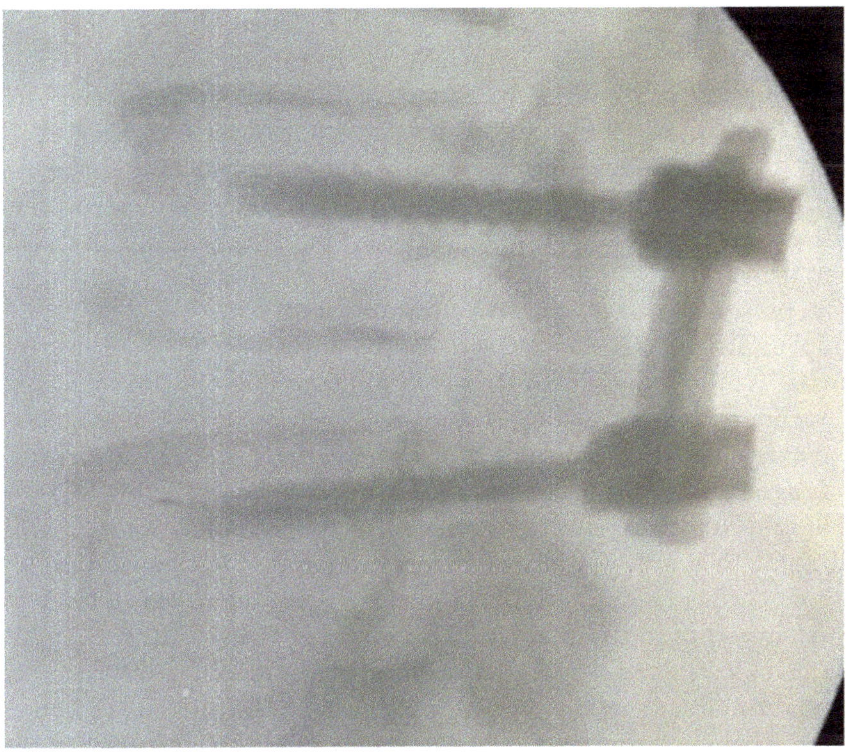

Figure 8. Post-operative sagittal X-ray check—patient code: 5BML4L501.

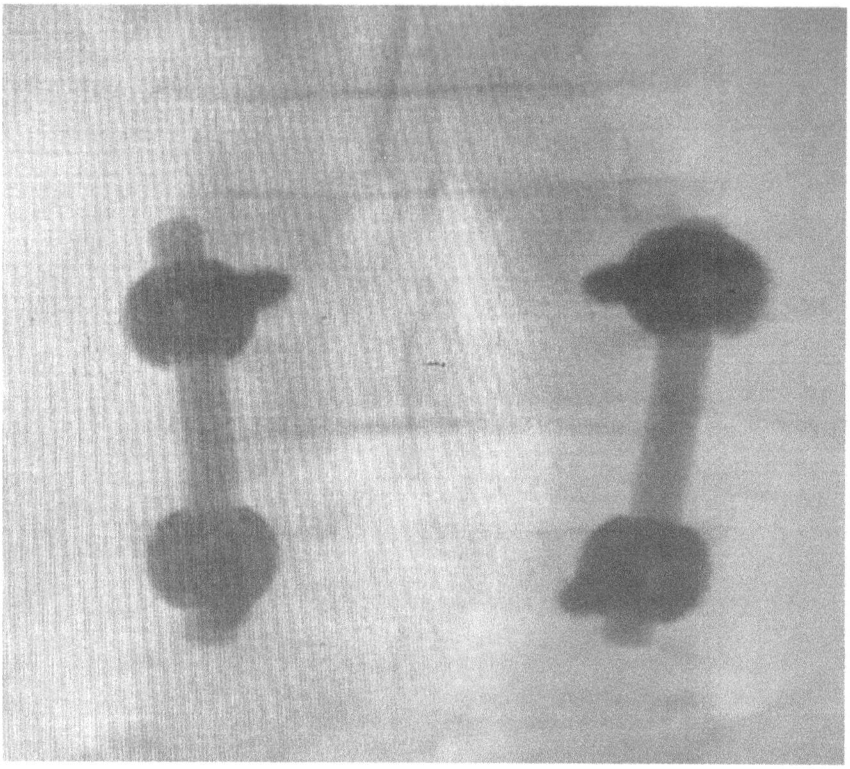

Figure 9. Post-operative coronal X-ray check—patient code: 5BML4L501.

5. Discussion and Perspectives

The standard freehand procedure for pedicle screw insertion is normally characterized by a long learning curve, and the success of the surgery depends on the surgeon's experience. The surgical device presented is an aid that optimizes the standard procedure. Under this point of view, it becomes an alternative to the very expensive navigation systems that involve additional personnel and equipment.

A patented algorithm finds optimal insertion directions and defines length and diameter of the screws based on a custom-made CAD model, obtained via RE. In order to avoid incorrect relative positioning between the template and the vertebra surface, the proposed template features a novel shape that makes its placement univocal and comfortable for the surgeon. An innovative contact surface between template and vertebra has been designed improving the coupling between the template itself and the vertebras, avoiding possible mismatching. Moreover, the device is designed to disengage the template from the bone surface, making it completely innovative.

The production of a 3D-printed template takes, on average, 1.5 man-hours using the RP machine. Since the template design is based on the use of a patented algorithm [11,12,15], the authors are already working on a modelling system that will allow the semi-automatization of the template design based on the 3D model of the spine. Nevertheless, the surgeon will continue to interact with template designers in order to explain to them his/her preferences about the entry point (for which the surgeon remains responsible) and the template's size and anchorage.

This device, which gives the surgeon the optimal screw trajectories and provides information regarding the length and diameter of the screws, significantly reduces the risk that the screws get out of the vertebra surface, damaging the vascular and/or the nervous system, and at the same time risking to fracture the bone. Moreover, the duration of the arthrodesis surgery is significantly shortened. Accordingly, the patient's bleeding, the quantity of drugs, as well as the staff members' stress levels, are significantly reduced. There is also an important reduction of the harmful X-rays.

For this type of research, it is important to highlight the percentage reduction of both the average insertion time for a single screw and the corresponding number of X-ray shots, measured with and without the surgical guide.

The averaging of the results of interest taken from the surgeries are shown below:

- Standard procedure (no template): 27 min for the insertion of one screw and a total of 25 X-rays shots per screw;
- Novel procedure (with template): 10 min for the insertion of one screw with the aid of the template and 2 X-rays shots per screw.

The proposed novel device is experimental, and so the duration of the surgeries has been stretched, since the surgeons involved have payed closer attention to a procedure that was somewhat unfamiliar. Anyway, surgery execution times fell within the range stipulated by the Lazio region local health trust [18].

The use of the proposed novel device achieved improvements in terms of precision, duration and safety, even though the surgical procedure remained the same.

The procedure itself and the use of templates showed some limitations that can be highlighted as the limitation of the study. First of all, the use of templates needs for excellent bone skeletonization of the interface area of the surgical template; in positioning and use of the template, the support of a second staff unit is preferable to ensure that the template is kept in position; nevertheless, surgeons are used to having secondary staff to help the surgery. In order to avoid any kind of mismatch or error in surgery, the surgical template cannot be used if the surgeon wrongly removes part of the bone or if the ligaments to be removed are calcified (not detectable by X-ray). In those cases, the standard procedure has to be performed. This aspect is a limitation, but is also a safety-exit for surgeons who, in case of error, have no problem continuing and completing the procedure by using their standard knowledge and practice.

Finally, the proposed procedure cannot be used for emergency surgeries, as it takes time for 3D reconstruction and redesign.

6. Conclusions

This paper is focused on the design of a novel custom-made surgical template for the optimization of pedicle screw insertion during arthrodesis surgeries. The design is based on both RE and RP techniques, but the surgeon remains responsible for choosing the entry point of the screws.

To summarize briefly, the time spent on the insertion of pedicle screws via the proposed surgical template was cut down by about 63%, while the number of X-ray shots was reduced by about 92%. Precision in surgery outcomes was the same or higher in all of the tests performed.

Future developments will concern the treatment of more complex vertebral shapes. These will entail the introduction of innovative devices for anchoring the surgical template on the vertebra. A new trial has been planned to surgically treat cases with hard scoliosis.

Finally, the template approach will allow a new methodology to be developed for mini-invasive template-based surgery that will bring new methods for percutaneous approaches.

Author Contributions: All authors contributed to the study conception and the design of the presented medical device. In vivo trial was performed by N.N. Data collection and analysis were performed by E.C., and N.C. The first draft of the manuscript was written by A.N. and F.N. and all authors commented on previous versions of the manuscript. All authors have read and agreed to the published version of the manuscript.

Compliance with Ethical Standards: All procedures were performed in accordance with the ethical standards of current Italian law and were in line with the 1964 Helsinki Declaration and its later amendments or comparable ethical standards. The surgery-trial was approved by the Ethical Review Board of the San Giovanni di Dio e Ruggi d'Aragona University Hospital in Salerno, where the trial/tests were conducted. The trial itself and the proposed procedure have been approved by the Ethical Committee of Italian Health Ministry (Campania regional district). The principal investigator, responsible for the clinical trial, is Dr. Nicola Narciso, co-author of this paper.

Informed Consent: All participants were informed about the experiment protocol, the nature of the medical implements used and risks and benefits linked to the new surgical device. Informed consent was signed by the patients.

References

1. Popescu, D.; Anania, D.; Amza, C.G.; Cicic, D. Design and rapid manufacturing of patient-specific spinal surgical guides: A survey. *Proc. Manuf. Syst.* **2012**, *7*, 111–115.
2. Ma, T.; Xu, Y.Q.; Cheng, Y.B.; Jiang, M.Y.; Xu, X.M.; Xie, L.; Lu, S. A novel computer-assisted drill guide template for thoracic pedicle screw placement: A cadaveric study. *Arch. Orthop. Trauma. Surg.* **2012**, *132*, 65–72. [CrossRef] [PubMed]
3. Kashani, J.; Abdul Kadir, M.R.; Arabshahi, Z. A surgical drill guide for pedicle screw placement. *Int. Conf. Biomed. Eng.* **2012**, 305–307. [CrossRef]
4. Merc, M.; Drstvensek, I.; Vogrin, M.; Brajlih, T.; Recnik, G. A multi-level rapid prototyping drill guide template reduces the perforation risk of pedicle screw placement in the lumbar and sacral spine. *Arch. Orthop. Trauma. Surg.* **2013**, *133*, 893–899. [CrossRef] [PubMed]
5. Wiker, R.B.; Tedla, B. Methods and Systems for Imageguided Placement of Implants. U.S. Patent US10448263, 9 December 2004.
6. Pacheco, H.O. Method for Determining Size and Placement of Pedicle Screw in Spinal Surgery. CN Patent 1960680B, 8 September 2010.
7. Popescu, D.; Parpala, R.; Laptoiu, D.; Antoniac, I. Computer-aided technique for determining spinal pedicle screw size and optimal insertion trajectory. *Ann. DAAAM Proc.* **2010**, *1*, 527–533.
8. Naddeo, F.; Cataldo, E.; Naddeo, A.; Cappetti, N.; Narciso, N. An automatic and patient-specific algorithm to design the optimal insertion direction of pedicle screws for spine surgery templates. *Med. Biol. Eng. Comput.* **2017**, *55*. [CrossRef] [PubMed]
9. Solitro, G.F.; Amirouche, F. Innovative approach in the development of computer assisted algorithm for spine pedicle screw placement. *Med. Eng. Phys.* **2016**, *38*, 354–365. [CrossRef] [PubMed]
10. Kim, S.B.; Won, Y.; Sin, L.J.; Rhee, J.M.; Lee, S.W.; Lee, G.S. Unilateral Spinous Process Noncovering Hook Type Patient-specific Drill Template for Thoracic Pedicle Screw Fixation: A Pilot Clinical Trial and Template Classification. *Spine* **2017**, *42*, E1050–E1057. [CrossRef] [PubMed]
11. Techno Design Srl; Naddeo, A.; Cataldo, E.; Naddeo, F.; Cappetti, N.; Ruggeri, R. Metodologia per L'individuazione Della Direzione Ottima e del Diametro Massimo di una Vite Peduncolare Affinché la Vite non Fuoriesca dal Peduncolo Durante L'inserimento. Italian Patent ITUB20152877, 22 January 2017 (priority on 22 July 2015).
12. Techno DESIGN Srl; Naddeo, A.; Cataldo, E.; Naddeo, F.; Cappetti, N.; Ruggieri, R. Techno DESIGN Srl; Method for Identifying the Optimal Direction and Maximum Diameter of a Pedicle Screw. European Patent EP3120797A3, 25 January 2017 (priority on 22 July 2015).
13. Zanoli, G. Outcome assessment in lumbar spine surgery. *Acta Orthop.* **2005**, *76*, 2–47. [CrossRef]
14. Cappetti, N.; Naddeo, A.; Naddeo, F.; Solitro, G. Finite elements/Taguchi method based procedure for the identification of the geometrical parameters significantly affecting the biomechanical behavior of a lumbar disc. *Comput. Methods Biomech. Biomed. Engin.* **2015**, *19*, 1–8. [CrossRef] [PubMed]
15. Techno DESIGN Srl; Naddeo, A.; Cataldo, E.; Naddeo, F.; Cappetti, N.; Ruggieri, R. Dima di Foratura Direzionale per Chirurgia Vertebrale. Italian Patent ITNA20150019, 14 November 2016 (priority on 14 May 2015).
16. Naddeo, F.; Fontana, C.; Naddeo, A.; Cataldo, E.; Cappetti, N.; Narciso, N. Novel design for a customized, 3D-printed surgical template for thoracic spinal arthrodesis. *Int. J. Med. Robot. Comput. Assist. Surg.* **2019**. [CrossRef] [PubMed]
17. Kaneyama, S.; Sugawara, T.; Sumi, M.; Higashiyama, N.; Takabatake, M.; Mizoi, K. A novel screw guiding method with a screw guide template system for posterior C-2 fixation: Clinical article. *J. Neurosurg. Spine* **2014**, *21*. [CrossRef] [PubMed]
18. Agrillo, U. UOC Neurochirurgia in ASL ROMA 2. 2013. Available online: http://www.aslromab.it/cittadini/ospedali/pertini/dip_chirurgia/UOC_neurochirurgia.php (accessed on 25 July 2019).

5

Regenerative Models for the Integration and Regeneration of Head Skeletal Tissues

Warren A. Vieira and Catherine D. McCusker *

Department of Biology, University of Massachusetts Boston, Boston, MA 02125, USA; Warren.Vieira@umb.edu
* Correspondence: catherine.mccusker@umb.edu

Abstract: Disease of, or trauma to, the human jaw account for thousands of reconstructive surgeries performed every year. One of the most popular and successful treatment options in this context involves the transplantation of bone tissue from a different anatomical region into the affected jaw. Although, this method has been largely successful, the integration of the new bone into the existing bone is often imperfect, and the integration of the host soft tissues with the transplanted bone can be inconsistent, resulting in impaired function. Unlike humans, several vertebrate species, including fish and amphibians, demonstrate remarkable regenerative capabilities in response to jaw injury. Therefore, with the objective of identifying biological targets to promote and engineer improved outcomes in the context of jaw reconstructive surgery, we explore, compare and contrast the natural mechanisms of endogenous jaw and limb repair and regeneration in regenerative model organisms. We focus on the role of different cell types as they contribute to the regenerating structure; how mature cells acquire plasticity in vivo; the role of positional information in pattern formation and tissue integration, and limitations to endogenous regenerative and repair mechanisms.

Keywords: regenerative medicine; transplantation; jaw regeneration; limb regeneration; positional information; zebrafish; axolotl

1. Introduction

The skeletal bones of the face and head play multiple roles that are essential to our survival. They encase and protect our fragile brain tissue from injury. They are essential for respiration, the intake and mastication of food, and verbal communication. They separate our eyes and ears at an appropriate distance, so that we can achieve binocular vision and resolve the spatial origin of sound, respectively. Given these diverse and essential functions of the head skeleton, traumatic injury to these tissues can have a profound impact on our health and quality of life. Although humans have limited regenerative capacity of these structures, different surgical and regenerative treatments have been developed to repair these injuries. However, the outcome of these treatments can vary greatly depending on the age of the patient and the location and size of the injury. In this review we will discuss (1) the most recent advances in regenerative technologies to replace or repair damaged cranioskeletal tissues with a focus on the jaw, (2) how endogenous regeneration of the jaw occurs in regenerative model organisms, and (3) how we can apply what is known about endogenous regeneration of the jaw and other skeletal elements in the body to develop more effective regenerative therapies.

2. Current Regenerative Therapies for the Jaw

Damage to the human mandibular and maxillary jaw bones can occur through a variety of mechanisms, including diseases, such as cancers, or direct trauma. Moreover, tooth loss or extraction will lead to the alveolar ridge exhibiting atrophy, both in height and width, which impedes implantation; although, the basal processes of the mandible and maxilla will remain unaffected [1]. Therefore, bone maintenance and/or regeneration under these circumstances is essential to ensure jaw functionality and allow for the restoration of dentation by implantation where necessary.

A variety of different methods have been pursued to replace or repair damaged jaw tissue, with varying degrees of success. One method that has worked well for repairing missing jaw tissue in some patients has been through distracting the remaining mandibular bone. Distraction is the process whereby new bone is generated by applying stress (stretching) to the bone. Some positive aspects of using distraction are (1) that the new bone tissue is fully integrated and (2) there is an expansion of the other surrounding tissues, including skin, muscle, nerve, blood vessels, periosteum, and cartilage. Additionally, since this method utilizes endogenous tissue, the issues of tissue rejection can be avoided. Distractors can be internal or external and are directly fixed on the bone. The method of distraction has been used successfully on children with congenital craniofacial deformities [2], as well as reconstructing mandibular defects [3]. However, in instances where there is not enough of the mandible to distract, for example in some cancer and trauma patients, this method of treatment is not an option.

In circumstances where minimal alveolar or mandibular bone remains, many studies have tried repairing the damaged jaw tissue by using implants or tissue transplants from different anatomical locations. Some of the earlier attempts involved alloplastic implants of a structure composed of an inert metal such as steel, titanium, or chrom-colbalt steel. One of the many issues with these types of implants is that the material is not composed of cells, and so the implant is incapable of healing and fully integrating with the surrounding tissues. Not surprisingly, these implants had a high failure rate and were removed as a result. Hybrid implants consisting of metal trays with "cancellous bone" were also tested and associated with similar, poor outcomes (reviewed in [4]).

Over the last few decades, much work has focused on the development of different synthetic bone substitutes, many of which have led to good healing outcomes (reviewed in [5]). Implants composed of these substitutes have the advantage that they alleviate the need to harvest bone from a different region of the patient's body, and can be "tunable" to the needs of a particular injury site. For example, the porocity and topography [6] of these scaffolds can be easily manipulated, biologically active molecules such as specific extracellular matrix molecules or growth factors [7–10] can be added, and specific cell types such as osteoblasts [11], mesencymal stem cells [12] and endothelial cells [13] can be seeded to generate patient and need-specific implants.

Osteomyocutaneous flaps, which are composed of vascularized muscle (ex. trapezius or latissimus muscle) that sometimes includes a portion of the underlying bone, have been used for head, neck, and jaw defects. These transplantations have been moderately successful in repairing the damaged tissue; however, patients often suffer from complications associated with the removal of the donor tissue. Vascularized bone flaps, also known as free flaps, where the graft tissues have been harvested from a variety of locations including ribs, iliac crest, fibula, or metatarsals have also been used. Early trials resulted in high morbidity, surgical complications, and a total or partial bone loss of the graft. More recent trials with the fibula with fixed plates to the mandible have been relatively successful, with remarkable integration reported between the tissue transplant and the mandibular defect [14,15]. Similar results have been reported from iliac crest and scapular spine implants [16].

Currently, the most frequently preformed methods for jaw repair involve autologous bone grafts; and is associated with 100–76.4% success and 100–86.9% survival rates [17,18]. Common procedures in this context involves either the direct implantation of the donor bone, or grinding thereof, and subsequently seeding the resultant particulate matter into a scaffold, prior to implantation (also referred to as bone graft substitutes). The latter procedure is beneficial when donor tissue is limited and would require remodel into an appropriate shape for implantation.

Multiple aspects appear to contribute to the success of autologous bone transplantation in the context of jaw repair. Donor tissue has been derived from intraoral (maxilla, mandible) or more distal (iliac crest, pelvic or calvarial) sites [19]; however, they are not equivalent in terms of their restorative capacities. Calvarial bone grafts, for example, show better stability after oral implantation relative to iliac bone, but graft segments are thinner and exhibits worse vertical bone growth [20]. Jaw-derived grafts are associated with better graft survival, osteogenic activity and less volume loss relative to iliac bone [19]; and better mineralization, albeit less than the original jaw tissue, compared to pelvic grafts [21]. These donor site differences in regenerative capabilities may, in part, be due to the fact that mammalian bone mesenchymal stem cells exhibit skeletal site-specific variations in terms their osteogenic potential [22,23]. In humans and rodents, maxilla and mandible bone derived mesenchymal stem cells (MSCs) exhibit greater proliferative and survival properties, and significantly higher in vitro and in vivo osteogenic capacity, relative to iliac crest and tibia derived counterparts [22,23]. In rodents, direct implantation of mandible derived MSCs, seeded onto a scaffold, into a mandible defect resulted in more new bone formation relative to tibia derived MSCs or scaffold-alone grafts [23].

In the case of alveolar bone regeneration, local augmentation by guided bone regeneration is commonly employed with success. This has been extensively reviewed elsewhere [24,25] but briefly, this surgical protocol involves the implantation of a resorbable membrane into the defected area which mechanically allows for the invasion of osteogenic but no other competing non-osteogenic tissues. Although non-resorbable membranes show poor soft tissue compatibility, their use is associated with a reduction in new bone resorption and the generation of harder, stiffer and more mineralized osteoblast-derived matrices relative to its resorbable counterpart. Irrespective of the degradability of the membrane, growth factors, bone, or bone-derived materials are frequently used in conjunction with this technique [24,25]. Growth factors, such as bone morphogenetic proteins and platelet-rich plasma, aid regeneration by recruiting and stimulating proliferation of osteogenic tissue [24]. The use of bone derived material in this context has varying outcomes. For example, cortical bone grafts exhibit far more resorption relative to cancellous block grafts; with the latter also exhibiting superior revascularization and strengthening during the healing process as well [25].

There is also evidence that transplantations may stimulate an endogenous regenerative response in younger patients. Striking regeneration, where a *de novo* jaw joint is formed, has been reported in an adolescent patient that was treated with a costochondral graft into a mandibular resection [26]. Still, although the outcome at treatment site was improved, patients need to recover from the removal of the harvested tissue and any complications that are involved with the loss of that tissue at the site of harvest.

More recently, researchers have attempted stem cell-based therapies. Stem cells, and differentiated osteoblasts thereof, are valuable sources of donor tissue, as it negates the risk of donor site morbidity which have been associated with bone graft harvesting [27–29]. Bioabsorable poly (L-lactide) (PLLA) mesh scaffolds with bone marrow have been tested for jawbone regeneration. This method had an 84% success rate but does not work well with post radio-therapy patients or elderly people who have diminished bone precursor cells [30]. A combination of buccal fat pad stem cells (from the cheek) with iliac bone grafts has been used to treat maxillomandibular atrophy, and a resultant increased bone width was reported in the experimental group [30,31]. Similarly, allogenic chord stem cells or cranial derived bone marrow stem cells combined with alloplastic graft material for mandibular reconstruction has demonstrated some bone regeneration [22,23]. Dental pulp stem/progenitor cells can be employed for jaw restoration as well. When seeded into a collagen sponge scaffold and implanted into mandible, patients exhibited vertical repair of alveolar bone and restoration of periodontal tissue [30]. Some of the major challenges of these treatments are the formation of structures with the appropriate bone pattern (without ectopic bone formation), and the integration of the newly regenerated bone with the existing bone and the surrounding soft tissues.

In summary, although both reconstructive and regenerative methods have been developed with moderate success, not all of these methods will work for all patients. Future therapies will need to focus on either improving the integration of tissue transplantations, or the stimulation of an endogenous regenerative response for better patient outcomes. In this review, we will explore the mechanisms by which regenerative model organisms perfectly integrate transplanted tissue or endogenously regenerate missing jaw tissue to identify potential targets that can be explored for regenerative therapies for humans.

3. The Patterning and Development of the Cranial-Facial Skeleton

Many similarities exist between how the head skeleton is formed during embryogenesis, and how these structures can reform during regeneration. Thus, we will first discuss how the cranial-facial skeleton develops so that comparisons can be more easily made with the regenerative mechanisms.

The skeletal structures in the cranium are derived from a tissue in the developing embryo known as the cranial neural crest (CNC). The CNC is a transient population of multipotent cells that is located lateral to the neural plate on the dorsal side of the anterior end of all vertebrate embryos. During neurulation, the CNC cells delaminate from the neural folds and migrate ventrally between the ectodermal and endodermal germ layers. Depending on where the CNC cells are located on the A/P axis in the developing head they will express different positional markers, migrate on discreet pathways, and differentiate into different skeletal elements.

During early development the hindbrain is segmented into anterior/posterior compartments known as rhombomeres, and CNC migration is directed by these underlying compartments (as reviewed in [32]). The CNC migrates in a ventral direction along three major pathways, the mandibular, the hyoid, and the proximal pharyngeal (branchial) arches. The mandibular arch migrates around the optic vesicle, will fuse at the region below the optic vesicle, and will generate most of the cartilage and membranous bone of the face and jaw. The CNC cells from the hyoid arch will migrate ventrally and differentiate into a small number of skeletal elements in the middle ear and the hyoid bone. The most posterior CNC segments migrate to populate the pharyngeal pouches, and differentiate into the "gill" and pharyngeal cartilages in the neck skeleton.

Each arch of the CNC expresses specific patterning genes, and the expression of these genes plays an important role in the formation of specific skeletal elements in the head. The mandibular (neurocranial) arch arises from the Otx-expressing region of the hindbrain, and does not express Homeobox (*Hox*) genes. As the cells that form this arch migrate, they express distal-less homeobox genes (*Dlx*) *Dlx1/2* and *Dlx1/2/5/6* in a dorsal ventral gradient and further subdivide into the maxillary and mandibular processes, respectively [33–35]. The hyoid and branchial streams arise from the *Hox-2* and *Hox-3* expressing regions of the hindbrain, respectively. The alteration of the expression of these genes results in homeotic transformations. For example, the disruption of *Hoxa-2* expression in the rostral branchial (hyoid) region of the head in developing mice results in the loss of hyoid cartilages and the formation of duplicated mandibular arch-derived skeletal structures [36,37]. The reverse manipulation of overexpressing *Hox-2* in the normally Hox-negative mandibular arch cells results in the loss of jaw elements and duplication of hyoid skeletal elements [38,39].

Interestingly, grafts of cells from the mandibular (*Hox* negative) to the hyoid (*Hox* positive) arch in avian species results in the formation of ectopic skeletal tissue from the mandibular segment in the host location [40]. Thus, the lack of *Hox* expression in these cells does not preclude their identity as the mandibular segment. However, a community effect also plays an important role in determining whether or not these cells maintain their original, arch-specific identities. Transplantation of either single cells or small groups of cells from one arch to another during an early stage of CNC development in zebrafish results in the transformation of *Hox* expression from the original to the host location, and the contribution of the grafted cells to the host structures [41]. This plasticity is, however, dependent on how differentiated the cells are. Performing the same grafting manipulations in later staged embryos, where the CNC cells have differentiated, results in the grafted population maintaining their original *Hox* expression profile and facilitating the development of structures consistent with the original location from which the graft was derived [41]. Similar results have also been reported in the mouse model system [42].

Once the CNC cells reach their destination in the embryo and cease migrating they will differentiate into their fated tissue identities. Evidence indicates that the cells that are fated to become skeletal tissue provide positional cues to the surrounding cell types. For example, grafts of the mandibular segment to the hyoid segment in developing avian embryos doesn't just result in the formation of ectopic mandibular skeleton in the hyoid segment, but also reorganizes the surrounding mesoderm to pattern and differentiate into the mandibular musculature, which integrates with the ectopic skeletal tissue [40]. The transplanted CNC cells also provide instructional cues to other non-neural crest populations including those that generate the avian beak, feathers, and tendons [43]. However, it is also clear that the surrounding epithelium is providing patterning cues to the *Hox* negative mandibular arch. Removal of the endoderm close to this arch results in the loss of cranial skeletal elements, and the addition of grafted endoderm results in the formation of ectopic cranial skeletal elements [44,45]. Thus, and interplay of patterning cues between the epithelial cells and the CNC are required for the development of this tissue.

4. Differentiation of the Head Skeleton

As opposed to the more posteriorly located trunk neural crest, the cranial neural crest cells contribute to skeletal tissues of the head. This ability appears to depend, at least in part, on their low *Hox* expression status [46,47]. The most caudal (anterior) CNC arch is *Hox* negative and will form most of the skeletal elements in the head and face. The hyoid arch expresses *Hox2* genes, and will only form the small hyoid and middle ear skeletal elements. Last, the posterior pharyngeal arches express both group 2 and 3 *Hox* genes, and has only a small contribution to the neck skeleton. Loss of *Hox* expression can force trunk neural crest cells to differentiate into skeleton [48].

The mechanism of osteogenesis depends on the cranium skeletal element considered (as reviewed in [49]). The flat bones of the skull that form the top and sides of the brain case, as well as the facial bones, form through a process of intramembranous ossification, whereby mesenchymal cells are converted directly into bone. The bones that compose the floor of the brain case form via endochondrial ossification, where a cartilage intermediate forms first, and acts as a scaffold for the osteogenic precursors.

Multiple molecular signaling events play an important role in the differentiation of the head skeleton. Endothelin-1 (Et-1) secretion from the epithelium and mesenchyme surrounding the pharyngeal arch, instructs the formation of dorsal/ventral skeletal elements in the head [50–52]. Loss of function studies in mice and zebrafish indicate that the concentration of Et-1 dictates whether a dorsal or ventral skeletal element is induced; high concentrations of Et-1 result in the formation of ventral structures, whereas low concentrations result in the formation of dorsal skeletal elements [50,53,54]. *FGF* expression is linked to CNC cell survival, migration, and also activates the expression of genes that promote CNC-specific cell differentiation, including the skeleton [55]. Additionally, high concentrations of FGF promote cartilage and bone differentiation, and can result in the formation of ectopic cartilage elements. In summary, the interplay of signaling events between the different tissues in the developing head plays an essential role in the differentiation of the craniofacial skeleton.

5. Vertebrate Model Systems to Study for Jaw Regeneration

While the embryonic mechanisms underlying the development of the craniofacial skeleton are mostly conserved, regenerative capabilities are highly variable amongst different vertebrate species; fish and amphibians exhibit extensive regenerative abilities of complex tissues and structures, whereas mammals and birds exhibit limited, minimal responses. As reviewed elsewhere, zebrafish [56] are commonly employed as model systems for both cardiac and neurological regeneration, while Urodele amphibians (newts and salamanders) are typically used to study limb [57] as well neurological regeneration [58]. The phenomenon of jaw regeneration has also been documented in these model organisms; however, it is less extensively studied. Interestingly, this specific phenomenon is absent in most anuran species, such as the adult African Clawed frog [59], but appears to present in at least some reptile species, such as the Marsh crocodile [60].

To facilitate better comparisons between these model organisms we will provide a brief description of the basic anatomical structure of the zebrafish and Urodele jaw. We will then discuss current findings (Table 1), interpretations, and limitations of jaw regeneration associated with the use of these different model systems. Focus will be placed on lower jaw regeneration, which has been more extensively studied relative to the upper jaw; however, work by Ghosh 1994 has shown that upper and lower jaw regeneration occur by identical process in the adult newt [61].

Table 1. Comparison of regenerative and fracture healing responses across vertebrate species in the lower jaw. n/a—not applicable; w/m—whole mount staining; µCT—Micro computed tomography, hst—histology.

Process		Mammalian	Avian	Urodele	Teleost
Regeneration	Capacity	No	No	Yes	Yes
	Mechanism	n/a	n/a	Epimorphic regeneration	Epimorphic regeneration
	Pattern relative to original	n/a	n/a	Juvenile = identical (based on w/m), Adult = different (based on w/m, µCT)	Different (based on w/m)
	Integration with stump	n/a	n/a	Juvenile = fully integrated (based on w/m) Adult = incomplete (based on w/m, hst)	Incomplete (based on w/m, hst)
Fracture healing	Capacity	Yes	Yes	Yes	Yes
	Mechanism	Secondary ossification	Secondary ossification	Absence of secondary ossification	Absence of secondary ossification
	Pattern relative to original	Poor (based on hst, µCT)	Poor (based on hst)	Poor (based on hst)	Poor (based on hst)
	Integration with stump	Poor (based on hst, µCT)	Poor (based on hst)	Poor (based on hst)	Poor (based on hst)

6. The Anatomy of the Lower Jaw in Regenerating Species

The lower jaws of adult zebrafish and Urodele amphibian are anatomically similar and comprises of the mandible, hyoid apparatus, brachial arches as well as the associated mandibular muscles and connective tissues. These structures are similar to those of the mammalian counterpart; however, distinct differences do exist.

In the zebrafish and amphibian, two dermal bones, pre-articular (present on the lingual side only) and dentary, enclose a cartilaginous rod, known as Meckel's cartilage, to form the mandible. Dorsally and ventrally the mandible curves inwards, with the distal ends joined by the median symphysis, a cartilaginous structure [59,61–68]. In the adult newt, the dentary bone of the mandible, which stretches from the basal articulation to the median symphysis, possess mature, bicuspid teeth that are arranged towards the outer, dorsal margin of the bone. Immature teeth, which will develop and migrate out with time to replace the mature teeth in the event of tooth loss, are located in the inner border of this tissue [59,61,66,68,69]. The pre-articular bone serves as a site of masticatory muscle attachment [61]. Far less ossification is present in the lower jaw of the larval amphibian, with the mandible being constituted by an elongated cartilaginous rod that becomes surrounded by bone, in a proximal to distal direction, with time. Once the dentary bone has been established, monocuspid teeth will erupt [61].

Relative to the amphibian and fish, the tissue composition of the human jaw is different. The U-shaped human mandible is formed early during embryogenesis, initially constituted by hyaline cartilaginous tissue and thick perichondral fibrous mesenchyme, derived from Meckel's cartilage [70]. As development progresses, ossification produces intramembranous bone adjacent to the Meckel's cartilage, which forms the architecture of the mandibular body. Endochondral ossification is associated with the mandibular condyle. By 12 weeks post-fertilization, the Meckel's cartilage has diminished in size, and only a small portion of it, located in the mandible close to the midline near the symphysis, remains unossified and forms two nodules of fibrous tissue that occupies the dorsal surface of the symphysis [71]. Human dentition is both heterodont and diphyodont; with the eruption of the deciduous teeth being delayed till after birth and subsequently replaced, at a later time point, by permanent dentation (as reviewed by the authors of [72]).

7. Endogenous Regeneration of the Jaw

Regenerative mechanisms can take different forms depending on the organism and the organ or tissue that is being regenerated (as reviewed in Lismaa [73]). These mechanisms are generally divided into four categories, epimorphosis, morphallaxis, stem cell mediated, and compensatory regeneration. Compensatory regeneration occurs when differentiated cells divide but maintain their differentiated function to replace missing or damaged tissue. Human liver regeneration is an example of a regenerative process that heavily utilizes this mechanism. In stem cell mediated regeneration, stem cells generate the "building blocks" of the missing structures. The re-growth of hair shafts, from follicular stem cells, and the replacement of blood cells, from hematopoietic stem cells, are examples of this regenerative mechanism. Epimorphosis and morphallaxis are regenerative mechanisms that are generally reserved for the replacement of more complex structures. Morphallaxis occurs when the remaining undamaged tissue reorganizes into the pattern of the missing structure(s). This type of regeneration has been well documented in hyrax species that utilize morphallaxis to regenerate complete heads. Last, epimorphic regeneration occurs when mature cells dedifferentiate into progenitor cells known as blastema cells, which divide, re-pattern, and re-differentiate into the missing structure(s). Amphibian limb regeneration is an example of epimorphic regeneration. Many regenerative processes do not exclusively use one regenerative mechanism, but often use a combination of mechanisms.

8. Jaw Blastema Formation

Jaw regeneration in appears to occur mostly by epimorphosis, where the surrounding tissue dedifferentiates and contributes to the formation of the regenerative organ known as the blastema. Distal transverse amputation of the lower jaw in zebrafish as well as Urodele species including the Eastern Newt, the Japanese fire belly newt, the Northern dusky salamander, the Red-backed salamander, the Northern two-lined salamander, the Marbled salamander, and the Tiger salamander (*Nofophthalmus viridescens, Triturus viridescens, Cynops pyrrhogaster, Desmognathus juscus, Plethodon cinereus, Eurycea bislineata; Ambystoma opacum, Ambystoma Tigrinum*) induces a regenerative response (Figure 1). The initial response to this type of injury appears to be conserved, not only between species but also between body-structures (Figure 2). Prior to blastema formation, soft tissue [61,62,74], including muscle [59,64]) and dental lamina [74], retract at the plane of amputation [61,74,75], and a wound epithelium is quickly established over the site of injury [62,74]. Work by Zhang et al. 2015 suggests that in zebrafish jaw regeneration foxi1-foxo1b-pou3f1 signaling promotes wound epithelium formation. *Foxo1* is also upregulated in the early (24 h) stages of axolotl limb regeneration and appears to also be linked to the wound healing response in this organism as well [76].

This initial process of tissue degradation and wound epithelium formation is akin to that documented during limb regeneration in Urodele amphibians (as reviewed in [77]; however, unlike limb regeneration, no prominent innervation of the wound epithelium is apparent [61,62,64]), or required [63] for the continuation of the regenerative process. During limb regeneration, nerve-derived signaling in the wound site plays an essential role in blastema formation and growth; and nerve removal results in regenerative failure [78,79]. (reviewed in [80]). However, denervation of the already poorly innervated lower jaw of the adult newt has no effect on the regenerative process [63]. It is possible that direct nerve signaling is not necessarily required for regeneration, since salamander limbs that developed aneurogenically demonstrate regenerative abilities in response to amputation [69]. To explain the observations in these situations, the local tissues may compensate for low or absent innervation by the local production of sufficient regeneration-specific tropic factors [63]. More work is required to determine the necessity, nature, quantity and source of the trophic factors required for blastema formation in the context of jaw regeneration.

Early stages of limb regeneration in the newt and axolotl are relatively avascular, with the apical epithelial cap and initial blastema formation occurring in the absence of vascularization. As the blastema grows new vessels begin to invade from the proximal end, thus only later in blastema development is the entire structure fully vascularized [81]. Despite this delay in vascularization, one day post amputation transcriptional and gene ontology analysis indicates enrichment of genes relating to vasculature development in the regenerating axolotl [82]. This rapid vascular response in gene expression is also documented in the regenerating jaw, with transcriptional analyses suggesting that by two days post amputation blastemal angiogenesis and vasculogenesis is regulated by a pou5f1-cdx4-kdrl signaling pathway [83]. However, unlike the regenerating limb; new blood vessels sprouting from muscle tissue at the site of injury can be noted as early as 2 h post jaw amputation [83].

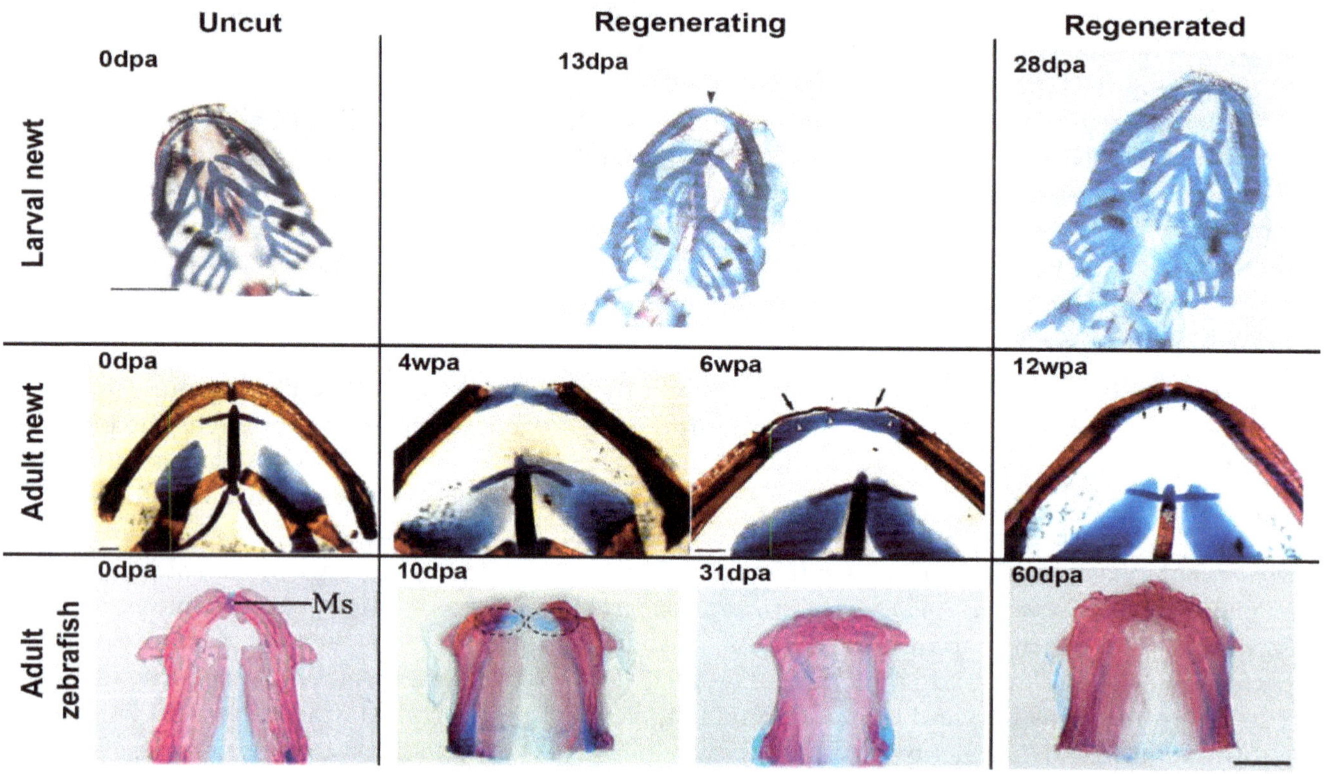

Figure 1. Whole mount preparations demonstrate the jaw-regenerative capacities of Urodeles and Zebrafish. Stage 40 newt larvae (top panel) exhibit more robust regenerative capabilities relative to their adult counter parts (middle panel) as well as to zebrafish (lower panel). In all three cases a cartilage rod is initially generated, fusing the two damaged ends of the mandible; however, this cartilage is replaced completely by bone in the zebrafish and results in the loss of the mandibular symphysis (MS). In the larval newt the regenerated pattern is identical to the original jaw; while in the adult regenerate is inappropriately patterned in terms of bone and cartilage relative to the original. Blue—cartilage staining, red—bone staining. Arrow in upper panel highlights the absence of dentary bone 13 dpa. Arrows in the middle panel highlights the dentary bone growing towards the mid-line 6wpa, and the absence of ossification on the lingual side of the jaw at 12 wpa. Dpa—days post amputation, wpa—weeks post amputation. (Images modified with permission from Ghosh et al. 1994 and Wang et al. 2012).

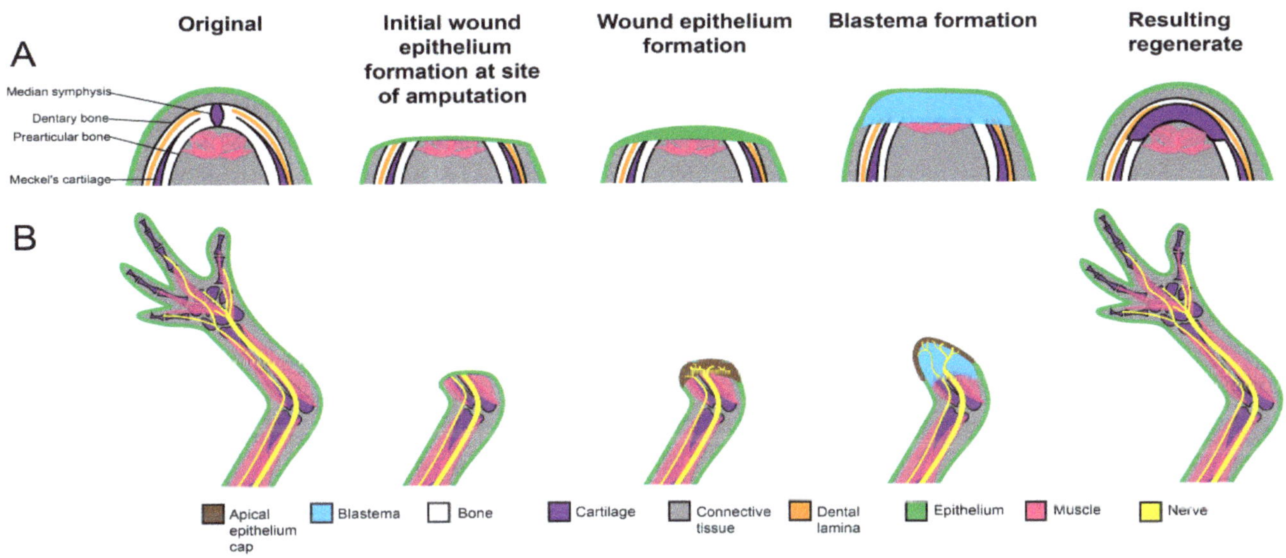

Figure 2. Differences and similarities in blastema and structure formation during adult Urodele jaw and limb regeneration. (**A**) The stages of jaw regeneration. The intact amphibian jaw consists of Meckel's cartilage, dentary and prearticular bone, and the median symphysis connecting both sides of the jaw. The hyoid and brachial skeletons have been removed for simplicity. Upon amputation, a wound epithelium forms over the remaining jaw stump tissue. Independent of nerve singling, blastema cells accumulate at the severed edge of the jaw, derived from a variety of mature stump tissues, and will proliferate, repattern, and differentiate into a structure similar to the original structure, but with notable differences. The medium symphysis is lost and the majority of regenerated skeleton is cartilaginous (connect with Meckel's cartilage), with only the dentary bone being restored. (**B**) The stages of limb regeneration. Limb regeneration also requires blastema formation, however its induction is slightly different from that of jaw regeneration. After amputation, a wound epithelium (WE) forms over the severed edge of the limb stump. The WE becomes innervated by the regenerating neurons, and establishes a specialized wound epithelium known as the Apical Epithelial Cap (AEC). The AEC is required for the dedifferentiation of the limb stump cells into blastema cells. The blastema cells, also derived from a variety of mature tissue, proliferate, pattern, and redifferentiate into all of the missing limb structures. The resulting limb regenerate is identical to the original.

During limb regeneration in the salamander, the blastema is derived from a variety of stump cells [84–86]; although, not all stump tissues contribute equally to this progenitor population. For example, cells of connective tissue origin contribute more substantially to the blastema than muscle cells, while skeletal elements (bone and cartilage) fail to contribute at all [66,86,87]. Additionally, the contribution of these progenitor cells to the ultimate regenerate is restricted in a lineage specific manner. For example, muscle and Schwann cell derived blastema cells only differentiate into muscle and Schwann cells respectively, while blastema cells of connective tissue origin exhibit great plasticity and differentiate into cartilage, connective tissue and tendons [84,86,88].

A thorough understanding of the origins and differentiation potential of jaw blastema cells is largely lacking; however, it would appear from histological analysis, limited cell linage identification, transcriptional analysis and BrdU studies, that similar to limb regeneration, a heterogeneous population of dedifferentiated cells is generated at the plane of amputation in the jaw. These cells are derived from a variety of mature stump tissues, including muscle [64], a portion of which are *Pax7* positive muscle progenitor cells in newt [59] and *Pax3a, Isl1* muscle positive progenitor cells in fish [62], periosteum [89], and Foxi1 positive neural crest derived cells [62]. The *Pax3a, Isl1* positive progenitor population in fish localize to the posterior region of the regenerating jaw and are believed to contribute to muscle regeneration [62]. The *Foxi1* progenitors, associated with *Sox9a* expression 5 days post amputation, are localized to the region of new cartilage formation, suggesting that these cells contribute to skeletal regeneration [62]. Additionally, about 50% of the newt jaw blastema was found to exhibit lineage marks for dental pulp and dermal fibroblasts markers [61].

Cells of connective tissue origin also contribute to the jaw blastema. During limb regeneration, the missing skeletal tissues are derived completely from cells of connective tissue origin except for bone and cartilage [86,89]. In contrast, it appears that a small number of cells within the cartilage of the mandible undergo proliferation in response to amputation and may therefore contribute to the jaw blastema [59]. Cell lineage tracking experiments are required to determine the identity of these cells, to ensure they are not of soft connective tissue origin, and then test whether they migrate into the growing blastema. However, if the mandibular cartilage does contribute to the blastema it may indicate that different skeletal populations have different propensities for contributing towards a regenerative response. Secondly, from the available data, jaw regeneration in the newt appears dependent on the presence of the mandible. Excision of the central portion of the lower jaw, such that the mandible is left intact, results in regeneration, whereas an amputation that removes the entire mandible inhibits regeneration completely [90].

It is possible that different regions of the mandible contribute in different ways to the regenerating jaw. Histological analysis reveals that only peripheral tissues that are attached to the inner edges of the mandibles contributed towards the growth of the blastema, while little to no direct cellular contribution comes from posterior soft tissues [68]. Additionally, connective tissues cells play multiple roles during epimorphic regeneration. During limb regeneration, connective tissue cells not only contribute to all of the various connective tissues in the limb (dermis, tendons, periosteum, cartilage, bone) but they also play an essential role in the patterning of the blastemal cells into the missing limb structures, and provide positional cues to the surrounding cells to integrate the regenerated tissues [86] (reviewed in [77]). In newts, amputations have been performed along the length of the jaw; as the site of amputation approaches the proximal end of the jaw regenerative capacity diminishes, along with pattern [64]. Since the periosteum of the mandible has been shown to contribute to the regenerating jaw [74,89], it is therefore plausible that the periosteum of the mandible is necessary for pattern formation in jaw regeneration as well.

In summary, jaw regeneration requires the contribution of multiple cell types, derived from the underlying stump tissues, to the blastema. Mandibular tissue appears to be specifically required for the patterning and regeneration of the missing mandibular skeleton. We will further discuss the implications of these observations and how they can apply to regenerative therapies for humans below.

9. Jaw Blastema Cell Differentiation

9.1. Skeleton Formation

As the newt jaw blastema grows, the first differentiated cell type to arise is the chondrocyte. These cells produce a dense collagen matrix to establish a cartilaginous mass at the inner margins of the pre-articular bone of the stump, which is not continuous with the dentary bone or the Meckle's cartilage [64,89]. As the cartilage grows outwards in a mediodistal direction, it fuses at the midline in a curved fashion to restore the general shape of the jaw [64]. At this later stage of regeneration in the adult and juvenile newt, the new cartilage finally becomes continuous with the Meckel's cartilage, [64]. The cartilage bridge that ultimately spans the jaw, acts as a scaffold for mandibular bone formation. However, bone formation is distinctly different between fish and newts during jaw regeneration.

In zebrafish the entire cartilage scaffold is ossified through the process intramembranous ossification. No Meckle's cartilage persists, and the median symphysis is absent due to the two mandibular bones fusing directly [62,89]. The remaining un-amputated portion of jaw however still retains cartilage, suggesting that any signals or stimuli responsible for the aberrant ossification pattern documented during jaw regeneration, relative to the original jaw, is restricted spatially to the regenerated tissue alone. At a molecular level, cartilage formation and subsequent ossification during regeneration in the zebrafish is, at least in part, dependent on Indian hedge homology a (*Ihha*) [89]. This is particularly interesting as *Ihha* is dispensable for zebrafish jaw development, where the only obvious defect in *Ihha* mutants was a delay in perichondral bone formation [89]. Therefore, the involvement and role of specific molecular signals involved in jaw skeleton regeneration may, in part, be different relative to their developmental counterparts.

Age and/or metamorphosis appear to alter the regenerative capacity during newt jaw regeneration. In the juvenile newt, the cartilaginous mandible has both dentary and prearticular bone form around it, such that it resembles the original jaw exactly. After the ossification of the dentary bone a complete row of monocuspid teeth develop [61]. In the post-metamorphic adult newt, a thin layer of bone is formed along the ventral and lateral side in a proximo-distal direction of the regenerated cartilage scaffold, through intramembranous ossification, which fuses at the midline. Once dental lamina restoration is complete, bicuspid tooth development is observed in the newly formed dentary bone [61]. Intriguingly, no ossification occurs on the lingual side of the jaw [61]. Additionally, neither the pre-articular bone nor lingual dentary bone appear to regenerate [61]. Similarly, regenerates of the upper jaw which were missing parts of the nasal bone and the vomer are replaced with cartilage and not bone [61]. The molecular basis for this unusual ossification pattern, relative to the original jaw, is unknown; although, it is plausible that ossification of the outstanding cartilaginous skeletal structures may occur at some later stage. Together this data indicates that although newts retain impressive regenerative abilities as adults, the regeneration of a complete jaw structure occurs only in younger animals.

Last, there are clear limitations in the regenerative and restoration capabilities of different skeletal elements within the jaw. In addition to the mandibular skeleton, the lower jaw of the fish and amphibians is also constituted by the more proximally located branchial and hyoid skeletons. Studies involving the removal of portions of the branchial and hyoid skeletal elements are limited to adult newts and indicate that these structures cannot be regenerated [64,78]. In the axolotl, cartilage formation in response to a tissue puncture through the hyoid apparatus in the tongue is also incomplete [91]. To our knowledge, the regenerative capacities of the branchial and hyoid skeletons have not been considered in the zebrafish or juvenile Urodeles. Thus, whether regeneration of these elements is related to organism age or is species specific remains to be resolved experimentally.

9.2. Teeth Restoration

Tooth development begins around the time of mandible bone formation [61]; however, the dental lamina required for this process is not generated *de novo* during regeneration. Instead, stump dental lamina migrates into the regenerating tissue to repopulate the new jaw [74]. If the stump is devoid of dental lamina, an edentulous jaw is generated [74]. Quarter jaw amputations have revealed that immigration of dental lamina cells into the adult regenerate is directional, only occurring from the posterior stump towards the anterior of the regenerate [74]. This directional mechanism is age specific, as identical amputations in juvenile newt species are associated with migration of dental lamina cell into the regenerate from both the anterior and posterior stump tissue [74]. The mechanisms controlling and restricting this directional migration of dental lamina is unknown. An important note to make is that newt dentation is restored in an age appropriate manner during regeneration, with the adult jaw regenerating bicuspid and the juvenile jaw monocupsid teeth. It is thought that the morphology of the dentation is hormonally regulated [61].

10. Pattern Formation and Positional Identity

Although the regenerated jaws in the zebrafish and adult newt are functionally restored, aesthetically they are not. The general, curved shape of the jaw is reformed in both model organisms, with dentation when appropriate, but the dimensions, precise pattern and proportions of the regenerate are frequently distorted relative to the original [64,89]. Micro computed tomography (μCT) scans of these regenerated jaws demonstrate an irregular and rough pattern, unlike that of the original [59,89]. μCT scans have not been used to assess the regenerate of larval newts; however, based on whole mount staining the regenerate matches the original mandible identically [61]. The reason for this patterning difference between larval and adult newts is unknown, but may be a consequence of metamorphosis-related cellular alterations or differences in mandible structure and tissue composition at these different life stages. Identification of the mechanisms responsible for this age-related patterning defect, and subsequent manipulation thereof, will be of great value in the context of human regenerative medicine.

Hox Gene Re-Expression and Positional Plasticity

There is great value associated with understanding the transcriptional profile of blastema cells, and the regulatory mechanisms thereof, as these cells re-pattern, re-differentiate and integrate. The spatiotemporal differential expression patterns have been documented for a plethora of genes in this context, including those involved in wound healing and development [80,82,92–94]. These studies implicate multiple signaling pathways and transcription factors during pattern formation in the regenerate. Here we will focus on patterning genes, including the *Hox* genes, because they have been well documented to play an important role in both pattern formation and the retention of positional memory in mature adult cells [95,96].

The *Hox* transcription factors are expressed sequentially along the length of the body axis and participate in body patterning and the establishment of positional identity during embryogenesis [97]. The concept of positional identity is well described in this context; however, a paucity of understanding on this topic exists in adult tissues. Available data indicates that mammalian and amphibian cells of connective tissue origin retain positional information throughout adulthood [86,88,95,98,99]. Adult human fibroblasts, being the most-well characterized cell type in this context, stably retain the expression of specific *Hox* genes, even if placed in cell culture, in a pattern similar to that document in the developing embryo [95,98,100]. A variety of epigenetic mechanisms control this phenomenon [96].

As we have described previously, connective tissue cells are essential for the patterning of the missing structures. Moreover, these cells provide positional cues to the surrounding tissues during both embryogenesis and regeneration ([101] and reviewed in [77]). However, little information is known about how connective tissue cells communicate positional formation to each other or other cells types. In humans, dermal fibroblasts communicated positional information to epidermal cells through the secretion of Wnt molecules [100]. Additionally, some data indicates that heparin sulfate proteoglycans communicate positional information between connective tissue cells in the axolotl [86,102]. Thus, more research is required to understand how cells with positional memory use this memory to pattern the regenerating structures.

While connective tissue cells must retain positional memory during homeostasis, these cells must also exhibit the capacity of positional re-programing, such that they can adopt new positional information as they contribute to more distant structures in the regenerate. In support of this hypothesis, positional plasticity has been documented during axolotl limb regeneration. By grafting differently staged blastemas to different locations on the limb it was observed that early blastemas patterned and expressed molecular markers consistent with the new location. Late staged blastemas, however, retained memory of their original location and patterned according to the site of origin. These observations indicate that early stage blastema tissue is positionally plastic, while late staged blastema tissue, that is beginning to undergo differentiation, has a new positional identity already established [103].

Furthermore, plasticity in tissue polarity has also been exhibited during both jaw and limb regeneration. If salamander the autopod (hand) is attached to the salamander flank, and the limb is amputated, the remaining stump tissue has a reverse proximal/distal polarity. The resulting limb regenerate does not have a reversed polarity however, it regenerates with a normal proximal distal axis, indicating that proximal distal polarity in the limb is plastic (Figure 2) [104]. A similar process occurs in the adult newt jaw. When a quarter jaw fragment is flipped, relative to the host site, and transplanted from the left to the right mandible and amputated, the newly regenerated jaw will have the appropriate polarity based on the new host location [74]. Moreover, the dental lamina, which normally migrates into the regenerate in only the posterior to anterior direction, will also migrate according to the new host location (Figure 3). This suggests that the polarity of the dental lamina has also been reprogrammed at the site of amputation [74]. The mechanisms for this reprogramming event are, however, unknown but it can be postulated to involve changes at an epigenetic level.

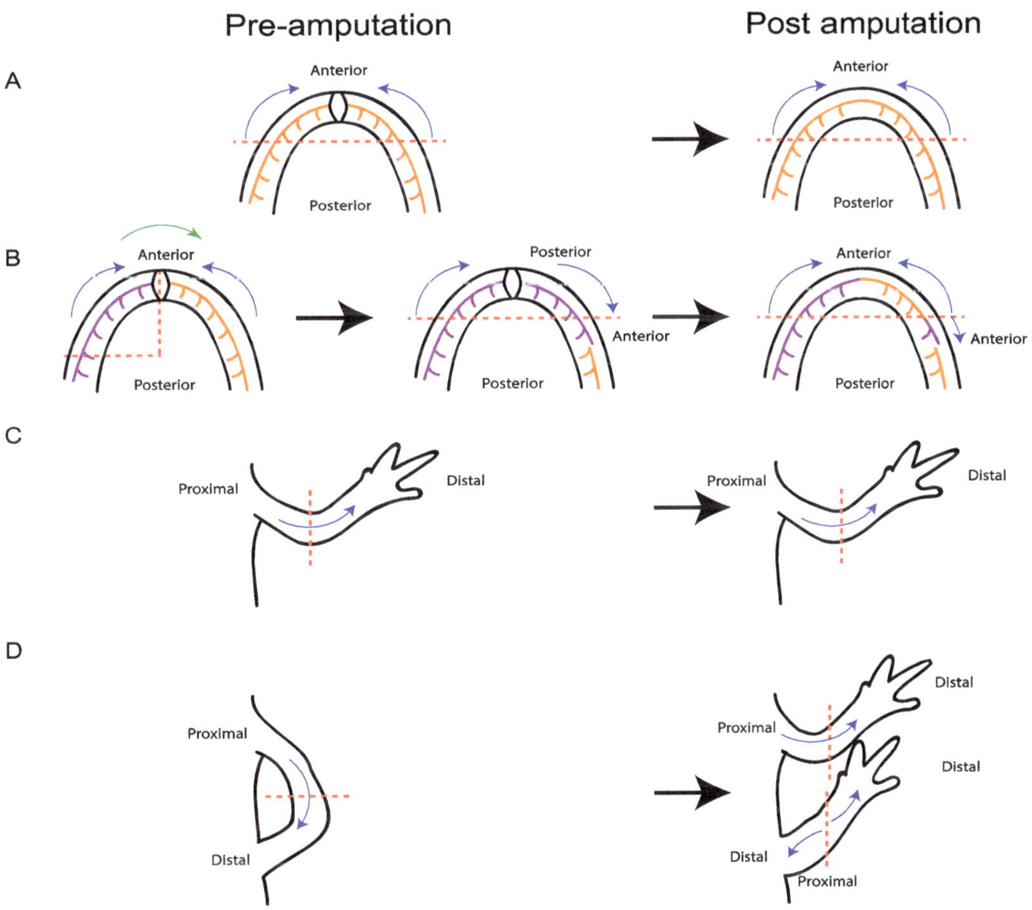

Figure 3. Plasticity of tissue polarity during jaw and limb regeneration is conserved. (**A**) Jaw regeneration normally occurs with a posterior to anterior polarity; (**B**) When a portion of the jaw is reversed along its anterior-posterior axis and amputated, rather than generating structures that are posterior to the amputation plane, the blastema cells reverse their polarity so that they only regenerate structures anterior to the amputation plane. Dental lamina migrates into the adult jaw regenerate in a unidirectional manner, from posterior to anterior; however, the dental lamina migrates into the regenerate in the appropriate direction, despite the grafted tissue being rotated relative to the host site and regenerate; (**C**) During normal limb regeneration, the regenerate retains the proximal/distal polarity of the original limb; (**D**) Limbs with reversed proximal/distal axes can be generated by attaching the autopod to the flank. When the limb is amputated, the part of the limb that remains attached to the flank has the reverse proximal/distal orientation. However, rather than regenerating limb structures proximal to the wound site, the blastema reverses its polarity such that it regenerates tissue distal to the amputation plane. Therefore, there is a conserved mechanism, which prevents regeneration in a proximal direction. Red dashed lines represent the plane of amputation. Blue arrows indicate the direction of tissue polarity. Purple and orange lines represent dental lamina. Green arrow represents tissue grafting. Black arrows represent amputation and regeneration time.

As part of this re-programing event, adult cells would need to assume location-appropriate *Hox* expression profiles; and various studies have demonstrated dramatic changes in transcriptional profile of *Hox* genes during regeneration (Figure 4). In the regenerating axolotl (*Ambystoma mexicanum*) and larval newt (*Notophthalmus viridescens*) limb, Hox genes involved in normal patterning of the limb bud during development—*Hoxa9, Hox13, Hoxb13, Hoxc6, Hoxd8, Hoxd10,* and *Hoxd11*—were re-expressed in the blastema [105–107]. In the zebrafish, several caudal fin specific *Hox* genes, including *dlx4a* and *dlx5a*, were expressed in the blastema during the regeneration of this structure as well [94,108]. In the case of the zebrafish, molecular analysis correlates this re-expression pattern with a loss in H3K27me3 marks near the start site of these genes [94].

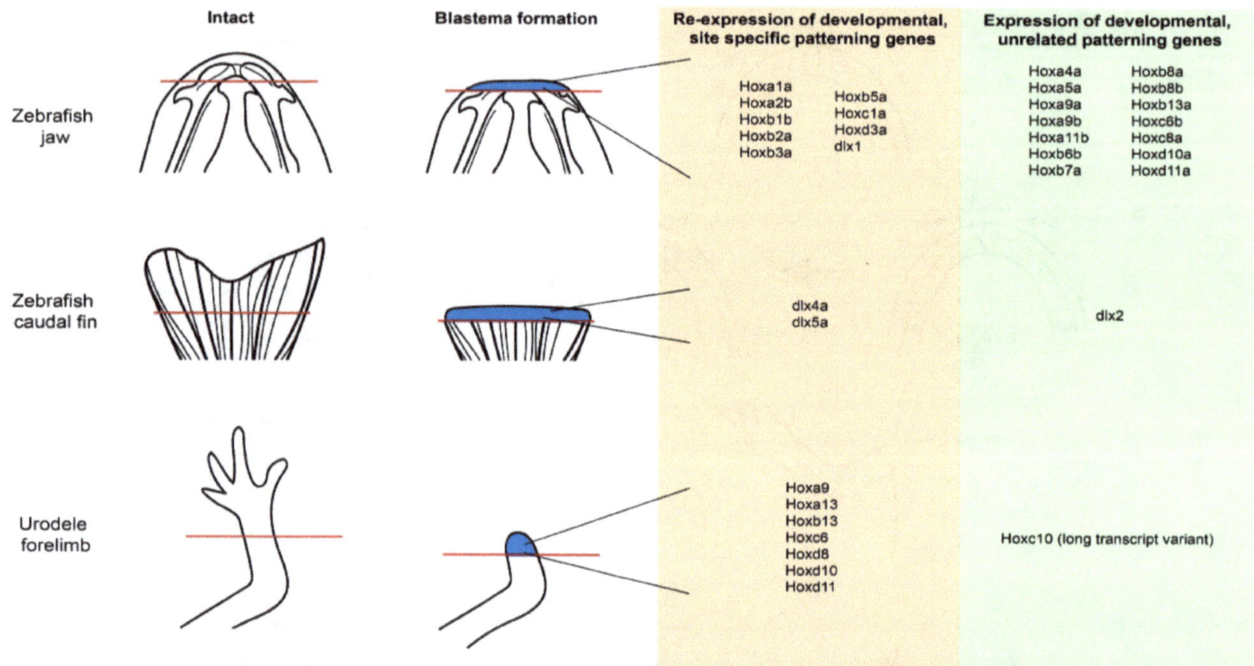

Figure 4. Hox gene re-expression is a characteristic of regeneration shared between species and anatomical locations. Jaw, limb and tail blastema tissue exhibit the re-expression of both developmentally related and unrelated Hox genes. Red line indicates plan of amputation; blue tissue indicates blastema tissue.

Alterations in *Hox* gene expression have also been documented in the regenerating mandible. In response to amputation of the distal third of the lower jaw in zebrafish, 22 of the annotated Hox genes were also found to be differentially activated [62,83]. As early as 2 h post amputation the expression of *Hoxb2a, Hoxb5a, Hoxa9a* and *Hoxb13a* was elevated; with the remaining genes upregulated by day 5. This expression pattern is somewhat surprising considering that the mandibular arch is *Hox* negative during early embryogenesis. However, it was also observed that *dlx1*, a homeobox gene specifically expressed in the mandibular arch of the CNC, expression is increased in the fish jaw blastema. RNA in situ hybridization indicates that *Hoxa2b* was expressed in the blastema mesenchyme, localized most strongly in the chondrogenic zone [62]. Additionally, 5′ *Hox* genes (including *Hoxa4a, Hoxa5a, Hoxa9a, Hoxa9b, Hoxb13a, Hoxa11b* and *Hoxd11a*), associated with patterning of posterior structures, were also expressed [62]. Fish hematopoietic progenitors express these 5′ *Hox* genes; thus, invading blood cells may in part explain the elevated expression of these genes within the blastema. However, RNA in situ hybridization indicates that *Hox11* was broadly expressed in the blastema mesenchyme, concentrated near the wound epithelium as well as adjacent the stump muscle [62]. This activation of positionally-unrelated *Hox* genes has been documented during limb and tail regeneration as well [94,106] and may be a consequence of the positional reprogramming that is required for re-patterning to occur.

The capacity of cells to assume new positional information is largely limited to a regeneration permissive environment. However, in the context of stem cell grafts, *Hox*-negative cells can assume new identities while *Hox*-positive populations cannot (Figure 5). In the developing murine limb bud, *Hoxa11* is expressed in the mesenchyme, and this expression is retained in the adult murine tibia, specifically in periosteum and osteocytes, even in response to injury and subsequent repair. This is unlike the mandible, where the skeleton retains a *Hox11a*-negative status after development, even in response to injury. When *Hox11a* positive tibia derived periosteum was grafted into the *Hox11a*-negative mandibular environment, *Hox11a* expression was retained in the grafted population. These cells failed to differentiate into osteoblasts and thus did not integrate with the host tissue. Instead a cartilaginous callus was generated as the junction site [109]. The reciprocal grafting experiment, however, gave a very different outcome. *Hox11a*-negative mandible derived periosteum grafted into the *Hox*-positive tibia resulted in appropriate intramembranous bone formation, with the grafted cells expressing *Hoxa11* and integrating with the surrounding host tissue seamlessly [109]. These observations indicate that the Hox11a-negative (mandibular) population is more positionally plastic than the *Hox11a* positive (tibia) population, and that this plasticity promotes the integration of the transplantation into the host site. However more studies are required to test this hypothesis. For example, a complete *Hox* expression analysis should be performed to determine whether the up-regulation of other *Hox* genes occurs in the injured mouse mandible, in a similar manner as the zebrafish. It would also be very interesting to observe changes in the epigenetic landscape of the mouse mandibular and tibia transplants before and after transplantation to determine whether the tibia transplants are resistant to epigenetic alterations.

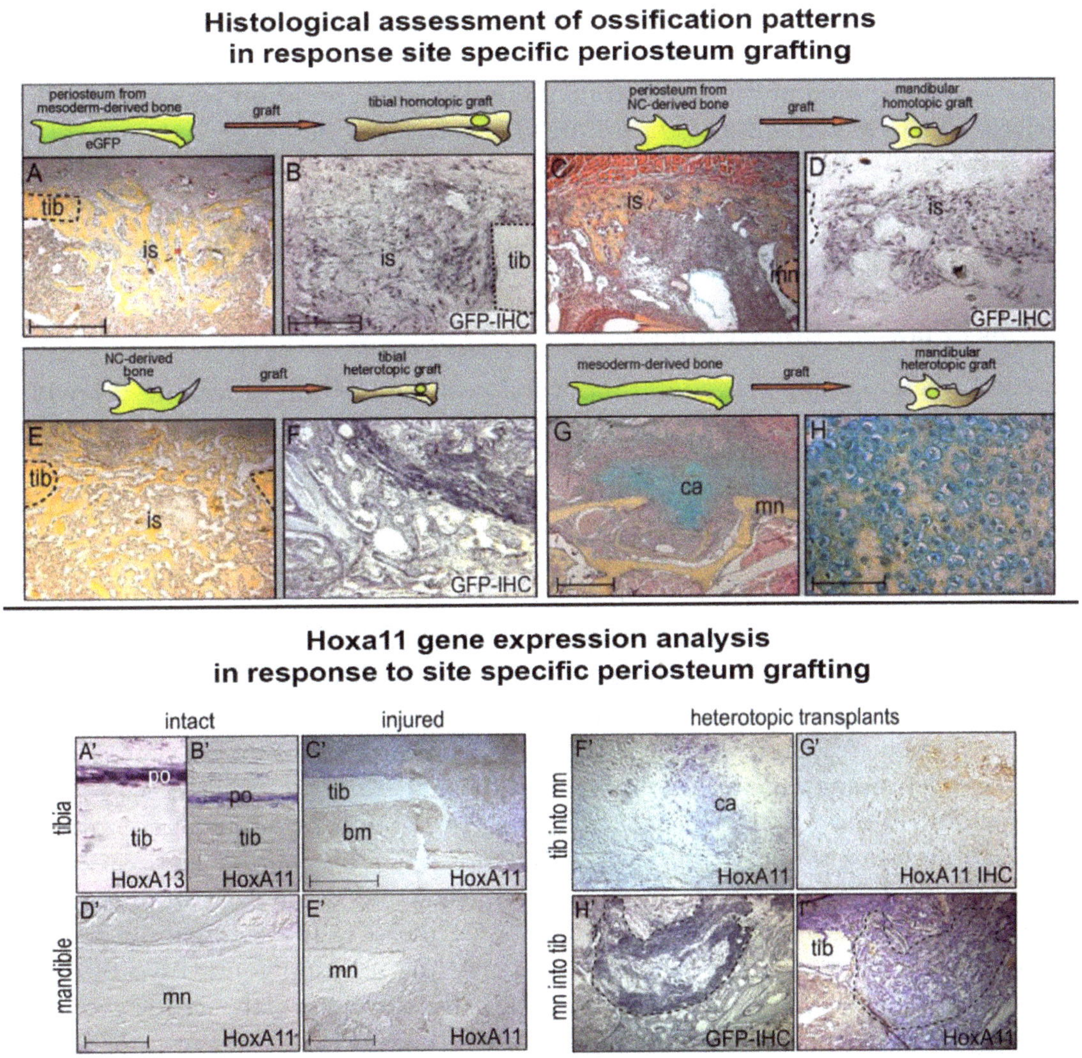

Figure 5. The capacity of bone derived mesenchymal cells to participate in bone restoration is dependent on both the donor and recipient site. Top panel: Robust tibia bone repair, whereby pentachrome staining

indicates intramembranous ossification (**A**), is facilitated directly by the homographic translation, survival and differentiation of GFP-positive tibial periosteum at the site of injury (**B**, GFP immunohistochemistry). A similar response is documented in mandibular sites (**C**) transplanted with GFP-positive mandibular periosteum (**D**). Although intramembranous bone is generated in tibial sites (**E**) in response to engraftment, survival and differentiation of GFP positive mandibular derived periosteum cells (**F**); tibial periosteum transplanted into the mandible exhibits failed integration due to inappropriate endochondral ossification (**G**) and cartilage condensation (**H**, high magnification). ca, cartilage; is, injury site; mn, mandible; tib, tibia. Scale bar: 200 μm in A, C, E; 100 μm in B, D, F; 400 μm in G; 50 μm in H. Lower panel: Periosteum derived from the adult tibia expresses *Hoxa13* (**A'**) and *Hoxa11* (**B'**) under homeostatic conditions, and *Hoxa11* in response to injury (**C'**). *Hoxa11* expression is absent in mandibular periosteum under both normal and injury conditions (**D'**,**E'** respectively). Tibia periosteum retains *Hoxa11* expression when transplanted into the Hox-negative mandibular environment (**F'**,**G'**), while GFP-positive mandibular periosteum (**H'**, GFP expression encompassed by dashed lines) grafted into the tibia exhibits *Hoxa11* expression (I, mandibular cells encompassed by dashed lines) bm, bone marrow; ca, cartilage; mn, mandible; po, periosteum; tib, tibia. Scale bar: 50 μm in A, B, D, F, G; 100 μm in E; 200 μm in C, H, I. (Images republished with permission from Leucht et al. 2008).

There are, however, limitations to this reprogramming response; which apparently prevents tissues from assuming positional identities of distant, unrelated body locations. For example, in the axolotl, when head-derived full thickness skin or dermis alone was grafted into the limb and the limb was then amputated at the site of transplantation, regeneration was inhibited or impeded respectively [66]. Head derived cells did contribute to the blastema; however, in the case of regeneration failure the structure never developed beyond the early bud stage [66].

Altogether, this data indicates that achieving plasticity of positional memory plays an important role in the regeneration of the jaw. It is likely that future regenerative therapies will need to recapitulate this process to promote endogenous regeneration in the jaw.

11. Mechanisms of Jaw Fracture Healing

As opposed to endogenous regeneration of the jaw, the healing of fractured jawbones occurs poorly in both mammalian and regenerative model organisms (Table 1). Multiple studies in rodent and avian models indicate that skull and jaw fractures heal using secondary ossification where the fractured ends of the bones become connected through a fibrous callus [110–112]. Cartilage and bone formation at the fractured bone ends is documented in the chick, generated by periosteal cells as well as bone derived osteoblasts or osteocyte [112]. In the rodent, cartilage formation is absent but bone formation is achieved by proliferating parietal bone-derived osteoblasts that invade the callus; however, this invasion is also restricted to sites adjacent the damaged bone ends [110,111]. This limited invasion of skeleton-derived cells is thought be due to the fibrotic nature of callus [111]. Interestingly, increased inflammation correlates to increased bone formation during fracture repair in the rodent [111]. Since the callus fails to align the fractured ends of the bones, the integration of the new and old tissue is poor and prevents the restoration of the original pattern [110–112].

While regenerative models do not heal bone fractures perfectly, their regenerative response is more robust than mammalian or avian species. In *Ambystoma maculatum*, periosteal cells respond to the initial injury, covering the fractured ends of the bone and ultimately joining the dentary and prearticular sides of the fracture with a bony bridge. A cartilage callus is generated separately to this bridge, and appears to be derived by metaplasia of the surrounding connective tissue rather than being derived from the Meckle's cartilage or bone directly. Over time, the callus grows to unite the two fractured portions of the jawbone and ossifies. Although this healing response is more robust relative to that of mammals and birds, this structure is not well integrated with the original jaw. The bony barrier that divides the callus cartilage and Meckle's cartilage is retained and jaw misalignment is frequently documented [113]. Similarly, acellular and cellular fish skeletons responds similarly to injury; and lower jaw fractions are resolved by the formation of a cartilaginous callus with limited ossification [114]. Interestingly, the efficiency of callus formation is species dependent and strongly affected by diet, water quality and temperature [114].

12. Tissue Integration

Tissue integration is an essential but under-appreciated topic in context of regenerative medicine. Bone as well as other jaw tissues, including muscle and nerves, need to integrate seamlessly with one another during regeneration or after a tissue engraftment, to restore functionality of the resulting structure. For example, the regeneration of missing portions of the mandible that effectively restores the shape of the jaw but fails to reconnect appropriately with the stump tissue, would impede, if not hinder, its use in mastication and speech.

Tissue integration and regeneration are often considered synonymous events; however, the two process can be uncoupled (as reviewed in [115]). This observation suggests that distinct molecular processes must underlay each phenomenon individually. Additional support for this idea comes from situations where regenerative responses at different locations, in the same animal, exhibit differential capacities for integration. For example, limb regeneration in the Urodele naturally exhibits full integration of the regenerate with the stump tissue (as reviewed by [115]), while the adult jaw does not. The initial cartilaginous structure regenerated within the post-metamorphic newt jaw does become continuous with the Meckel's cartilage; but no pre-articular bone nor lingual dentary bone are generated [61,64], thus preventing appropriate connections between the stump pre-articular and lingual dentary bones to the regenerate. Interestingly, pre-metamorphic newts not only regenerate all of the missing jaw structure, but they also appear to be integrated perfectly with the stump structures [61]. Thus, metamorphosis and/or aging induces changes in the cells that inhibits integration. Understanding these changes will help us understand how we can promote better integration of new jaw structures in mammals.

Jaw fracture repairs in the newt exhibits even worse integration, relative to jaw regeneration, with the misaligned bony union at the site of injury being separated by a bony barrier from the jaw bone [113]. Integration failure in this context appears to be conserved, with mammalian fractures also exhibiting callus formation that does not restore appropriate pattern or tissue connections [110–112]. Despite the importance of integration to regeneration, the molecular pathways and mechanisms for this phenomenon still need to be elucidated.

13. On the Development of New Regenerative Therapies: Conserved Mechanisms of Endogenous Regeneration

13.1. Positional Plasticity

Ideally, the repair of damaged or missing patient jaw tissue would occur through the induction of an endogenous regenerative response. Endogenous regeneration alleviates the need to harvest tissue from the patient or a donor, and avoids additional issues such as the rejection of the tissue transplant. Furthermore, in regenerative models, endogenous regenerative responses result in the formation of a structure that is similar in pattern to the original structure, and is better integrated with the original tissues including the surrounding muscles, nerves, and vasculature. Here we have reviewed how jaw regeneration occurs in multiple regenerative species, and have compared these mechanisms with amphibian limb regeneration to help identify unified regenerative mechanisms.

One of the most important unifying properties of regenerating limbs and jaws appears to be the plasticity of positional information. Evidence indicates that plasticity not only plays an important role in establishing the pattern of the missing structures, but also in the integration of the new tissue with the existing tissue. Positional plasticity is achieved naturally in a regenerating environment, but little is known about how it is established. In regenerating limbs, there is evidence that nerve-derived signals help maintain positional plasticity in blastema cells [80,93,103], and that cells that are differentiated or are differentiating are not positionally plastic [103,116]. Both the jaw and limb blastemas appear to re-express patterning genes, including patterning genes that are not expressed in these tissues during embryogenesis, although more experimentation will be required to understand the full extent of these expression patterns in multiple model systems. This reactivation of patterning genes is likely due, in part, to large scale opening up of the chromatin landscape in the blastemal cells. Although this has not been looked at in detail in the jaw, increased presence of euchromatin has been well-established in the limb regenerate [117,118]. Additionally, multiple epigenetic modifications have been observed in different species and regenerating structures, and appear to play a role in regenerative ability.

How can positionally plastic human cells be generated? In tissue culture, tissue plasticity can be induced in adult mammalian fibroblasts through the transfection of specific combinations of pluripotent transcription factors, which converts the cells into induced Pluripotent Stem Cells (iPSCs) [119]. Interestingly, however, Hox genes are differentially expressed in iPSCs that have been generated from different somatic sources, indicating that these cells retain some positional memory [65,67]. One possibility is to generate iPSCs from a source of cells that are known to be positionally plastic. For example, in mice, transplants of mandibular tissue adopt the new Hox code of the host site, indicating that these cells are inherently plastic. This is exciting, because it poses the jaw as a structure that could be uniquely well suited for the generation of positionally plastic jaw progenitor cells in vivo.

To date, multiple cell types have been converted to iPSCs in vivo [120–126]. In vivo reprograming of mesenchymal cells into iPSCs that differentiate into epithelial tissue has been used to heal skin ulcers in mice [126]. The use of this technology has also been applied with some success in regenerating missing neurons in damaged adult brains, although the efficacy of reprogramming and the survival of the differentiated neurons depends largely on the in vivo environment and type of injury [122]. However, concerns of the use of iPSCs and their tumorigenic potential need to be resolved before this technology can be safely used for in vivo regeneration in humans. Additionally, it should be noted that during endogenous regeneration, cells are reprogramed to a progenitor-like state as opposed to a pluripotent embryonic-like state, yet are able to establish positional plasticity. Thus, there appears to be unique mechanisms in the erasure of tissue identity versus positional identity to make blastema cells plastic. Further research focused on understanding how blastema cells attain positional plasticity while remaining restricted in their potential lineages will provide valuable insight into the development of endogenous regeneration technologies.

13.2. Imperfect Fracture Repair

One surprising observation is that both regenerative models and poorly regenerating species, including mammals, do not heal jaw fractures well. Although regenerative species heal fractures better than humans, the integration of the fractured ends of the jaw is not perfect. In these species it appears that larger injuries that require an endogenous regenerative response do a better job of seamlessly connecting the new tissue with the existing tissue. This could be due, in part, due to the cells that help heal jaw fractures versus those that contribute to a regenerative response. The cells that contribute to jaw fracture repair appear to be derived mostly from the periosteum and bones. Jaw regeneration however recruits multiple cell types, including different connective tissues, muscle progenitors, cranial neural crest derived cells, and dental pulp cells. It is possible that a more diverse contribution is required for improved integration.

Another potentially important aspect is that *de novo* pattern formation occurs during endogenous regenerative responses, but is unlikely to occur during jaw fracture repair. No blastema forms during fracture repair, and it seems that this response is more attune to a compensatory regenerative response as opposed to epimorphic regeneration. However, a more detailed analysis of *Hox* gene expression patterns needs to be performed during jaw fracture healing in different species to fully understand how pattern information might be modulated during fracture repair. Regardless, the signaling events that occur during pattern formation are unlikely to be present in fractures, and this could also explain why fractures integrate poorly.

13.3. Age-Related Changes in Regenerative Capacity

Another unifying property associated with better regenerative outcomes is young age. This has been well documented with human patients that have received reconstructive jaw surgeries, where the new tissue is well integrated, and sometimes appears to stimulate an endogenous regenerative response. It is also observed in vertebrate regenerative models such as the newt, where juveniles replace and integrate the missing jaw tissue perfectly, while adult newts only replace some of the missing jaw structures. It has been previously hypothesized that the presence of a sufficient supply of bone precursor cells is a major contributor to the improved outcomes in younger patients. However, as we have learned from organisms that regenerate endogenously, the establishment of cellular plasticity as well as the recruitment of a more diverse cell population during a regenerative response may also be contributing factors.

13.4. Transplantations

While being able to endogenously regenerate damaged or missing jaw tissue would be ideal, there is still a lot we need to learn about the basic biology underlying these mechanisms before we can apply this to human medicine. Bone transplantation methodologies have been well developed over the years, and have a relatively high success rate. Due to the large number of bone grafting procedures conducted (estimated to be more than 500,000 in America annually) (AAOS, 2010), there is sufficient evidence to support idea that an effective bone graft should not only fill in the deficit but also promote new bone formation on its surface (osteoconduction) and within itself (osteogensis); stimulate the adjacent, host tissue stem cell population to generate new bone cells (osteoinduction), and integrate with the host bone without any intervening fibrotic layer [127,128]. Of autologous, allogenic and synthetic bone grafts, only the former fulfills all these requirements and is therefore considered the "gold standard", in addition to being histocompatible (as reviewed in [129]).

One feature that appears to play a role in the efficacy of an autologous transplantation is the location from which the grafted tissue was harvested. Evidence indicates that bone harvested from the head (cavarial and mandible) exhibits better integration and stimulates more bone growth when transplanted into the jaw compared to bones harvested from more distant regions in the body (iliac or tibia). It is possible that this is due to the increased positional plasticity of head bone cells, as we have described previously, compared to bones from other regions. It may also be related to how these bones naturally form during embryogenesis. The mandible and cavarial bones develop via intramembranous ossification, while the iliac and long bones develop via endochondrial ossification. While callus formation appears to be a conserved mechanism of bone repair regardless of location, physiological differences in these bones, and which cells contribute to bone repair may play a role in how compatible they will be as a transplant for jaw repair.

Along with tissue viability, the healing and integration of the transplanted bone with the existing bone is potentially the greatest challenge to a successful outcome. While increased viability will depend on the health of the transplantation tissue and the host site, it is also likely that integration will play a role because the vasculature and neural connections in the host location will need to integrate with the engrafted tissue for its survival. One potential way to facilitate this process is by combining the induction of an endogenous regenerative response in the host location by inducing pluripotency in vivo along with an autologous transplant from the head skeleton. In theory, this would deconstruct the surrounding tissues and make the cells more plastic, and thus more likely to integrate with the bone transplant. Testing this method in regenerative and non-regenerative model organisms will help us determine whether this is a feasible method for jaw-related regenerative therapies.

14. Conclusions

Unlike humans, multiple vertebrate organisms, including the zebrafish, newt, and axolotl, naturally exhibit profound capabilities in terms of regenerating injured or missing jaw tissue. Utilizing these model systems, we can begin to understand as well as identify conserved mechanisms underlying regeneration, including, but not limited to, the mechanisms of dedifferentiation, positional plasticity, *de novo* pattern formation, and tissue integration. Translating this knowledge into the mammalian system will allow us to engineer better regenerative therapies for humans suffering from a variety of jaw aliments, and in some cases it already has. Future research is additionally required to thoroughly compare and contrast the mechanisms and outcomes of jaw injury and transplantation in regenerative and non-regenerative models so to determine and understand the pathways that can potentially be deployed to facilitate a more robust regenerative response in non-regenerative species.

References

1. Cawood, J.I.; Howell, R.A. A classification of the edentulous jaws. *Int. J. Oral Maxillofac. Surg.* **1988**, *17*, 232–236. [CrossRef]
2. McCarthy, J.G. The role of distraction osteogenesis in the reconstruction of the mandible in unilateral craniofacial microsomia. *Clin. Plast. Surg.* **1994**, *21*, 625–631. [PubMed]
3. Shwyrkow, M.B.; Shamsudinov, A.K. Methods of simultaneous treatment of the mandible defects and the adjacent soft tissues. *Acta Chir. Plast.* **1989**, *31*, 226–235. [PubMed]
4. Komisar, A. *Mandibular Reconstruction*; Thieme: Stuttgart, Germany, 1997; ISBN 313103811X.
5. Glenske, K.; Donkiewicz, P.; Kowitsch, A.; Milosevic-Oljaca, N.; Rider, P.; Rofall, S.; Franke, J.; Jung, O.; Smeets, R.; Schnettler, R.; Wenisch S, S.; Barbeck, M. Applications of Metals for Bone Regeneration. *Int. J. Mol. Sci.* **2018**, *19*, 826. [CrossRef] [PubMed]
6. Gong, T.; Xie, J.; Liao, J.; Lin, S.; Lin, Y. Nanomaterials and bone regeneration. *Bone Res.* **2015**, *3*, 15029. [CrossRef] [PubMed]
7. Bae, S.E.; Choi, J.; Joung, Y.K.; Park, K.; Han, D.K. Controlled release of bone morphogenetic protein (BMP)-2 from nanocomplex incorporated on hydroxyapatite-formed titanium surface. *J. Control. Release* **2012**, *160*, 676–684. [CrossRef] [PubMed]
8. Wang, J.; Guo, J.; Liu, J.; Wei, L.; Wu, G. BMP-functionalised coatings to promote osteogenesis for orthopaedic implants. *Int. J. Mol. Sci.* **2014**, *15*, 10150–10168. [CrossRef] [PubMed]
9. Fernandez-Yague, M.A.; Abbah, S.A.; McNamara, L.; Zeugolis, D.I.; Pandit, A.; Biggs, M.J. Biomimetic approaches in bone tissue engineering: Integrating biological and physicomechanical strategies. *Adv. Drug Deliv. Rev.* **2015**, *84*, 1–29. [CrossRef] [PubMed]
10. Faruq, O.; Kim, B.; Padalhin, A.R.; Lee, G.H.; Lee, B.-T. A hybrid composite system of biphasic calcium phosphate granules loaded with hyaluronic acid-gelatin hydrogel for bone regeneration. *J. Biomater. Appl.* **2017**, *32*, 433–445. [CrossRef] [PubMed]
11. Florencio-Silva, R.; Sasso, G.R.D.S.; Sasso-Cerri, E.; Simões, M.J.; Cerri, P.S. Biology of Bone Tissue: Structure, Function, and Factors That Influence Bone Cells. *Biomed. Res. Int.* **2015**, *2015*, 421746. [CrossRef] [PubMed]
12. Diomede, F.; Gugliandolo, A.; Scionti, D.; Merciaro, I.; Cavalcanti, M.; Mazzon, E.; Trubiani, O. Biotherapeutic Effect of Gingival Stem Cells Conditioned Medium in Bone Tissue Restoration. *Int. J. Mol. Sci.* **2018**, *19*, 329. [CrossRef] [PubMed]
13. Santos, M.; Unger, R.; Sousa, R.; Reis, R. Crosstalk between osteoblasts and endothelial cells co-cultured on a polycaprolactone–starch scaffold and the in vitro development of vascularization. *Biomaterials* **2009**, *30*, 4407–4415. [CrossRef] [PubMed]
14. Hidalgo, D.A. Fibula free flap mandible reconstruction. *Microsurgery* **1994**, *15*, 238–244. [CrossRef] [PubMed]
15. Sanger, J.R.; Matloub, H.S.; Yousif, N.J. Sequential connection of flaps: A logical approach to customized mandibular reconstruction. *Am. J. Surg.* **1990**, *160*, 402–404. [CrossRef]

16. Tang, Y.B.; Hahn, L.J. Major mandibular reconstruction with vascularized bone graft. *J. Formos. Med. Assoc.* **1990**, *89*, 34–40. [PubMed]
17. Nkenke, E.; Neukam, F.W. Autogenous bone harvesting and grafting in advanced jaw resorption: Morbidity, resorption and implant survival. *Eur. J. Oral Implantol.* **2014**, *7*, S203–S217. [PubMed]
18. Sakkas, A.; Wilde, F.; Heufelder, M.; Winter, K.; Schramm, A. Autogenous bone grafts in oral implantology—Is it still a "gold standard?" A consecutive review of 279 patients with 456 clinical procedures. *Int. J. Implant Dent.* **2017**, *2*, 23. [CrossRef] [PubMed]
19. Kang, Y.H.; Kim, H.M.; Byun, J.H.; Kim, U.K.; Sung, I.Y.; Cho, Y.C.; Park, B.W. Stability of simultaneously placed dental implants with autologous bone grafts harvested from the iliac crest or intraoral jaw bone. *BMC Oral Health* **2015**, *15*, 172. [CrossRef] [PubMed]
20. Mertens, C.; Decker, C.; Seeberger, R.; Hoffman, J.; Sander, A.; Freier, K. Early bone resorption after vertical bone augmentation—A comparison of calvarial and iliac grafts. *Clin. Oral Implants Res.* **2012**, *24*, 820–825. [CrossRef] [PubMed]
21. Schlegel, K.A.; Schultze-Mosgau, S.; Wiltfang, J.; Neikam, F.W.; Rupprecht, S.; Thorwarth, M. Changes of mineralization of free autogenous bone grafts used for sinus floor elevation. *Clin. Oral Implants Res.* **2006**, *17*, 673–678. [CrossRef] [PubMed]
22. Akintoye, S.O.; Lam, T.; Shi, S.; Brahim, J.; Collins, M.T.; Robey, P.G. Skeletal site-specific characterization of orofacial and iliac crest human bone marrow stromal cells in same individuals. *Bone* **2006**, *38*, 758–768. [CrossRef] [PubMed]
23. Dong, W.; Ge, J.; Zhang, P.; Fu, Y.; Zhang, Z.; Cheng, J.; Jiang, H. Phenotypic characterization of craniofacial bone marrow stromal cells: Unique properties of enhanced osteogenesis, cell recruitment, autophagy, and apoptosis resistance. *Cell Tissue Res.* **2014**, *358*, 165–175. [CrossRef] [PubMed]
24. Tonelli, P.; Duvina, M.; Barbato, L.; Biondi, E.; Nuti, N.; Brancato, L.; Delle Rose, G. Bone regeneration in dentistry. *Clin. Cases Miner. Bone Metab.* **2011**, *8*, 24–28. [PubMed]
25. Khojasteh, A.; Kheiri, L.; Motamedian, S.; Khoshkam, V. Guided bone regeneration for the reconstruction of alveolar bone defects. *Ann. Maxillofac. Surg.* **2017**, *7*, 263. [CrossRef] [PubMed]
26. Castellon, L.; Jerez, D.; Mayorga, J.; Fuenzalida, C. Remodeling of Costochondral Graft After Mandibular Reconstruction. *J. Oral Maxillofac. Surg.* **2017**, *75*, 226.e1–226.e7. [CrossRef] [PubMed]
27. Almaiman, M.; Al-Bargi, H.; Manson, P. Complication of Anterior Iliac Bone Graft Harvesting in 372 Adult Patients from May 2006 to May 2011 and a Literature Review. *Cranial Maxillofac. Trauma Reconstruct.* **2013**, *6*, 257–266. [CrossRef] [PubMed]
28. Dosoglu, M. Enterocutaneous Fistula: A Complication of Posterior Iliac Bone Graft Harvesting not Previously Described. *Acta Neurochir.* **1998**, *140*, 1089–1092. [CrossRef] [PubMed]
29. Younger, E.; Chapman, M. Morbidity at bone graft donor sites. *J. Orthop. Trauma* **1989**, *3*, 192–195. [CrossRef] [PubMed]
30. Kinoshita, Y. Regenerative Medicine for Jawbone. *JMAJ* **2004**, *47*, 294–297.
31. Manimaran, K.; Sharma, R.; Sankaranarayanan, S.; Perumal, S.M. Regeneration of mandibular ameloblastema defect with the help of autologous dental pulp stem cells and buccal pad of fat stromal vascular fraction. *Ann. Maxillofac. Surg.* **2016**, *6*, 97–100. [PubMed]
32. Knight, R.D.; Schilling, T.F. Cranial neural crest and development of the head skeleton. *Adv. Exp. Med. Biol.* **2006**, *589*, 120–133. [PubMed]
33. Depew, M.J.; Lufkin, T.; Rubenstein, J.L.R. Specification of jaw subdivisions by *Dlx* genes. *Science* **2002**, *298*, 381–385. [CrossRef] [PubMed]
34. Jeong, J.; Li, X.; McEvilly, R.J.; Rosenfeld, M.G.; Lufkin, T.; Rubenstein, J.L. *Dlx* genes pattern mammalian jaw primordium by regulating both lower jaw-specific and upper jaw-specific genetic programs. *Development* **2008**, *135*, 2905–2916. [CrossRef] [PubMed]
35. Minoux, M.; Rijli, F.M. Molecular mechanisms of cranial neural crest cell migration and patterning in craniofacial development. *Development* **2010**, *137*, 2605–2621. [CrossRef] [PubMed]
36. Rijli, F.M.; Mark, M.; Lakkaraju, S.; Dierich, A.; Dolle, P.; Chambron, P. A Homeotic Transformation Is Generated in the Rostra1 Branchial Region of the Head by Disruption of Hoxa-2, Which Acts as a Selector Gene. *Cell* **1993**, *75*, 1333–1349. [CrossRef]
37. Gendron-Maguire, M.; Mallo, M.; Zhang, M.; Gridley, T. Hoxa-2 mutant mice exhibit homeotic transformation of skeletal elements derived from cranial neural crest. *Cell* **1993**, *75*, 1317–1331. [CrossRef]

38. Pasqualetti, M.; Ori, M.; Nardi, I.; Rijli, F.M. Ectopic Hoxa2 induction after neural crest migration results in homeosis of jaw elements in Xenopus. *Development* **2000**, *127*, 5367–5378. [PubMed]
39. Hunter, M.P.; Prince, V.E. Zebrafish Hox Paralogue Group 2 Genes Function Redundantly as Selector Genes to Pattern the Second Pharyngeal Arch. *Dev. Biol.* **2002**, *247*, 367–389. [CrossRef] [PubMed]
40. Noden, D.M. The role of the neural crest in patterning of avian cranial skeletal, connective, and muscle tissues. *Dev. Biol.* **1983**, *96*, 144–165. [CrossRef]
41. Schilling, T.F.; Prince, V.; Ingham, P.W. Plasticity in Zebrafish hox Expression in the Hindbrain and Cranial Neural Crest. *Dev. Biol.* **2001**, *231*, 201–216. [CrossRef] [PubMed]
42. Trainor, P.A.; Krumlauf, R. Patterning the cranial neural crest: Hindbrain segmentation and Hox gene plasticity. *Nat. Rev. Neurosci.* **2000**, *1*, 116–124. [CrossRef] [PubMed]
43. Schneider, R.A.; Helms, J.A. The cellular and molecular origins of beak morphology. *Science* **2003**, *299*, 565–568. [CrossRef] [PubMed]
44. Couly, G.; Creuzet, S.; Bennaceur, S.; Vincent, C.; le Douarin, N.M. Interactions between Hox-negative cephalic neural crest cells and the foregut endoderm in patterning the facial skeleton in the vertebrate head. *Development* **2002**, *129*, 1061–1073. [PubMed]
45. David, N.B.; Saint-Etienne, L.; Tsang, M.; Schilling, T.F.; Rosa, F.M. Requirement for endoderm and FGF3 in ventral head skeleton formation. *Development* **2002**, *129*, 4457–4468. [PubMed]
46. Creuzet, S.; Couly, G.; Vincent, C.; le Douarin, N.M. Negative effect of Hox gene expression on the development of the neural crest-derived facial skeleton. *Development* **2002**, *129*, 4301–4313. [PubMed]
47. Abzhanov, A.; Tzahor, E.; Lassar, A.B.; Tabin, C.J. Dissimilar regulation of cell differentiation in mesencephalic (cranial) and sacral (trunk) neural crest cells in vitro. *Development* **2003**, *130*, 4567–4579. [CrossRef] [PubMed]
48. McGonnell, I.M.; Graham, A. Trunk Neural Crest Has Skeletogenic Potential. *Curr. Biol.* **2002**, *12*, 767–771. [CrossRef]
49. Opperman, L.A. Cranial sutures as intramembranous bone growth sites. *Dev. Dyn.* **2000**, *219*, 472–485. [CrossRef]
50. Miller, C.T.; Schilling, T.F.; Lee, K.; Parker, J.; Kimmel, C.B. Sucker encodes a zebrafish Endothelin-1 required for ventral pharyngeal arch development. *Development* **2000**, *127*, 3815–3828. [PubMed]
51. Kimmel, C.B. Endothelin 1-mediated regulation of pharyngeal bone development in zebrafish. *Development* **2003**, *130*, 1339–1351. [CrossRef] [PubMed]
52. Miller, C.T. Two endothelin 1 effectors, hand2 and bapx1, pattern ventral pharyngeal cartilage and the jaw joint. *Development* **2003**, *130*, 1353–1365. [CrossRef] [PubMed]
53. Clouthier, D.E.; Hosoda, K.; Richardson, J.A.; Williams, S.C.; Yanagisawa, H.; Kuwaki, T.; Kumada, M.; Hammer, R.E.; Yanagisawa, M. Cranial and cardiac neural crest defects in endothelin-A receptor-deficient mice. *Development* **1998**, *125*, 813–824. [PubMed]
54. Kurihara, Y.; Kurihara, H.; Suzuki, H.; Kodama, T.; Maemura, K.; Nagai, R.; Oda, H.; Kuwaki, T.; Cao, W.H.; Kamada, N.; et al. Elevated blood pressure and craniofaclal abnormalities in mice deficient in endothelin-1. *Nature* **1994**, *368*, 703–710. [CrossRef] [PubMed]
55. Ferguson, C.A.; Tucker, A.S.; Sharpe, P.T. Temporospatial cell interactions regulating mandibular and maxillary arch patterning. *Development* **2000**, *127*, 403–412. [PubMed]
56. Gemberling, M.; Bailey, T.J.; Hyde, D.R.; Poss, K.D. The zebrafish as a model for complex tissue regeneration. *Trends Genet.* **2013**, *29*, 611–620. [CrossRef] [PubMed]
57. Song, F.; Li, B.; Stocum, D.L. Amphibians as research models for regenerative medicine. *Organogenesis* **2010**, *6*, 1–10. [CrossRef]
58. Tazaki, A.; Tanaka, E.M.; Fei, J.-F. Developmental Biology. *Dev. Biol.* **2017**, *432*, 63–71. [CrossRef] [PubMed]
59. Kurosaka, H.; Takano-Yamamoto, T.; Yamashiro, T.; Agata, K. Comparison of molecular and cellular events during lower jaw regeneration of newt (*Cynops pyrrhogaster*) and West African clawed frog (*Xenopus tropicalis*). *Dev. Dyn.* **2007**, *237*, 354–365. [CrossRef] [PubMed]
60. Brazaitis, P. Maxillary Regeneration in a Marsh Crocodile, *Crocodylus palustris*. *J. Herpetol.* **1981**, *15*, 360. [CrossRef]
61. Ghosh, S.; Thorogood, P.; Ferretti, P. Regenerative capability of upper and lower jaws in the newt. *Int. J. Dev. Biol.* **1994**, *38*, 479–490. [PubMed]
62. Wang, X.; He, H.; Tang, W.; Zhang, X.A.; Hua, X.; Yan, J. Two Origins of Blastemal Progenitors Define Blastemal Regeneration of Zebrafish Lower Jaw. *PLoS ONE* **2012**, *7*, e45380. [CrossRef] [PubMed]

63. Finch, R.A. The influence of the nerve on lower jaw regeneration in the adult newt, *Triturus viridescens*. *J. Morphol.* **1969**, *129*, 401–413. [CrossRef] [PubMed]
64. Goss, R.J.; Stagg, M.W. Regeneration in lower jaws of newts after excision of the intermandibular regions. *J. Exp. Zool.* **1958**, *137*, 1–11. [CrossRef] [PubMed]
65. Chen, J.; Lin, M.; Foxe, J.J.; Pedrosa, E.; Hrabovsky, A.; Carroll, R.; Zheng, D.; and Lachman, H.M. Transcriptome Comparison of Human Neurons Generated Using Induced Pluripotent Stem Cells Derived from Dental Pulp and Skin Fibroblasts. *PLoS ONE* **2013**, *8*, e75682. [CrossRef] [PubMed]
66. Tank, P.W. The Effect of Nonlimb Tissues on Forelimb Regeneration in the Axolotl, Ambystoma-Mexicanum. *J. Exp. Zool.* **1987**, *244*, 409–423. [CrossRef]
67. Kim, K.; Zhao, R.; Doi, A.; Ng, K.; Unternaehrer, J.; Cahan, P.; Huo, H.; Loh, Y.H.; Aryee, M.J.; Lensche, M.W.; et al. Donor cell type can influence the epigenome and differentiation potential of human induced pluripotent stem cells. *Nat. Biotechnol.* **2011**, *29*, 1117–1119. [CrossRef] [PubMed]
68. Goss, R.J.; Stagg, M.W. Regeneration of lower jaws in adult newts. *J. Morphol.* **1958**, *102*, 289–309. [CrossRef]
69. Yntema, C.L. Regeneration in sparsely innervated and aneurogenic forelimbs of *Amblystoma larvae*. *J. Exp. Zool.* **1959**, *140*, 101–123. [CrossRef] [PubMed]
70. Lee, S.K.; Kim, Y.S.; Oh, H.S.; Yang, K.H.; Kim, E.C.; Chi, J.G. Prenatal Development of the Human Mandible. *Anat. Rec.* **2001**, *263*, 314–325. [CrossRef] [PubMed]
71. Rodriguez-Vazques, J.F.; Merida-Velasco, J.R.; Merida-Velasco, J.A.; Sanchez-Montesinos, I.; Espin-Ferra, J.; Jimenez-Collado, J. Development of Meckel's Cartilage in the Symphyseal Region in Man. *Dev. Biol.* **1997**, *249*, 249–254. [CrossRef]
72. Hovorakova, M.; Lesot, H.; Peterka, M.; Peterkova, R. Early development of the human dentition revisited. *J. Anat.* **2018**, *233*, 135–145. [CrossRef] [PubMed]
73. Lismaa, S.E.; Kaidonis, X.; Nicks, A.M.; Bogush, N.; Kikuchi, K.; Naqvi, N.; Harvey, R.P.; Husain, A.; Graham, R.M. Comparative regenerative mechanisms across different mammalian tissues. *npj Regen. Med.* **2018**, *3*, 6.
74. Graver, H.T. Origin of the dental lamina in the regenerating salamander jaw. *J. Exp. Zool.* **1974**, *189*, 73–84. [CrossRef] [PubMed]
75. Ghosh, S.; Thorogood, P.; Ferretti, P. Regeneration of lower and upper jaws in urodeles is differentially affected by retinoic acid. *Int. J. Dev. Biol.* **1996**, *40*, 1161–1170. [PubMed]
76. Dwaraka, V.B.; Smith, J.J.; Woodcock, M.R.; Voss, S.R. Comparative transcriptomics of limb regeneration_ Identification of conserved expression changes among three species of Ambystoma. *Genomics* **2018**. [CrossRef]
77. McCusker, C.; Bryant, S.V.; Gardiner, D.M. The axolotl limb blastema: Cellular and molecular mechanisms driving blastema formation and limb regeneration in tetrapods. *Regeneration* **2015**, *2*, 54–71. [CrossRef] [PubMed]
78. Singer, M. On the Nature of the Neurotrophic Phenomenon in Urodele Limb Regeneration. *Integr. Comp. Biol.* **1978**, *18*, 829–841. [CrossRef]
79. Mullen, L.M.; Bryant, S.V.; Torok, M.A.; Blumberg, B.; Gardiner, D.M. Nerve dependency of regeneration: The role of Distal-less and FGF signaling in amphibian limb regeneration. *Development* **1996**, *122*, 3487–3497. [PubMed]
80. McCusker, C.D.; Athippozhy, A.; Diaz-Castillo, C.; Fowlkes, C.; Gardiner, D.M.; Voss, S.R. Positional plasticity in regenerating Amybstoma mexicanum limbs is associated with cell proliferation and pathways of cellular differentiation. *BMC Dev. Biol.* **2015**, *15*, 45. [CrossRef] [PubMed]
81. Smith, A.R.; Wolpert, L. Nerves and angiogenesis in amphibian limb regeneration. *Nature* **1975**, *257*, 224–225. [CrossRef] [PubMed]
82. Voss, S.R.; Palumbo, A.; Nagarajan, R.; Gardiner, D.M.; Muneoka, K.; Stromberg, A.J.; Athippozhy, A.T. Gene expression during the first 28 days of axolotl limb regeneration I: Experimental design and global analysis of gene expression. *Regeneration* **2015**, *2*, 120–136. [CrossRef] [PubMed]
83. Zhang, H.; Wang, X.; Lyu, K.; Gai, G.; Wang, G.; Fan, C.; Zhang, X.A.; Yan, J. Time Point-Based Integrative Analyses of Deep-Transcriptome Identify Four Signal Pathways in Blastemal Regeneration of Zebrafish Lower Jaw. *Stem Cells* **2015**, *33*, 806–818. [CrossRef] [PubMed]
84. Kragl, M.; Knapp, D.; Nacu, E.; Khattak, S.; Maden, M.; Epperlein, H.H.; Tanaka, E.M. Cells keep a memory of their tissue origin during axolotl limb regeneration. *Nature* **2009**, *460*, 60–65. [CrossRef] [PubMed]

85. Kragl, M.; Roensch, K.; Nusslein, I.; Tazaki, A.; Taniguchi, Y.; Tarui, H.; Hayashi, T.; Agata, K.; Tanaka, E.M. Muscle and connective tissue progenitor populations show distinct Twist1 and Twist3 expression profiles during axolotl limb regeneration. *Dev. Biol.* **2013**, *373*, 196–204. [CrossRef] [PubMed]
86. McCusker, C.D.; Diaz-Castillo, C.; Sosnik, J.; Phan, A.Q.; Gardiner, D.M. Cartilage and bone cells do not participate in skeletal regeneration in Ambystoma mexicanum limbs. *Dev. Biol.* **2016**, *416*, 26–33. [CrossRef] [PubMed]
87. Muneoka, K.; Fox, W.F.; Bryant, S.V. Cellular contribution from dermis and cartilage to the regenerating limb blastema in axolotls. *Dev. Biol.* **1986**, *116*, 256–260. [CrossRef]
88. Nacu, E.; Glausch, M.; Le, H.Q.; Damanik, F.F.R.; Schuez, M.; Knapp, D.; Khattak, S.; Richter, T.; Tanaka, E.M. Connective tissue cells, but not muscle cells, are involved in establishing the proximo-distal outcome of limb regeneration in the axolotl. *Dev. Stem Cells* **2013**, *140*. [CrossRef] [PubMed]
89. Paul, S.; Schindler, S.; Giovannone, D.; de Millo Terrazzani, A.; Mariani, F.V.; Crump, J.G. Ihha induces hybrid cartilage-bone cells during zebrafish jawbone regeneration. *Development* **2016**, *143*, 2066–2076. [CrossRef] [PubMed]
90. Thornton, C.S. The histogenesis of the regenerating fore limb of larval Amblystoma after exarticulation of the humerus. *J. Morphol.* **1938**, *62*, 219–241. [CrossRef]
91. Charbonneau, A.M.; Roy, S.; Tran, S.D. Oral-Facial Tissue Reconstruction in the Regenerative Axolotl. *J. Exp. Zool. (Mol. Dev. Evol.)* **2017**, *326*, 489–502. [CrossRef] [PubMed]
92. Padhi, B.K.; Joly, L.; Tellis, P.; Sith, A.; Nanjappa, P.; Chevrete, M.; Ekker, M.; Akimenko, M.A. Screen for genes differentially expressed during regeneration of the zebrafish caudal fin. *Dev. Dyn.* **2004**, *231*, 527–541. [CrossRef] [PubMed]
93. Monaghan, J.R.; Athippozhy, A.; Seifert, A.W.; Putta, S.; Stromberg, A.J.; Maden, M.; Gardiner, D.M.; Voss, S.R. Gene expression patterns specific to the regenerating limb of the *Mexican axolotl*. *Biol. Open* **2012**, *1*, 937–948. [CrossRef] [PubMed]
94. Stewart, S.; Tsun, Z.-Y.; Belmonte, J.C.I. A histone demethylase is necessary for regeneration in zebrafish. *Proc. Natl. Acad. Sci. USA* **2009**, *106*, 19889–19894. [CrossRef] [PubMed]
95. Rinn, J.L.; Bondre, C.; Gladstone, H.B.; Brown, P.O.; Chang, H.Y. Anatomic Demarcation by Positional Variation in Fibroblast Gene Expression Programs. *PLoS Genet.* **2006**, *2*, e119. [CrossRef] [PubMed]
96. Rinn, J.L.; Kertesz, M.; Wang, J.K.; Squazzo, S.L.; Brugmann, S.A.; Goodnough, L.H.; Helms, J.A.; Farnham, P.J.; Segal, E.; et al. Functional demarcation of active and silent chromatin domains in human HOX loci by noncoding RNAs. *Cell* **2007**, *129*, 1311–1323. [CrossRef] [PubMed]
97. Mallo, M.S. Reassessing the Role of Hox Genes during Vertebrate Development and Evolution. *Trends Genet.* **2018**, *34*, 209–217. [CrossRef] [PubMed]
98. Chang, H.Y.; Chi, J.T.; Dudoit, S.; Bondre, C.; van de Rijn, M.; Botstein, D.; Brown, P.O. Diversity, topographic differentiation, and positional memory in human fibroblasts. *Proc. Natl. Acad. Sci. USA* **2002**, *99*, 12877–12882. [CrossRef] [PubMed]
99. Endo, T.; Bryant, S.V.; Gardiner, D.M. A stepwise model system for limb regeneration. *Dev. Biol.* **2004**, *270*, 135–145. [CrossRef] [PubMed]
100. Rinn, J.L.; Wang, J.K.; Allen, N.; Brugmann, S.A.; Mikels, A.J.; Liu, H.; Ridky, T.W.; Stadler, H.S.; Nusse, R.; Helms, J.A.; et al. A dermal HOX transcriptional program regulates site-specific epidermal fate. *Genes Dev.* **2008**, *22*, 303–307. [CrossRef] [PubMed]
101. Dhouailly, D.; Rogers, G.E.; Sengel, P. The specification of feather and scale protein synthesis in epidermal-dermal recombinations. *Dev. Biol.* **1978**, *65*, 58–68. [CrossRef]
102. Phan, A.Q.; Lee, J.; Oei, M.; Flath, C.; Hwe, C.; Mariano, R.; Vu, T.; Shu, C.; Dinh, A.; Simkin, J.; et al. Positional information in axolotl and mouse limb extracellular matrix is mediated via heparan sulfate and fibroblast growth factor during limb regeneration in the axolotl (Ambystoma mexicanum). *Regeneration* **2015**, *2*, 182–201. [CrossRef] [PubMed]
103. McCusker, C.D.; Gardiner, D.M. Positional Information Is Reprogrammed in Blastema Cells of the Regenerating Limb of the Axolotl (*Ambystoma mexicanum*). *PLoS ONE* **2013**, *8*, e77064. [CrossRef] [PubMed]
104. Butler, E.G. Regeneration of the urodele forelimb after reversal of its proximo-distal axis. *J. Morphol.* **1955**, *96*, 265–281. [CrossRef]

105. Gardiner, D.M.; Blumberg, B.; Komine, Y.; Bryant, S.V. Regulation of HoxA expression in developing and regenerating axolotl limbs. *Development* **1995**, *121*, 1731–1741. [PubMed]
106. Carlson, M.R.; Komine, Y.; Bryant, S.V.; Gardiner, D.M. Expression of Hoxb13 and Hoxc10 in developing and regenerating Axolotl limbs and tails. *Dev. Biol.* **2001**, *229*, 396–406. [CrossRef] [PubMed]
107. Khan, P.A.; Tsilfidis, C.; Liversage, R.A. Hox C6 expression during development and regeneration of forelimbs in larval *Notophthalmus viridescens*. *Dev. Genes Evol.* **1999**, *209*, 323–329. [CrossRef] [PubMed]
108. Rabinowitz, J.S.; Robitaille, A.m.; Wang, Y.; Ray, C.A.; Thummel, R.; Gu, H.; Djukovic, D.; Raftery, D.; Berndt, J.D.; Moon, R.T. Transcriptomic, proteomic, and metabolomic landscape of positional memory in the caudal fin of zebrafish. *Proc. Natl. Acad. Sci. USA* **2017**, *114*, E717–E726. [CrossRef] [PubMed]
109. Leucht, P.; Kim, J.B.; Amasha, R.; James, A.W.; Girod, S.; Helms, J.A. Embryonic origin and Hox status determine progenitor cell fate during adult bone regeneration. *Development* **2008**, *135*, 2845–2854. [CrossRef] [PubMed]
110. Lim, J.; Lee, J.; Yun, H.-S.; Shin, H.-I.; Park, E.K. Comparison of bone regeneration rate in flat and long bone defects: Calvarial and tibial bone. *Tissue Eng. Regen. Med.* **2013**, *10*, 336–340. [CrossRef]
111. Pritchard, J.J. Repair of fractures of the parietal bone in rats. *J. Anat.* **1946**, *80*, 1–8.
112. Hall, B.K.; Jacobson, H.N. The repair of fractured membrane bones in the newly hatched chick. *Anat. Rec.* **1975**, *181*, 55–69. [CrossRef] [PubMed]
113. Hall, B.K.; Jacobson, H.N. Repair of Fractured Lower Jaws in the Spotted Salamander: Do Amphibians Form Secondary Cartilage? *J. Exp. Zool.* **1985**. [CrossRef]
114. Moss, M.L. Studies of the acellular bone of teleost fish. II. Response to fracture under normal an acalcemic conditions. *Cells Tissues Organs* **1962**, *48*, 46–60. [CrossRef]
115. Gardiner, D.M. *Regenerative Engineering and Developmental Biology*; CRC Press: Boca Raton, FL, USA, 2017.
116. McCusker, C.; Lehrberg, J.; Gardiner, D. Position-specific induction of ectopic limbs in non-regenerating blastemas on axolotl forelimbs. *Regeneration* **2014**, *1*, 27–34. [CrossRef] [PubMed]
117. Hay, E.D. The fine structure of differentiating muscle in the salamander tail. *Cell Tissue Res.* **1963**, *59*, 6–34. [CrossRef]
118. Sosnik, J.; Vieira, W.A.; Webster, K.A.; Siegfried, K.R.; McCusker, C.D. A new and improved algorithm for the quantification of chromatin condensation from microscopic data shows decreased chromatin condensation in regenerating axolotl limb cells. *PLoS ONE* **2017**, *12*, e0185292. [CrossRef] [PubMed]
119. Takahashi, K.; Yamanaka, S. Induction of pluripotent stem cells from mouse embryonic and adult fibroblast cultures by defined factors. *Cell* **2006**, *126*, 663–676. [CrossRef] [PubMed]
120. Niu, W.; Zang, T.; Zou, Y.; Fang, S.; Smith, D.K.; Bachoo, R.; and Zhang, C.L. In vivo reprogramming of astrocytes to neuroblasts in the adult brain. *Nat. Cell Biol.* **2013**, *15*, 1164–1175. [CrossRef] [PubMed]
121. Torper, O.; Pfisterer, U.; Wolf, D.A.; Pereira, M.; Lau, S.; Jakobsson, J.; Bjorklund, A.; Grealish, S.; Parmar, M. Generation of induced neurons via direct conversion in vivo. *Proc. Natl. Acad. Sci. USA* **2013**, *110*, 7038–7043. [CrossRef] [PubMed]
122. Grande, A.; Sumiyoshi, K.; Lopez-Juarez, A.; Howard, J.; Sakthivel, B.; Aronow, B.; Campell, K.; Nakafuku, M. Environmental impact on direct neuronal reprogramming in vivo in the adult brain. *Nat. Commun.* **2013**, *4*, 2373. [CrossRef] [PubMed]
123. Rais, Y.; Zviran, A.; Geula, S.; Gafni, O.; Chomsky, E.; Viukov, S.; Alfatah, A.; Caspi, I.; Krupalnik, V.; Zerbid, M.; et al. Deterministic direct reprogramming of somatic cells to pluripotency. *Nature* **2013**, *502*, 65–70. [CrossRef] [PubMed]
124. Abad, M.; Mosteiro, L.; Pantoja, C.; Canamero, M.; Rayon, T.; Ors, I.; Grana, O.; Megias, D.; Dominguez, O.; Martinez, D.; et al. Reprogramming in vivo produces teratomas and iPS cells with totipotency features. *Nature* **2013**, *502*, 340–345. [CrossRef] [PubMed]
125. Stadtfeld, M.; Maherali, N.; Borkent, M.; Hochedlinger, K. A reprogrammable mouse strain from gene-targeted embryonic stem cells. *Nat. Methods* **2010**, *7*, 53–55. [CrossRef] [PubMed]
126. Kurita, M.; Araoka, T.; Hishida, T.; O'Keefe, D.D.; Takahashi, Y.; Sakamoto, A.; Sakurai, M.; Suzuki, K.; Wu, J.; Yamamoto, M.; et al. In vivo reprogramming of wound-resident cells generates skin epithelial tissue. *Nature* **2018**, *561*, 243–247. [CrossRef] [PubMed]
127. Moore, W.R.; Graves, S.E.; Bain, G.I. Synthetic bone graft substitutes. *ANZ J. Surg.* **2001**, *71*, 354–361. [CrossRef] [PubMed]

6

High-Frequency Deep Sclerotomy, a Minimal Invasive Ab Interno Glaucoma Procedure Combined with Cataract Surgery: Physical Properties and Clinical Outcome

Bojan Pajic [1,2,3,4,*], Zeljka Cvejic [2], Kaweh Mansouri [5,6], Mirko Resan [4] and Reto Allemann [1]

1 Eye Clinic Orasis, Swiss Eye Research Foundation, 5734 Reinach AG, Switzerland; rallemann@gmail.com
2 Department of Physics, Faculty of sciences, University of Novi Sad, Trg Dositeja Obradovica 4, 21000 Novi Sad, Serbia; zeljka.cvejic@df.uns.ac.rs
3 Division of Ophthalmology, Department of Clinical Neurosciences, Geneva University Hospitals, 1205 Geneva, Switzerland
4 Faculty of Medicine of the Military Medical Academy, University of Defense, 11000 Belgrade, Serbia; resan.mirko@gmail.com
5 Glaucoma Center, Montchoisi Clinic, 1000 Lausanne, Switzerland; kwmansouri@gmail.com
6 Department of Ophthalmology, University of Colorado, Denver, CO 80014, USA
* Correspondence: bpajic@datacomm.ch.

Abstract: Background: The efficiency and safety of primary open-angle glaucoma with high-frequency deep sclerotomy (HFDS) combined with cataract surgery has to be investigated. Methods: Right after cataract surgery, HFDS was performed ab interno in 205 consecutive patients with open angle glaucoma. HFDS was performed with a custom-made high-frequency disSection 19 G probe (abee tip 0.3 × 1 mm, Oertli Switzerland). The bipolar current with a frequency of 500 kHz is applied. The nasal sclera was penetrated repetitively six times through the trabecular meshwork and consecutively through Schlemm's canal. Every time, a pocket of 0.3 mm high and 0.6 mm width was created. Results: Mean preoperative intraocular pressure (IOP) was 24.5 ± 2.1 mmHg (range 21 to 48 mmHg). After 48 months, the follow up average IOP was 15.0 ± 1.7 mmHg (range 10 to 20 mmHg). Postoperative IOP has been significantly reduced compared to preoperative IOP for all studied cases ($p < 0.001$). After 48 months, the target IOP less than 21 mmHg reached in 84.9%. No serious complications were observed during the surgical procedure itself and in the postoperative period. Conclusions: HFDS is a minimally invasive procedure. It is a safe and efficacious surgical technique for lowering IOP combined with cataract surgery.

Keywords: glaucoma; ab interno; minimally invasive glaucoma surgery; cataract surgery; high-frequency deep sclerotomy; intraocular pressure

1. Introduction

It is well known that glaucoma comes first in cases of irreversible vision loss and is the second leading cause of blindness worldwide [1]. Nowadays in developed countries, less than 50% of people are unaware of their diagnosis, mainly because of the asymptomatic nature of chronic glaucoma [2].

Trabeculectomy remains the gold standard for glaucoma surgery despite high rates of complications [3–5]. Choroidal effusions, hypotony, shallow anterior chambers, and hyphema are known as early postoperative complications [6–8]. Late complications are often bleb-related, including leakage, blebitis, and endophthalmitis. These complications are more common if antimetabolites like 5-Fluorouracil and Mitomycin C are used [9].

Outflow resistance is caused primarily by the juxtacanilicular trabecular meshwork and, especially, by the inner wall of the Schlemm's canal. This fact is used for the concept of the trabecular meshwork bypass [10]. It is presumed that 35% of the outflow resistance arises in the inner wall of the Schlemm's canal [11].

In addition to the procedures already mentioned, we focus in this work on an enhanced Schlemms canal (SC), which can be addressed both internally and externally. According to the current classification, the ab interno methods include trabectome, iStent, Hydrus, the results presented in this work, and high-frequency deep sclerotomy (HFDS) [12]. The trabectome was introduced in 2004 and has an electroablation of an arc of trabecular meshwork where direct access to the collector channels is given. The intraocular pressure (IOP) reduction of up to 40% is stated in the literature for this ab interno method [13,14]. Another approach for a micro-invasive glaucoma surgery (MIGS) from interno is the iStent. With this device, the aqueous humor is drained directly into the Schlemm's canal, thus avoiding the resistance of the trabecular meshwork [15]. Another representative of the ab interno procedure of the Schemm's canal microstent is the so-called hydrus. It is an 8 mm long crescent-shaped open structure that the bend and sludge canal adapts. It is introduced into the Schlemm's canal by a clear corneal incision [16]. The HFDS is an internally operative glaucoma method that was introduced in 1999. Initially, this surgical procedure was known as sclerothalamotomy ab interno (STT ab interno), and its name was only changed to HFDS in 2012. The aim of the new nomenclature was to describe the procedure more precisely. Regarding the procedure, there were no differences between STT ab interno and HFDS [17–20].

The aim of all MIGS is that, in addition to being effective, they can be carried out simply, quickly and inexpensively with the longest possible effect. The aim of this study is to show the clinical 4-year investigations of this trans-trabecular surgery using the Schlemm's canal as an outflow pathway combined with cataract surgery.

2. Materials and Methods

In this single center study from December 2012 till December 2016, 223 patients with insuffiently controlled primary open-angle glaucoma under maximal tolerated topical therapy without history of prior ocular surgery with significant cataract were included. Exlcusion criteria were monophthalmia, angle closure with or without glaucoma, missing willingness to attend follow-up examinations with randomization or any psychiatric disorder, and any condition that affects the optical system (severe alteration of cornea, anterior chamber, or retina). During the observation period of 48 months, 18 patients did not finish the follow up due to several reasons, so finally 205 patients were included in the study. HFDS was performed combined with cataract surgery, with cataract surgery first being performed. Both procedures were always performed by the same surgeon. A complete ophthalmological examination was carried out in each patient prior to surgery. Further ophthalmologic follow-up examinations were carried out postoperatively on days 1, 2, and 3, after 1 and 4 weeks, and then every 3 months until 48 months. Gonioscopy with a three-mirror goniolens was performed after 4 weeks to check the persistence of the sclerotomy. Tobramycin/dexamethasone and pilocarpin 2% eye drops were applied 3 times daily for 1 month. The tenets of the Declaration for Helsinki were followed in this study. The cantonal ethics committee of Aargau approved the study. According to the ethics committee, patient consent is not required for this retrospective study.

High-Frequency Diathermic Probe

The high-frequency diathermic probe (abee® Glaucoma Tip, Oertli Instrumente AG, Berneck, Switzerland) consists of an inner and outer coaxial electrode. Both electrodes are isolated, while the inner one is made by platinum.

The dimensions of platinum probe tips are 1 mm in length, 0.3 mm high, and 0.6 mm wide. The platinum probe tip is bent posteriorly at an angle of 150°. The probe external diameter is 0.9 mm. Electrical current is modulated at MF (~500 kHz) frequency. The temperature of approximately 130 °C at the tip of the probe is generated by alternating current, while target tissue temperature ranges from 90° to 100°. The tissue is heated by radio frequency-induced intracellular oscillation of ionized molecules, which leads to elevation of intracellular temperature. The very high temperatures cause breakdown of tissue molecules. Inhomogeneous electric field with high voltage and selective current flow conduct to electric arcs (Figure 1).

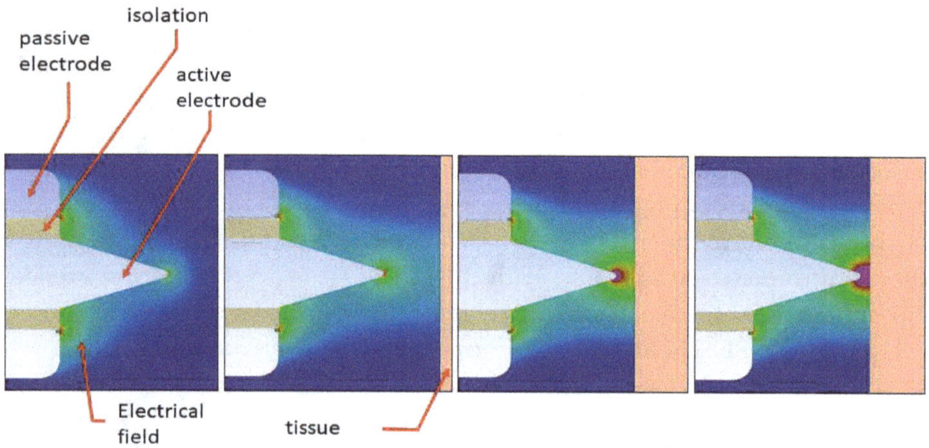

Figure 1. Inhomogeneous electric field, high voltage, and electric arc.

Bearing in mind that the vaporization or cutting process is the best accomplished with relatively low voltage, the coagulation is performed by arcing modulated high-voltage current to tissue. The electric arcs create cell bursts through the evaporation of cell content. By modulating the voltage, it is possible to cut and at the same time make locale coagulation. There is a galvanic separation between the power source and the surgery hand piece (Figure 2).

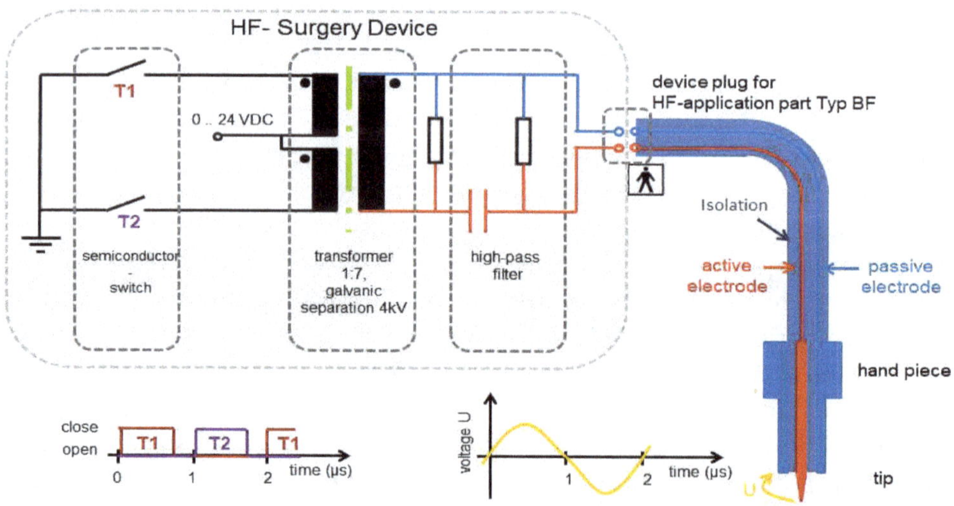

Figure 2. High-frequency (HF) generator.

First, the electrodes are placed away from the tissue, and then the gap between two electrodes is ionized. Due to ionization process, an electric arc discharge develops. In this approach, tissue burning is more superficial because the current is spread over the tissue area more than over the tip of electrode. The experimental set-up provides high-frequency power dissipation in the vicinity of the tip. This was demonstrated in the histological analysis by showing that there is more of a cutting effect in the tissue than coagulation, because there is no tissue nor cell denaturation in the cutting channel and surrounding tissue (Figure 3).

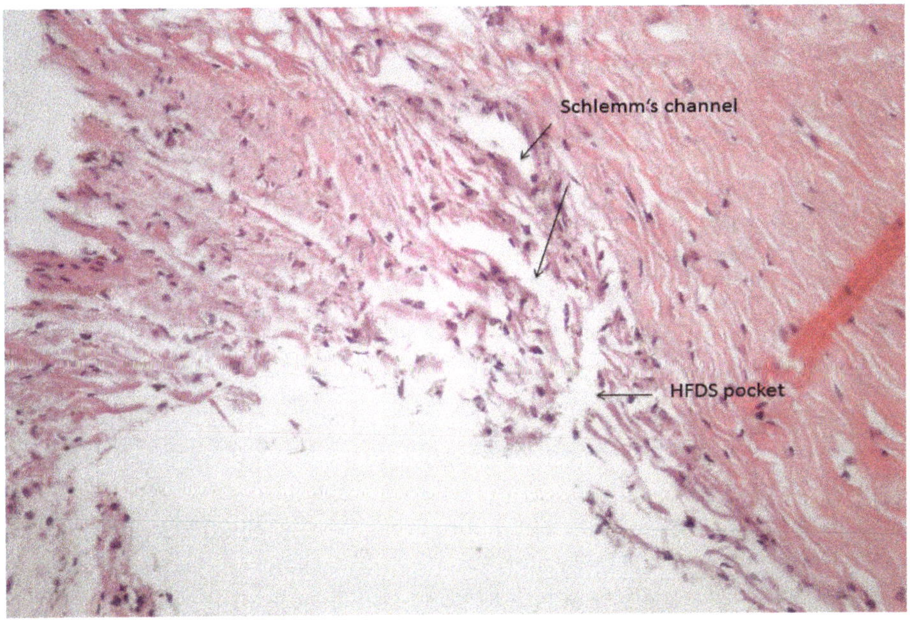

Figure 3. Histological analysis of a high-frequency deep sclerotomy (HFDS) cut (HE staining, human eye).

Two clear corneal incisions were used: one of 1.2-mm temporale or temporo-superior for introducing the abee tip and the other nasal with 0.8-mm created for cataract surgery. In the study, miochol (Acetylcholine chlorid 20 mg) was given intracamerally for the miosis. Anterior chamber was filled with a cohesive ophthalmic viscosurgical device (OVD). The standard high-frequency probe (Figure 4) as described above is consecutively inserted through the temporal paracentesis using a four mirror gonioscopic lens, until the probe is properly placed opposite nasally to the iridocorneal structure.

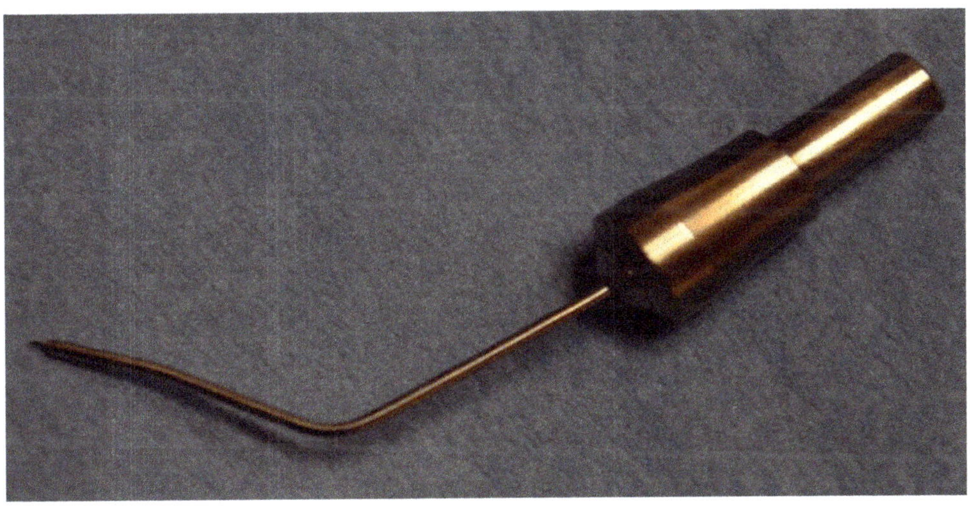

Figure 4. Abee® (HFDS) tip.

Then, six pockets were created consecutively in a row with approximately one tip length space between them. Recently, a new diathermic probe design was developed and used for all patients in the study. For all patients, six pockets were done. With the new abee tip design, three accesses to the anterior chamber are possible, i.e., temporal, superotemporal, or superonasal. The pockets can thus be placed nasally, nasally inferior, or nasally temporal. Consequent retreatments can be done easily. The external diameter is 0.9 mm. Oertli devices were used for the study, i.e., the Pharos and Catarhex 3, with the same setting.

The electric specifications of the probe remained unchanged. Pockets were created with the probe 1 mm through the trabecular meshwork, into Schlemm canal. The target was the insertion of a pocket of 1 mm into the sclera. The target deep sclerotomy pocket is approximatively 0.3 mm thick and 0.6 mm wide, resulting in a resorption surface area of 3.6 mm^2 (Figure 5a).

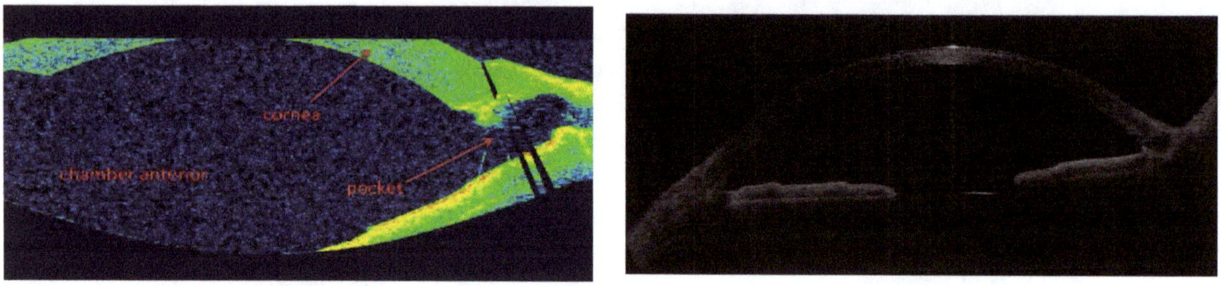

(a) (b)

Figure 5. (**a**) OCT image of the anterior chamber: Overview after HFDS procedure with a newly created pocket in the chamber angle (Visante OCT, Zeiss, Oberkochen, Germany). (**b**) OCT image of the anterior chamber of a normal angle anterior before HFDS surgery.

For comparison, it is shown a normal anterior chamber and angle anterior (Figure 5b).

The tip's dimensions and ab interno approach make it compatible with the stipulations of minimally invasive glaucoma surgery.

Statistical analysis: statistical calculation was done with SPSS Program Version 22. Two-tailed student t-test was used for statistical evaluation of parametric data. Significance was set at a p value of <0.05.

3. Results

Mean age of patients with open-angle glaucoma was 76.8 ± 11.1 years (range: 35–88 years). 103 patients (50.2%) were female, and 102 patients (49.8%) male. One eye of each patient was included. During the whole period of 48 months, no repeat-surgery was needed in any included patient.

Mean preoperative IOP in the study population of 205 patients was 24.5 ± 4.3 mmHg (range 18 to 48 mmHg). Decimalised Snellen visual acuity (VA) increased from 0.46 ± 0.27 preoperative to 0.68 ± 0.27 postoperative. For all patients, the follow-up was 48 months. After 10 days, a slight increase of IOP was detected but was not statistically significant. Mean IOP after 48 months was 15.0 ± 1.7 mmHg (range 10 to 20 mmHg). The IOP drop was statistically significant ($p < 0.001$) at all measured postoperative intervals (Figure 6).

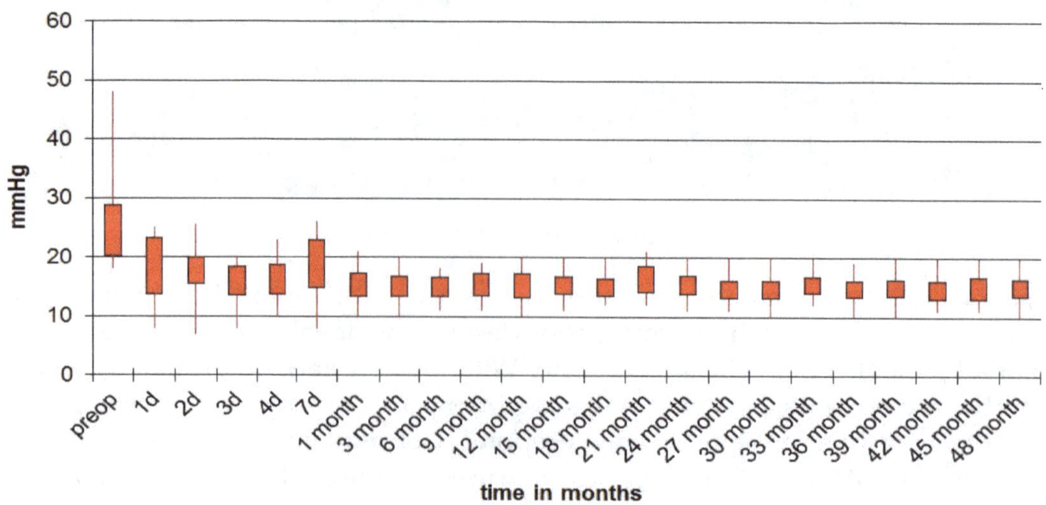

Figure 6. Intraocular pressure (IOP) follow-up of operated eyes during 48 months.

At month 48 after surgery, 54.7% of patients had an IOP < 15 mmHg, 77% had an IOP < 18 mmHg, and 84.9% had an IOP < 21 mmHg. Qualified success rate, defined as an IOP lower than 22 mmHg with medication, was 100% for all patients at 48 months (Figure 7).

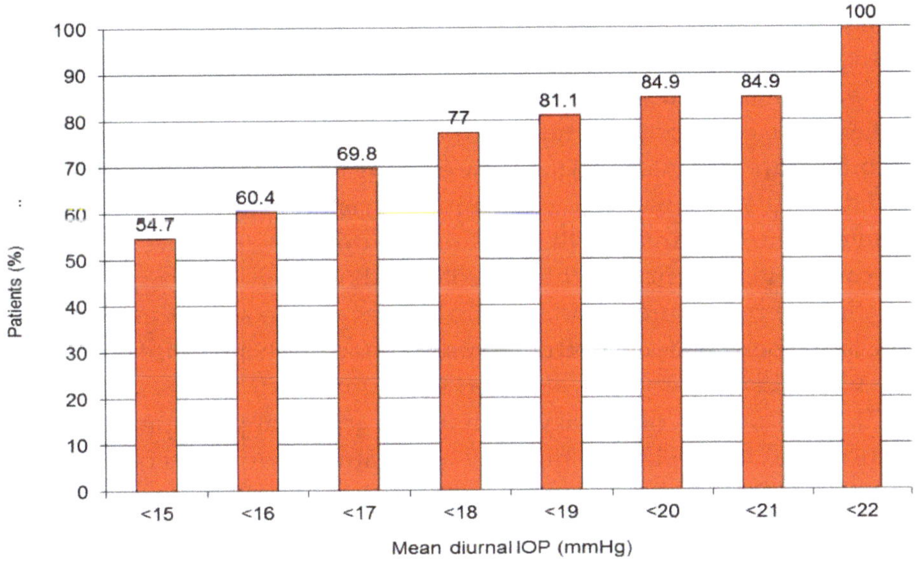

Figure 7. Qualified success rate after 48 months of follow-up.

The average preoperative administration of pressure-reducing number of antihypertensive eye agents was 2.6 ± 1.0. Following surgery, this value was decreased to 0.47 ± 0.59 after 1 month, 0.40 ± 0.54 after 3 months, 0.28 ± 0.62 after 6 months, 0.31 ± 0.49 after 12 months, 0.38 ± 0.57 after 24 months, 0.42 ± 0.83 after 36 months, and 0.48 ± 0.97 after 48 months (Figure 8).

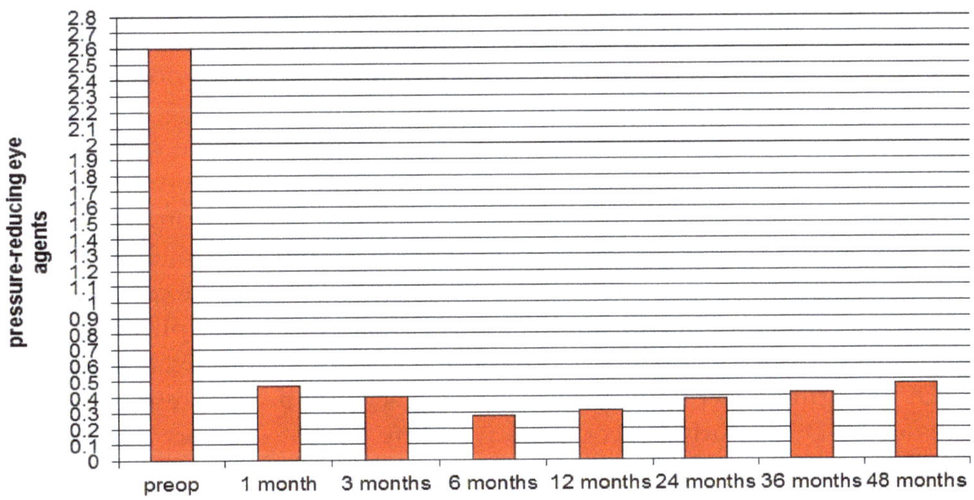

Figure 8. Progression of pressure-reducing eye agents pre-and postoperative during the 48 months, showing a marked and sustained postoperative reduction in numbers of agents needed.

There were no significant visual field changes (Octopus 900, Haag Streit, Switzerland) from baseline with a mean defect MD 7.06 ± 6.54 and loss of variance LV 26.4 ± 23.92. At 48 months, these values were MD 8.43 ± 2.11 and LV 24.1 ± 24.92 ($p = 0.22$ for MD, $p = 0.58$ for LV).

The mean excavation preoperative was 0.63 ± 0.22 and after 48 months 0.65 ± 0.21, which is not statistically significant ($p = 0.36$).

Temporary IOP elevation higher than 21 mmHg was observed in 18 of 205 eyes (8.7%). Four eyes (2%) showed transient fibrin formation. Fibrin was treated by topical dexamethasone and disappeared one day later.

4. Discussion

The present study has shown sustained IOP—lowering effect over 48 months using Schlemm's canal as an outflow pathway with a novel MIGS procedure. Looking into the past, the only possibility of glaucoma treatment was conservative medical management and more invasive glaucoma surgery. The advance MIGS procedure was intended to fill the existing gap regarding treatment. Early studies [19] have demonstrated its ability to lower IOP with minimal risk for mild to moderate glaucoma.

The HFDS ab interno method intends the creation of a direct channel between the anterior chamber and the Schlemm canal. Persistence of the sclerotomy has been investigated with a three-mirror goniolens 4 weeks after the procedures. The abee tip creates a deep sclerotomy with subsequent access of aqueous outflow to the scleral layer. Both aspects may facilitate a bypass effect of aqueous outflow. In an earlier study with deep sclerotomy ab interno, a significant IOP peak could be seen ten days postoperatively [17]. As shown in our study, with introduction of postoperative pilocarpine 2% eye drops application for the first 4 weeks, the high IOP peak amplitude could be avoided. This may have also been the case because the procedures were done combined with cataract surgery.

In general, MIGS procedures share five important features: ab interno approach, potential minimal trauma, ability to lower IOP, a high level of safety, and faster visual recovery. Hence, advantages of HFDS ab interno method, compared with trabeculectomy and perforating and nonperforating deep sclerectomy, seem to have a low rate of postoperative complications and a stable level of reduced IOP. Hypotension, a frequent finding in trabeculectomy, which is less frequently found in nonperforating deep sclerectomy, was not seen in the present population. The most frequent early complications in trabeculectomy are hyphaema (24.6%), shallow anterior chamber (23.9%), hypotony (24.3%), wound leak (17.8%), and choroidal detachment (14.1%). The most frequent late complications are iris incarceration (5.1%) and encapsulated bleb (3.4%) [21]. After HFDS, a transient IOP elevation was seen in 18 of 205 eyes (8.7%), on average occurring 10 days postoperatively. Four of 205 eyes (2%) had transient fibrin formation. Therefore, compared with penetrating or nonpenetrating techniques, HFDS seems to be a safe surgical technique [22–25].

An earlier study with deep sclerotomy ab interno had a complete success rate of 83% after 48 months [17,19] for open angle glaucoma. The present study shows that the success rate of 84.9% was similar. The slight improvement could be due to the fact that the procedures was carried out in combination with cataract surgery. It was particularly striking that the postoperative IOP range was significantly lower in the combined procedure. This effect could be explained by the additional reduction due to the cataract surgery, but also by the postoperative application of pilocarpine 2% during the first 4 weeks. If the postoperative IOP profile is analyzed, after 24 months there is a loss of the additional IOP-lowering effect from the cataract surgery will be apparent.

Advantages of HFDS include its comparative simplicity and short duration of the surgical procedure itself. Additionally, unlike ab externo filtering techniques, the technique avoids stimulation of episcleral and conjunctival tissues leading to fibroblast activation. Additionally, by comparing the histological alterations of HFDS with trabectome, another MIGS procedure, it has been shown that with trabectome tissue was damaged near the incision [26]. As trabectome was validated mainly in the pediatric population associated with long-term IOP control, recently a dual-blade device was developed for adult use but showing also smaller but still detectable damage to the tissue [27].

5. Conclusions

Although the number of six surgical pockets chosen was arbitrary, our results suggest that it may be sufficient to provide good long-term IOP-lowering efficacy and safety. With the introduction of the new abee-tip design, it is possible to perform surgical retreatment in the nasal and inferior quadrants of the trabecular meshwork. HFDS is a safe and minimally invasive method for glaucoma surgery with good long-term results. More studies are needed to confirm our findings in different populations and types of glaucoma.

Author Contributions: B.P. provided the treatment indication, developed the study design, acquired clinical data, and contributed to writing the paper. Z.C. contributed substantially to the development of the study design and substantially contributed to writing the paper. K.M. performed data analyses and substantially contributed advising regarding the paper contents. M.R. performed data anlysis and substantially contributed the study design. R.A. performed data analysis and contributed to writing the paper. All authors have read and agreed to the published version of the manuscript.

References

1. Flaxman, S.R.; Bourne, R.R.A.; Resnikoff, S.; Ackland, P.; Braithwaite, T.; Cicinelli, M.V.; Das, A.; Jonas, J.B.; Keeffe, J.; Kempen, J.H.; et al. Global causes of blindness and distance vision impairment 1990–2020: A systematic review and meta-analysis. *Lancet Glob. Health* **2017**, *5*, 1221–1234. [CrossRef]
2. Goh, Y.W.; Ang, G.S.; Azuara-Blanco, A. Lifetime visual prognosis of patients with glaucoma. *Clin. Exp. Ophthalmol.* **2011**, *39*, 766–770. [CrossRef] [PubMed]
3. Razeghinejad, M.R.; Fudemberg, S.J.; Spaeth, G.L. The changing conceptual basis of trabeculectomy: A review of past and current surgical techniques. *Surv. Ophthalmol.* **2012**, *57*, 1–25. [CrossRef] [PubMed]
4. Vinod, K.; Gedde, S.J.; Feuer, W.J.; Panarelli, J.F.; Chang, T.C.; Chen, P.P.; Parrish, R.K. Practice preferences for glaucoma surgery: A survey of the American Glaucoma Society. *J. Glaucoma* **2017**, *26*, 687–693. [CrossRef] [PubMed]
5. Gedde, S.J.; Chen, P.P.; Heuer, D.K.; Singh, K.; Wright, M.M.; Feuer, W.J.; Schiffman, J.C.; Shi, W.; Primary Tube Versus Trabeculectomy Study Group. The Primary Tube Versus Trabeculectomy Study: Methodology of a Multicenter Randomized Clinical Trial Comparing Tube Shunt Surgery and Trabeculectomy with Mitomycin, C. *Ophthalmology* **2018**, *125*, 774–781. [CrossRef] [PubMed]
6. Vaziri, K.; Schwartz, S.G.; Kishor, K.S.; Fortun, J.A.; Moshfeghi, D.M.; Moshfeghi, A.A.; Flynn, H.W., Jr. Incidence of postoperative suprachoroidal hemorrhage after glaucoma filtration surgeries in the United States. *Clin. Ophthalmol.* **2014**, *9*, 579–584.
7. Takihara, Y.; Inatani, M.; Ogata-Iwao, M.; Kawai, M.; Inoue, T.; Iwao, K.; Tanihara, H. Trabeculectomy for open-angle glaucoma in phakic eyes vs in pseudophakic eyes after phacoemulsification: A prospective clinical cohort study. *JAMA Ophthalmol.* **2014**, *132*, 69–76. [CrossRef]
8. Jeganathan, V.S.; Ghosh, S.; Ruddle, J.B.; Gupta, V.; Coote, M.A.; Crowston, J.G. Risk factors for delayed suprachoroidal haemorrhage following glaucoma surgery. *Br. J. Ophthalmol.* **2008**, *92*, 1393–1396. [CrossRef]
9. Gedde, S.J.; Herndon, L.W.; Brandt, J.D.; Budenz, D.L.; Feuer, W.J.; Schiffman, J.C. Surgical complications in the Tube Versus Trabeculectomy Study during the first year of follow-up. *Am. J. Ophthalmol.* **2007**, *143*, 23–31. [CrossRef]
10. Johnson, D.H.; Johnson, M. Glaucoma surgery and aqueous outflow: How does nonpenetrating glaucoma surgery work? *Arch. Ophthalmol.* **2002**, *120*, 67–70. [CrossRef]
11. Schuman, J.S.; Chang, W.; Wang, N.; de Kater, A.W.; Allingham, R.R. Excimer laser effects on outflow facility and outflow pathway morphology. *Investig. Ophthalmol. Vis. Sci.* **1999**, *40*, 1676–1680.
12. Shaarawy, T. Glaucoma surgery: Taking the sub-conjunctival route. *Middle East Afr. J. Ophthalmol.* **2015**, *22*, 53–58. [CrossRef] [PubMed]
13. Maeda, M.; Watanabe, M.; Ichikawa, K. Evaluation of trabectome in open-angle glaucoma. *J. Glaucoma* **2013**, *22*, 205–208. [CrossRef] [PubMed]
14. Minckler, D.S.; Baerveldt, G.; Alfaro, M.R.; Francis, B.A. Clinical results with the Trabectome for treatment of open-angle glaucoma. *Ophthalmology* **2005**, *112*, 962–967. [CrossRef] [PubMed]
15. Resende, A.F.; Patel, N.S.; Waisbourd, M.; Katz, L.J. iStent® Trabecular Microbypass Stent: An Update. *J. Ophthalmol.* **2016**, *2016*, 2731856. [CrossRef]
16. Pfeiffer, N.; Garcia-Feijoo, J.; Martinez-de-la-Casa, J.M.; Larrosa, J.M.; Fea, A.; Lemij, H.; Gandolfi, S.; Schwenn, O.; Lorenz, K.; Samuelson, T.W. A Randomized Trial of a Schlemm's Canal Microstent with

Phacoemulsification for Reducing Intraocular Pressure in Open-Angle Glaucoma. *Ophthalmology* **2015**, *122*, 1283–1293. [CrossRef]
17. Pajic, B.; Pajic-Eggspuehler, B.; Haefliger, I. New minimally invasive, deep sclerotomy ab interno surgical procedure for glaucoma, six years of follow-up. *J. Glaucoma* **2011**, *20*, 109–114. [CrossRef]
18. Abushanab, M.M.I.; El-Shiaty, A.; El-Beltagi, T.; Hassan Salah, S. The Efficacy and Safety of High-Frequency Deep Sclerotomy in Treatment of Chronic Open-Angle Glaucoma Patients. *BioMed Res. Int.* **2019**, *2019*, 1850141. [CrossRef]
19. Pillunat, L.E.; Erb, C.; Jünemann, A.G.; Kimmich, F. Micro-invasive glaucoma surgery (MIGS): A review of surgical procedures using stents. *Clin. Ophthalmol.* **2017**, *11*, 1583–1600. [CrossRef]
20. Edmunds, B.; Thompson, J.R.; Salmon, J.F.; Wormald, R.P. The National Survey of Trabeculectomy. III. Early and late complications. *Eye* **2002**, *16*, 297–303. [CrossRef]
21. Lindemann, F.; Plange, N.; Kuerten, D.; Schimitzek, H.; Koutsonas, A. Three-Year Follow-Up of Trabeculectomy with 5-Fluorouracil. *Ophthalmic Res.* **2017**, *58*, 74–80. [CrossRef] [PubMed]
22. Rodriguez-Una, I.; Rotchford, A.P.; King, A.J. Outcome of repeat trabeculectomies: Long-term follow-up. *Br. J. Ophthalmol.* **2017**, *101*, 1269–1274. [CrossRef] [PubMed]
23. Harju, M.; Suominen, S.; Allinen, P.; Vesti, E. Long-term results of deep sclerectomy in normal-tension glaucoma. *Acta Ophthalmol.* **2018**, *96*, 154–160. [CrossRef] [PubMed]
24. Bettin, P.; Di Matteo, F.; Rabiolo, A.; Fiori, M.; Ciampi, C.; Bandello, F. Deep Sclerectomy with Mitomycin C and Injectable Cross-linked Hyaluronic Acid Implant: Long-term Results. *J. Glaucoma* **2016**, *25*, 625–629. [CrossRef] [PubMed]
25. Pajic, B.; Pallas, G.; Gerding, H.; Böhnke, M. A novel technique of ab interno glaucoma surgery: Follow-up results after 24 months. *Graefes Arch. Clin. Exp. Ophthalmol.* **2006**, *244*, 22–27. [CrossRef] [PubMed]
26. Seibold, L.K.; Soohoo, J.R.; Ammar, D.A.; Kahook, M.Y. Preclinical investigation of ab interno trabeculectomy using a novel dual-blade device. *Am. J. Ophthalmol.* **2013**, *155*, 524–529. [CrossRef]
27. SooHoo, J.R.; Seibold, L.K.; Kahook, M.Y. Ab interno trabeculectomy in the adult patient. *Middle East Afr. J. Ophthalmol.* **2015**, *22*, 25–29. [CrossRef]

7

Scanning Electron Microscopy Analysis and Energy Dispersion X-Ray Microanalysis to Evaluate the Effects of Decontamination Chemicals and Heat Sterilization on Implant Surgical Drills: Zirconia vs. Steel

Antonio Scarano [1,2,3,*], Sammy Noumbissi [2,4], Saurabh Gupta [2,5], Francesco Inchingolo [6], Pierbiagio Stilla [1] and Felice Lorusso [7]

1 Department of Medical, Oral and Biotechnological Sciences and CeSI-Me, University of Chieti-Pescara, 3166100 Chieti, Italy
2 Zirconia Implant Research Group (Z.I.R.G.), International Academy of Ceramic Implantology, Silver Spring, MD 20901, USA
3 Department of Oral Implantology, Dental Research Division, College Ingà, UNINGÁ, Cachoeiro de Itapemirim 29312, Brazil
4 International Academy of Ceramic Implantology, Zirconia Implant Research Group (Z.I.R.G.), University of Chieti-Pescara, 3166100 Chieti, Italy
5 Private Practice Dentistry, Bangalore 560001, India
6 Department of Interdisciplinary Medicine, University of Bari "Aldo Moro", 70121 Bari, Italy
7 Department of Medical, Oral and Biotechnological Sciences, University of Chieti-Pescara, Via dei Vestini, 3166100 Chieti, Italy
* Correspondence: ascarano@unich.it

Featured Application: The control of the effect of drills wear and corrosion related to clinical use represents a critical factor in implantology, because it is strictly related to the bone cutting precision and heat generation during site preparation.

Abstract: Background: Drills are an indispensable tool for dental implant surgery. Today, there are ceramic zirconium dioxide and metal alloy drills available. Osteotomy drills are critical instruments since they come in contact with blood and saliva. Furthermore, they are reusable and should be cleaned and sterilized between uses. Depending on the material, sterilizing agents and protocols can alter the surface and sharpness of implant drills. The hypothesis is that cleaning and sterilization procedures can affect the surface structure of the drills and consequently reduce their cutting efficiency. **Methods:** Eighteen zirconia ceramic drills and eighteen metal alloy drills were evaluated. Within the scope of this study, the drills were not used to prepare implant sites. They were immersed for 10 min in human blood taken from volunteer subjects and then separately exposed to 50 cycles of cleansing with 6% hydrogen peroxide, cold sterilization with glutaraldehyde 2%, and autoclave heat sterilization. Scanning Electron Microscopy (SEM) and energy dispersion X-ray (EDX) microanalysis were conducted before and after each cycle and was used to evaluate the drill surfaces for alterations. **Results:** After exposure to the cleansing agents used in this study, alterations were seen in the steel drills compared to zirconia. **Conclusions:** The chemical sterilization products used in this study cause corrosion of the metal drills and reduce their sharpness. It was observed that the cycles of steam sterilization did not affect any of the drills. Zirconia drill surfaces remained stable.

Keywords: implant drills; zirconium dioxide; sterilization; disinfection; cleaning; corrosion; implant failure

1. Introduction

Drill wear is a phenomenon determined by the detachment of particles during the preparation of implant sites that can interfere with the process of bone healing. Considering that all materials are subject to wear and chemical attack by disinfectants, it would be desirable to have a biocompatible drill that is not susceptible to attack by the disinfectants used in clinical practice. The healing of peri-implant bone is a complex phenomenon that involves the proliferation and differentiation of pre-osteoblasts into osteoblasts. Periosteal and endosteal activity also contributes to the production of the osteoid matrix, which is followed by mineralization and organization of the bone–implant interface [1]. The success of implant surgery depends on the bone and soft tissue healing after the process of implant site preparation [2]. One of the key factors in implant success is to keep the osteotomy process as atraumatic as possible for fast, optimal recovery and healing. One of the most important factors in minimizing trauma during osteotomy is to control heat generation with irrigation, but also by utilizing drills that will cut through bone in an efficient and minimally invasive manner [3,4]. Even after a single use, drills will show signs of wear and start to lose their sharpness and cutting efficiency [5,6]. A slightly damaged or dulled drill will not only lose its cutting efficiency, but also overheat bone, leading to bone necrosis, poor healing, and an ill-defined osteotomy with a poor initial implant stability [7,8]. Among the materials used for the manufacturing of implant drills is steel, whose structural integrity can be affected by disinfectants and cleaning agents. When coming into contact with chemical disinfectants, an oxidation process takes place on the drill, giving rise to corrosion products and the release of metal particles and ions to the peri-implant tissues, which can cause inflammation, increased osteoclastic activity, and subsequent implant failure [9,10].

The phenomenon and mechanism by which the reuse of an implant drill can be a source of metal particles or ions in implant bed preparation have not been evaluated in the literature. Metal particles and ions are known to induce osteolysis, so it is important to avoid potential sources of metal ions and particles for the long-term survival of dental implants. The reuse of drills, repeated cleansing, and sterilization causes them to lose their sharpness and trigger the corrosion process. As a result, there is a loss of cutting efficiency, thus making it possible to leave metal particles and ions in the bone. Furthermore, the loss of cutting efficiency increases the friction between the bone and drills and elevates the osteotomy temperature, leading to bone cell death and implant failure. An alternative drill material to steel is zirconium dioxide, also known as zirconia, which is a ceramic and belongs to the category of materials called inert metal oxides. They are also used as dental implant materials [11]. Zirconia is bio-inert, and has excellent corrosion resistance, superior biocompatibility, high wear resistance, and high fracture resistance values [12,13]. Repeated disinfection and sterilization cycles can lead to undesirable changes in the physical properties of the instruments, such as a loss of structure, sharpness, and corrosion [5]. The purpose of this study is to analyze the effects of chemical disinfection and autoclave sterilization on zirconium oxide ceramic drills vs. steel drills by scanning electron microscopy and energy dispersion X-ray microanalysis. The null hypothesis of this study is that there will be no difference in surface alterations between zirconia and steel drills as a result of disinfection and sterilization procedures.

2. Materials and Methods

In this study, a total of 18 drills of zirconia (Dental Tech, Misinto, Milan) and 18 steel drills were used (Dental Tech, Misinto, Milan) (Figure 1).

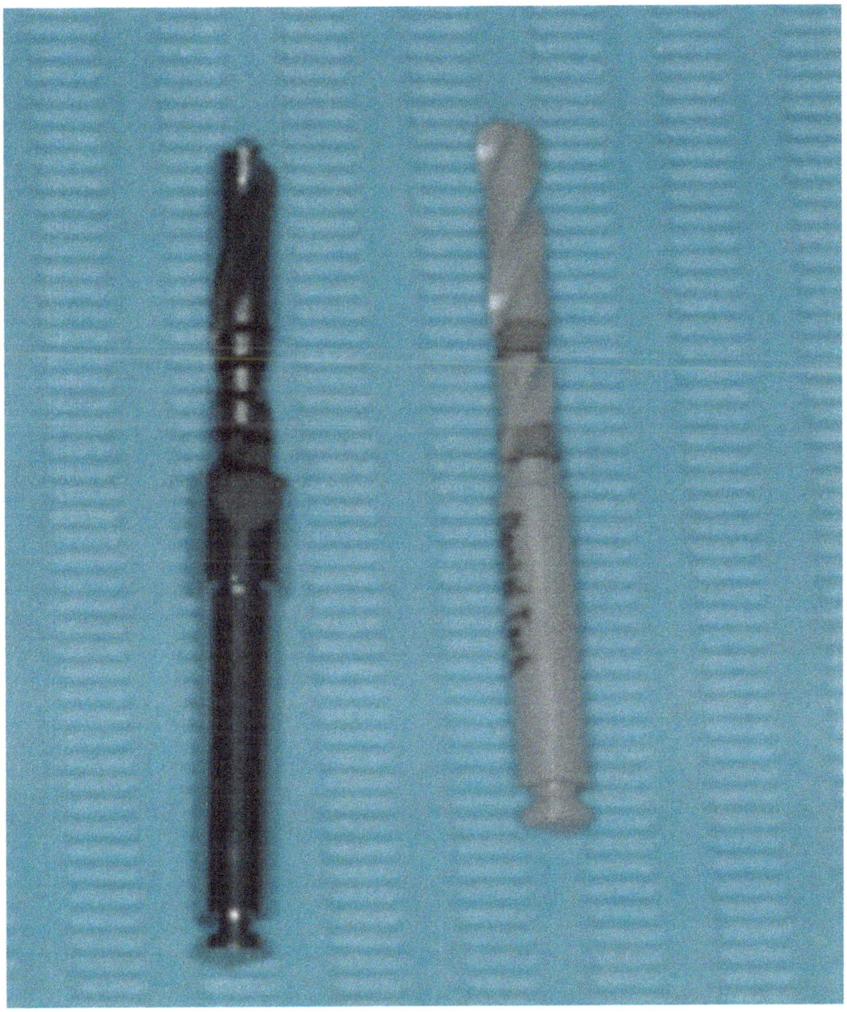

Figure 1. Macroscopic aspect of the steel drill (left) and zirconia drill (right) used in the present study.

Only 2 mm diameter helical conical drills were evaluated in order to analyze their response to disinfecting and cleansing agents, as well as autoclave sterilization. The steel drills presented the following chemical composition: 0.2% sulfur, 0.2% carbon, 0.6% silicon, 0.8% nickel, 1.2% molybdenum, 1.6% manganese, 16% chromium, 22% carbon, and balancing iron. The chemical composition shows the typical characteristics of a stainless-steel alloy. The drills studied were all externally irrigated and had three black laser markings with the function of guiding the surgeon in controlling the depth during osteotomy. In this investigation, chemical agents such as glutaraldehyde 2% (Dimexid, Amedics Ferrara, Italy) and hydrogen peroxide 6% (Sanibios, Noda, Balerna- Switzerland), were taken into consideration, and the effect of sterilization cycles was also observed. The drills were not subjected to the preparation of implant sites, but were immersed for 10 minutes in human blood taken from voluntary subjects and then underwent cycles of immersion in disinfectants without being subjected to autoclaving (approved by Inter Institutional Ethics Committee of UNINGÁ, No. 72105917.5.0000.5220). Before immersion, decontamination, or sterilization, the drills were rinsed in running water and scrubbed with a toothbrush made of nylon bristles in order to remove gross foreign material (e.g., organic material, clot). A total of 18 steel drills and 18 zirconia drills were used and allotted to 6 groups of 6 drills, with 6 in steel and 6 in zirconia for each group. Then, implant drills were assessed before and after the disinfection by Scanning Electron Microscopy (SEM). A disc of carborundum was used to separate the blades from the grips of the drills to be observed by SEM. Ten flat areas of 200 μm to 150 μm in diameter were evaluated for each drill and an image in JPEG format was created (Figure 2).

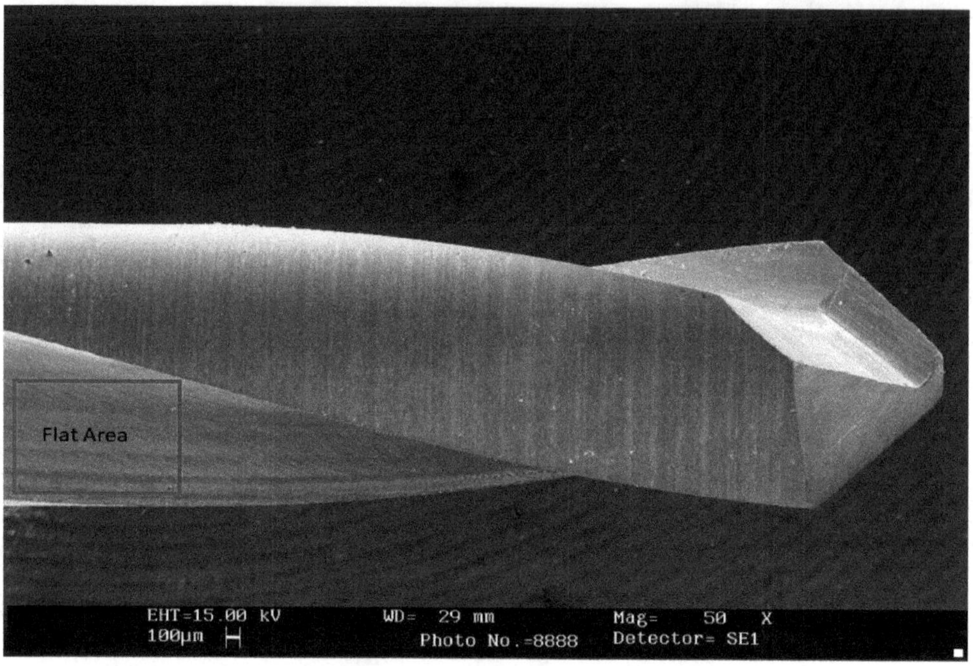

Figure 2. The flat area evaluated for each drill.

The drills were divided into the following groups:

Group 1: New non-sterilized Steel drill; Steel drills subjected to 50 cycles of 20 min sterilization immersion in glutaraldehyde;

Group 2: Steel drills subjected to 50 immersion cycles of 20 min immersion cleansing in hydrogen peroxide;

Group 3: Steel drills subjected to 50 cycles of heat sterilization in an autoclave at 134° C for 35 min at a pressure of 1.1 bar; New non-sterilized Zirconia drills;

Group 4: Zirconia drills subjected to 50 cycles of 20 min immersion sterilization in glutaraldehyde;

Group 5: Zirconia drills subjected to 50 immersion cycles of 20 min for cleansing in hydrogen peroxide;

Group 6: Zirconia drills subjected to 50 cycles of heat sterilization in an autoclave at 134° C for 35 min at a pressure of 1.1 bar (A-17 PLUS, ANTHOS, Imola, Italy).

All the solutions were poured into a plastic container in order to avoid interference between the liquid and metal. In accordance with the Italian legislation DMS of 28/9/90, the drills were immersed for 20 min in a liquid chemical sterilant. After 50 cycles of decontamination and cold sterilization immersion, the drills were rinsed in running water and then in demineralized water. They were then observed by a transmission electron microscope. The method of analysis followed the methodology proposed by Scarano et al. [5].

Previously calibrated examiners compared the micrographs before and after 50 cycles of disinfection and sterilization, respectively, with those obtained for the control group and assessed the percentage of surface covered by damage.

2.1. *SEM Observations*

In order to evaluate changes in the surface topography, we used a scanning electron microscope (SEM, JSM-6480LV; Jeol, Tokyo, Japan), with a solid-state backscattered detector operated at a 20 kV accelerating voltage. Each drill was attached to an aluminum stub with sticky conductive carbon tape. Images were taken in both secondary and backscattered electrons. The drills were mounted on aluminum stubs and gold-coated in Emitech K550 (Emitech Ltd., Ashford, UK). Pictures were recorded for each specimen to characterize the surface and presence of corrosion area. The pictures were processed with ImageJ (ImageJ, U.S. National Institute of Health, Bethesda, MD, USA).

2.2. *Energy Dispersive X-ray Spectroscopy (EDX)*

To detect possible drill alterations, the drills were examined before and after sterilization with a scanning electron microscope/energy dispersion X-ray microanalysis (SEM/EDX) using scanning electron microscopy (SEM, JSM-6480LV; Jeol, Tokyo, Japan) with the EDS QUANTAX-200 probe (Bruker Nano GmbH, Berlin, Germany).

2.3. *Statistical Evaluation*

Free software available on the site http://clincalc.com/stats/samplesize.aspx, was used to determine the number of drills needed to achieve statistical significance for quantitative analyses of drill surface damage. A calculation model was adopted for dichotomous variables (yes/no effect) by applying the effect incidence designed to caution the reasons, with values of 10% for zirconia drill and 95% for steel drill, and the alpha was set at 0.05 and power at 70%. The optimal number of specimens for analysis was six drills per group.

A normal data distribution was evaluated by the Shapiro–Wilk test and the differences between the groups were analyzed by one-way analysis of variance (ANOVA) followed by a Tukey post-hoc test. A p-value < 0.05 was considered statistically significant. Data processing and statistical analysis were performed by Excel origin and SPSS software (SPS, Bologna, Italy).

3. Results

Scanning Electron Microscopy Analysis and Energy Dispersion X-ray Microanalysis.

3.1. *Steel Drills*

New Non-Sterilized Drill

The spectroscopic analysis showed that the flat area of implant drills was composed of stainless-steel alloys with a high content of iron, nickel, and chromium (Figure 3).

Group 1

After 50 cycles of decontamination, the drills immersed in the glutaraldehyde showed traces of corrosion with deposits on the bottom of the container and traces of a rust color. The drills appeared to be macroscopically damaged and the laser depth markings were less distinctive, but still identifiable. The areas of corrosion were mostly present especially near the laser markings (Table 1). In total, 21 ± 3% of the drill surface in this group was covered by damage (Figure 4). None of the drills had surface damage over 30% of the total surface. The spectroscopic analysis of the drill surface showed a reduction in iron, nickel, and chromium and a comparable increase in oxygen (Figure 5).

Group 2

The drills immersed in hydrogen peroxide appeared to be macroscopically damaged, but the damaged surface areas were smaller and the laser depth marks remained clearly visible. A total of 12 ± 1% of the drill surface in the hydrogen peroxide group was covered by damage. No drill in this group had damage above 20% of the surface (Figure 6). Additionally, in this group, the spectroscopic analysis of the drill surface showed a decrease in iron levels and a comparable increase in oxygen.

Group 3

The steel drills that were subjected to 50 cycles of heat sterilization by steam neither caused areas of corrosion nor altered the depth notches (Table 1) (Figure 7). The spectroscopic analysis of the drill surface showed a smaller increase in oxygen and a decrease in the levels of iron, nickel, and chromium (Figure 8).

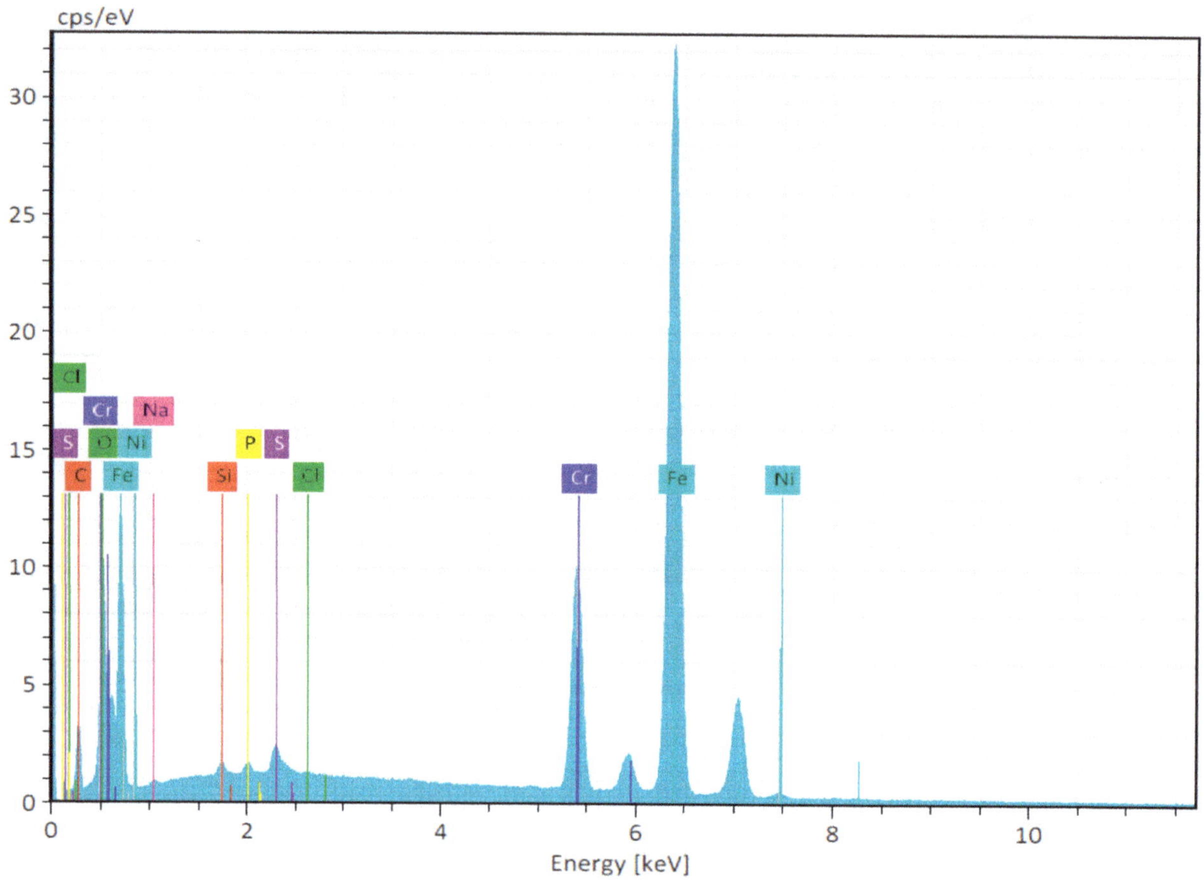

Figure 3. Spectra showing elemental peaks of the new drill surface.

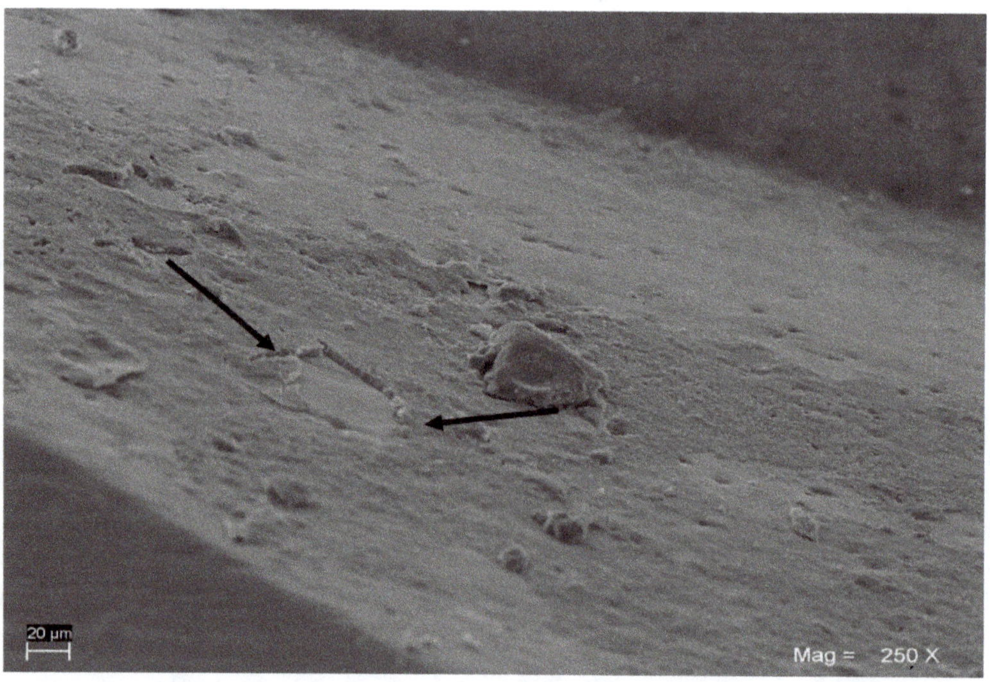

Figure 4. Group 1. Aspects of the steel drill after 50 disinfection cycles with glutaraldehyde, where zones of structural alteration can be observed.

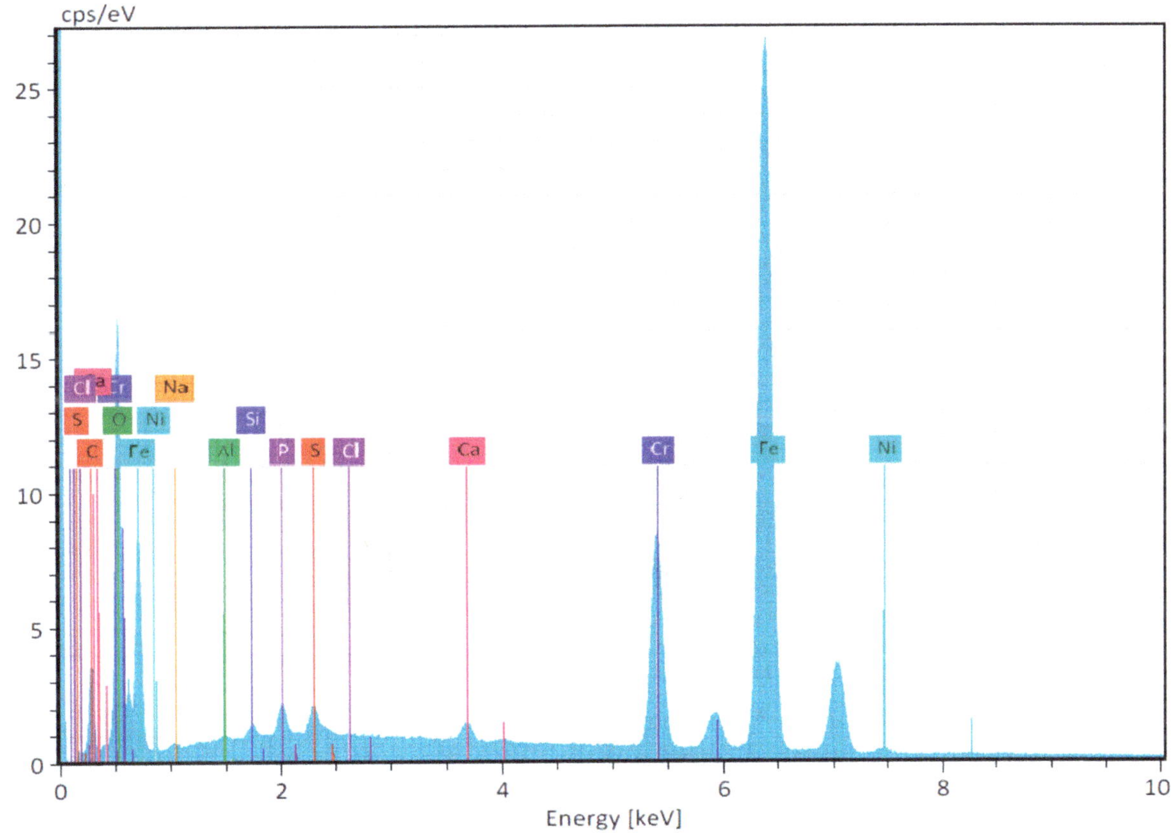

Figure 5. Group 1. The spectroscopic analysis of the drill surface after 50 disinfection cycles with glutaraldehyde showed a decrease in oxygen, iron, nickel, and chromium.

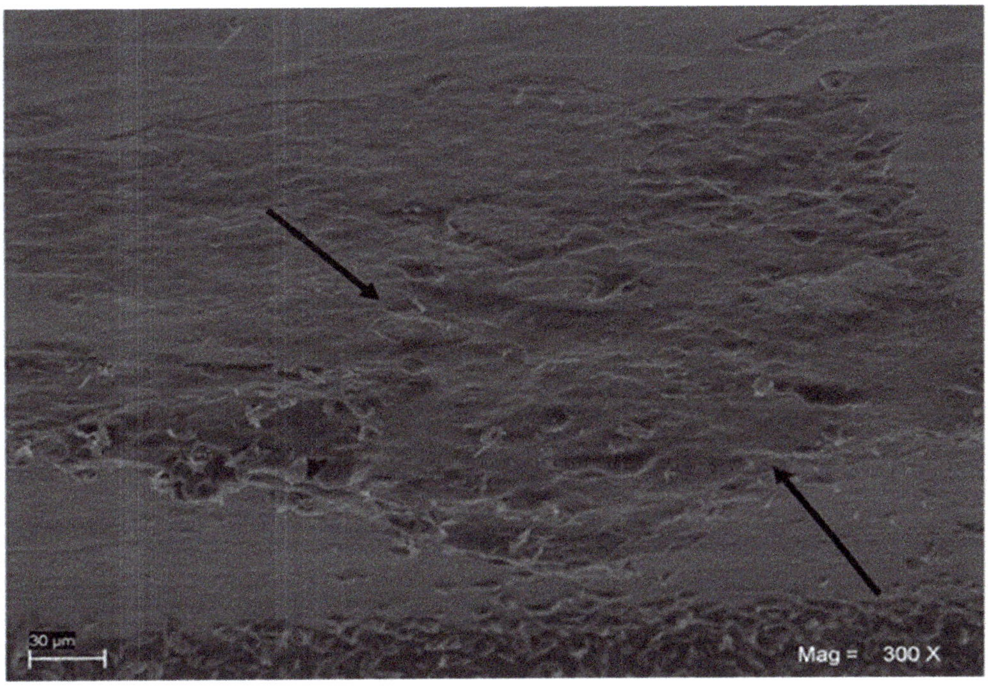

Figure 6. Group 2. After 50 disinfection cycles with hydrogen peroxide, zones of damage by the corrosive process were observed (arrows).

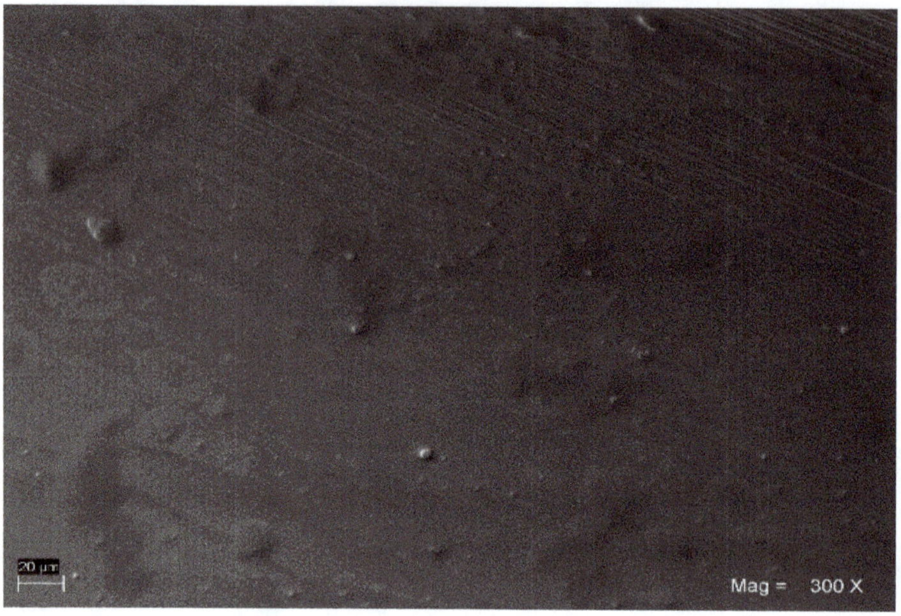

Figure 7. Group 3. After 50 steam autoclave cycles, no areas of corrosion were observed.

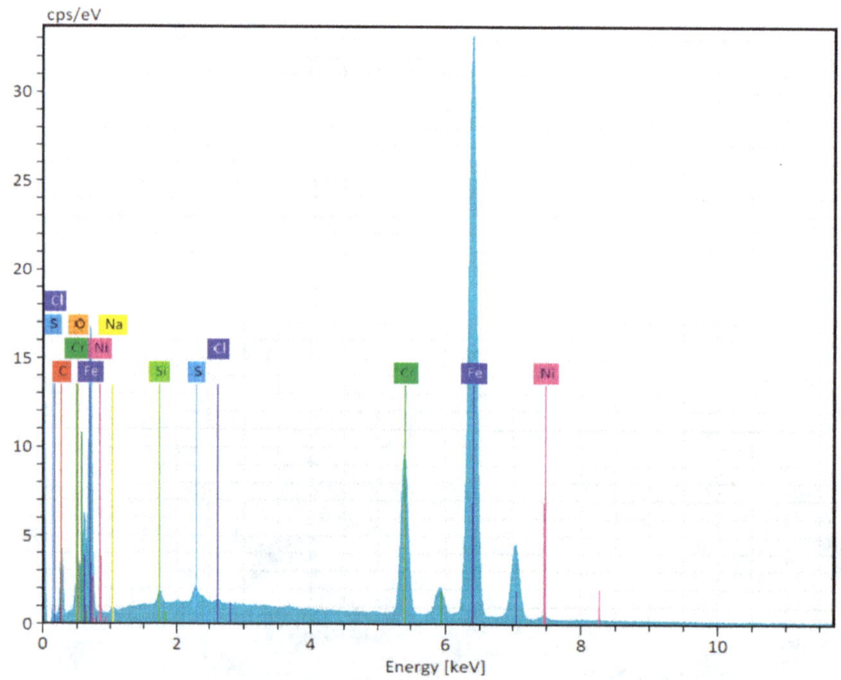

Figure 8. Group 3. The spectroscopic analysis of the drill surface after 50 steam autoclave cycles, where no changes in iron, nickel, and chromium levels and a smaller increase in oxygen where observed.

3.2. Zirconia Drills

New Non-Sterilized Drill

The spectroscopic analysis of the new unsterilized zirconia drill surface showed that the flat areas of implant drills were mainly composed of zirconia and carbon, oxygen, and aluminum (Figure 9).

Group 4

The zirconia ceramic drills observed after 50 cycles of immersion in the glutaraldehyde had the same appearance as the new non-sterilized drills and did not have residues of organic material (Figure 10). The spectroscopic analysis of the drill surface showed no change in the surface composition.

Group 5

The zirconia ceramic drills observed after 50 cycles of immersion in the hydrogen peroxide had the same appearance as the new non-sterilized drills and did not have residues of organic material (Figure 11). The spectroscopic analysis of the drill surface showed no change in the surface composition.

Group 6

No damage was detected after 50 cycles of heat sterilization in the autoclave, and there was no corrosion or alteration of the laser markings (Figure 12). No differences were observed between the different disinfection liquid immersions (glutaraldehyde and hydrogen peroxide). The black notches that showed the depth and the numbers printed on the drill shanks were intact and showed no signs of damage.

The spectroscopic analysis of the drill surface showed no change in the surface composition.

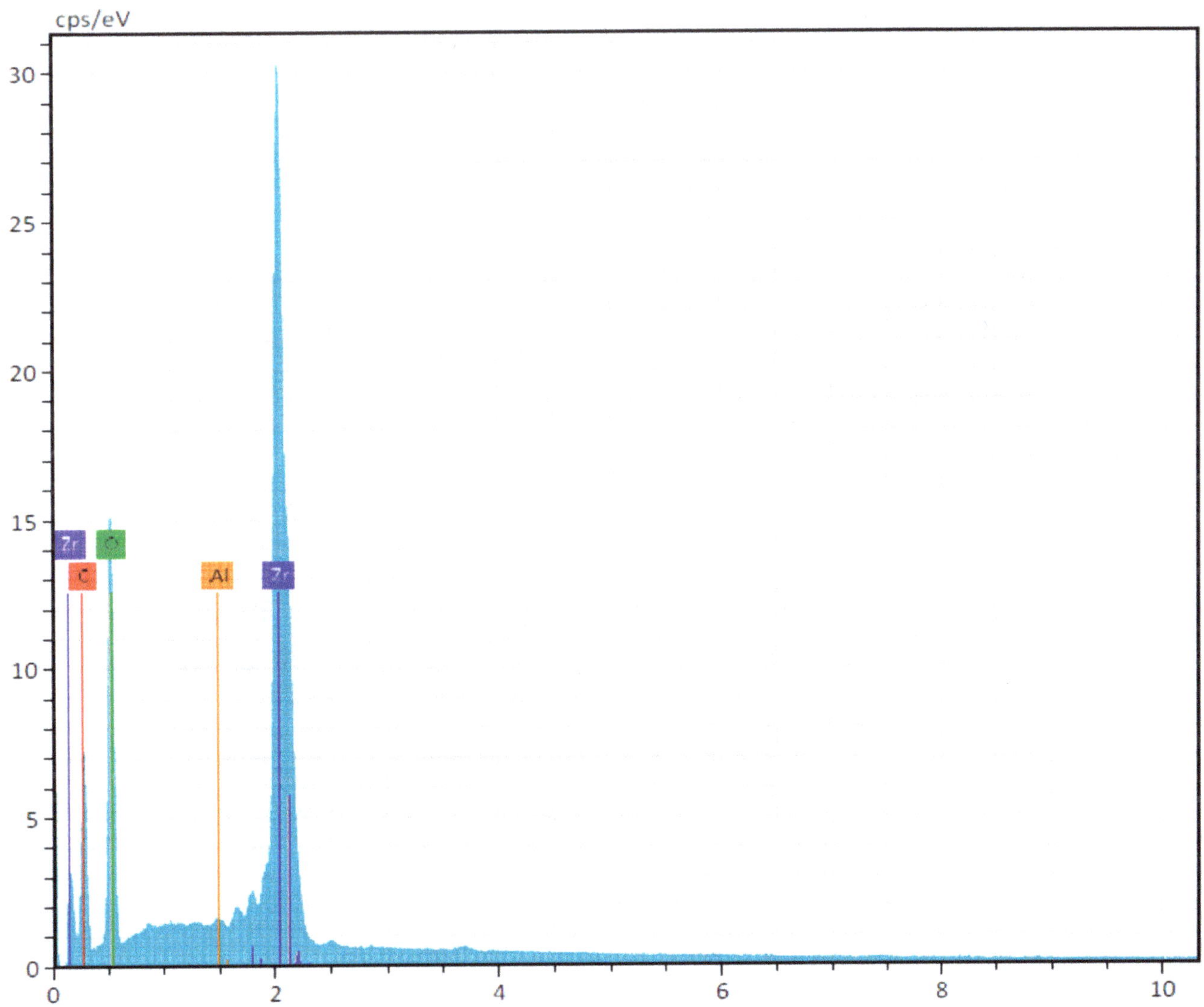

Figure 9. The spectroscopic analysis of the new zirconia drill surface showed that the flat area of implant drills was mainly composed of zirconia.

Figure 10. Group 4. The zirconia drill viewed under a scanning electron microscope after 50 disinfection cycles with glutaraldehyde. Sharp margins are free from defects.

Figure 11. Group 5. The zirconia drill after 50 disinfection cycles with hydrogen peroxide, where no damage was observed on the cutting edges or deposits of other substances.

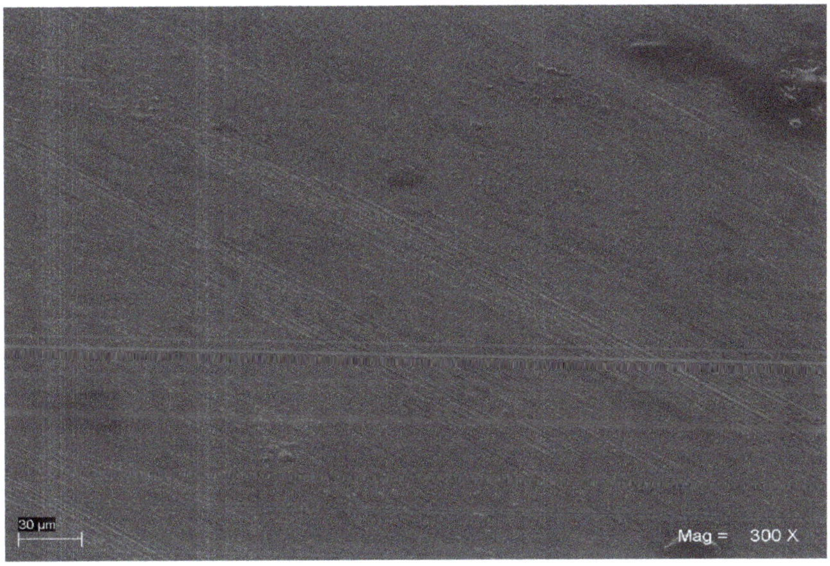

Figure 12. Group 6. After 50 steam autoclave cycles, no areas of corrosion were observed.

Table 1. Summary of the drills surface area damaged by the testing processes. The disinfection processes generated significant surface corrosion compared to the zirconia drills ($p < 0.01$). The autoclave sterilization did not cause any alteration to the different drill surfaces.

	STEEL DRILLS			ZIRCONIA DRILLS		
	Group I *(6 drills)*	**Group II** *(6 drills)*	**Group III** *(6 drills)*	**Group IV** *(6 drills)*	**Group V** *(6 drills)*	**Group VI** *(6 drills)*
Mean	21% **	12% **	No Damage **	No Damage **	No Damage **	No Damage **
SD	±3%	±2%	–	–	–	–

** $p < 0.01$.

3.3. *Statistical Analysis*

The SEM results showed the drill surface covered by damage and corrosion percentages for the steel drill. A statistically significant difference was found in the percentage of drill surface covered by damage and corrosion on the zirconia drill compared to the steel implant drills ($p = 0.000034$) (Figure 13).

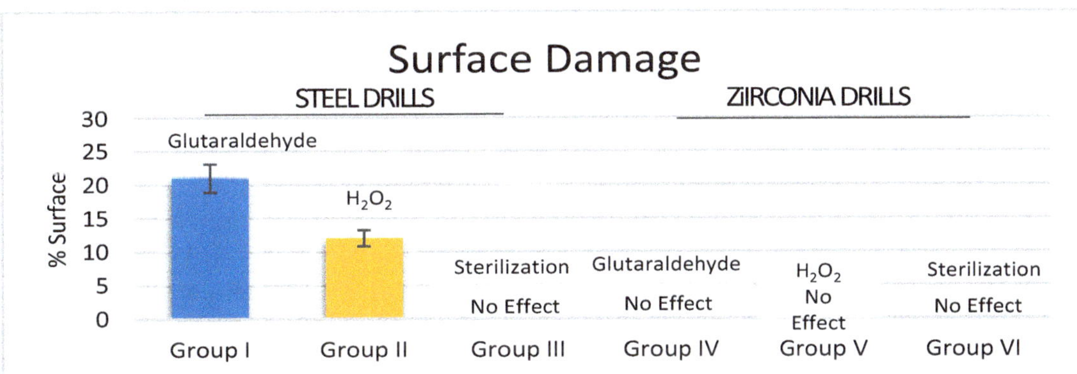

Figure 13. Differences in surface alteration occurred in the different study groups.

4. Discussion

In clinical practice, it is important to avoid cross-infection and it is for this reason that the drills should be treated with disinfectant chemicals, thoroughly rinsed, and submitted to autoclave heat sterilization.

In this study, we used two different disinfection chemicals, namely glutaraldehyde and hydrogen peroxide, which both provide high-level disinfection. The outcomes of the present research showed that zirconia drills are more resistant to the corrosive action of disinfecting chemicals. In fact, a greater difference was found in the percentages of drill covered by surface damage. SEM analysis demonstrated that repeated autoclave sterilization cycles had no effect on the zirconia and steel drills.

The purpose of the present investigation was to study the influence of disinfection and sterilization on the implant drill surfaces. The authors hypothesized that zirconia drills may offer a greater resistance to the action of disinfectants commonly used in clinical practice.

The contact with contaminated surfaces produces destructive hydroxyl free radicals that can attack DNA, membrane lipids, and other essential cell components. Glutaraldehyde is a saturated dialdehyde that has gained wide acceptance as a high-level disinfectant and chemical sterilant [14]. Aqueous solutions of glutaraldehyde are "activated" by using alkalinating agents to bring the pH to values between 7.5 and 8.5, which makes the solution sporicidal [15,16]. Glutaraldehyde (GAA) solutions are used for the sterilization of medical devices, such as endoscopes and fibroscopes. Hydrogen peroxide has good bactericidal, sporicidal, viricidal, and fungicidal properties [17]. However, both glutaraldehyde and hydrogen peroxide are corrosive to steel instruments.

Implant drills are reusable medical devices and implant bed preparation with drills is an invasive procedure involving contact of the drill with blood, bone, and other biological fluids. The major risk of all such procedures is the introduction of drill particles and transfer of pathogens, potentially leading to infection [18]. The main objective of disinfecting or sterilizing drills is to eliminate the transmission of pathogens by means of contaminated medical and surgical devices (e.g., HIV, HCV, *Mycobacterium tuberculosis*, and encephalopathies) [19,20]. Today, the disinfection of medical devices such as implant drills is very important for preventing the emergence of transmissible spongiform, such as the encephalopathies (TSEs), which is a prion protein less susceptible to denaturation by heat and is responsible for disease such as variant Creutzfeldt–Jakob [21]. Therefore, the predicable cleaning of implant drills is believed to be a key procedure for reducing the risks of onward transmission of infectious diseases and pathogens such as human immunodeficiency virus (HIV), hepatitis B and C, gram-negative and gram-positive bacteria, fungi, and preventing the risk of mycobacteria transmission. In addition to microbial inactivation, the removal of organic or inorganic debris is crucial as it may compromise subsequent disinfection or sterilization processes [22]. The cleaning of reusable implant drills is also important in order to ensure drill longevity and efficiency in cutting bone, also making the removal of organic and chemical residues important. The effect of liquid chemical sterilant depends on cleaning to eliminate organic and inorganic material, an optimal pH, concentration, contact time, and temperature are all paramount. During chemical disinfection, it is important that implant drills are not mixed with other drills, or other instruments of different material composition in order to avoid chemical corrosion. In this study, once chemical disinfection was completed, we proceeded to heat sterilization at 134 °C (273 °F) for 35 min.

It is known that the effect of disinfectants and sterilization can influence the cutting efficiency of drills [5,23]. The material that constitutes an osteotomy drill must also have a good resistance to corrosion, which is one of the factors responsible for the loss of cutting efficiency. The drills used for the preparation of implant sites must undergo decontamination and sterilization procedures before being reused on another patient. After every use, reusable medical devices must be rinsed, cleaned, and immediately immersed in an approved medical grade chemical disinfectant with a recognized effectiveness against HIV in accordance with Italian legislation art. 2 Ministerial Decree 28.09.90 [24]. The Ministerial Decree (DMS) imposes a set of rules for the protection of professionals from a broad range of infections in public and private health and care facilities. The objectives of these precautions are to prevent the transmission of pathogenic organisms through blood and biological fluids. The cleansing occurs as a result of the chemical actions of a detergent that must be used at recommended concentrations and contact times. It is necessary to frequently renew the solution in order to avoid the accumulation of debris and contamination, which both decrease the detergent efficacy.

Implant surgical procedures expose patients, surgeons, and staff to potential cross-infections if carried out without a series of cleaning and sterilization procedures aimed at preventing the spread of pathogens. Bone drills are classified as critical surgical objects according to the classification proposed by E.H. Spaulding [25] and from the DMS dated 28/9/90 as instruments that come in contact with bleeding tissues and body fluids. For this reason, implantology drills must also be subjected to decontamination and cleaning procedures using chemical substances before proceeding to heat sterilization with saturated steam in an autoclave. All these procedures and protocols can alter the cutting efficiency, as well as deteriorate the depth marks printed on the drills, thereby altering the references that the surgeon has during surgery to check the working depth of the osteotomy. The reduction in cutting efficiency has considerable repercussions for the preparation of the implant site because a loss of sharpness and cutting efficiency of the drill results in a large part of the cutting energy being transformed into heat. The consequences manifest themselves as poor organization of the clot, delayed healing, and poor quality of the tissues that form at the bone–implant interface [18,26]. As reported previously in another study [18], implant osteotomy drills can be reused up to 50 times since their loss of sharpness is directly proportional to the number of osteotomies made.

Chemical detergents can cause metal corrosion with alteration of the cutting edge of the drill blades, which is a process that can worsen when the drills are submitted to saturated steam sterilization. In the literature, there are several articles that have studied the degree of wear of osteotomy drills in relation to their reuse [26,27]. On the other hand, there is no published work investigating the problem of chemical decontamination or metal release in the bone from surgical drills. In the present work, we chose to separately study the effect on bone drills of the two different chemical agents and the effect of autoclave sterilization in order to understand which of these aspects of bone instrument care is the most critical and potentially damaging to the drills.

We observed that all the disinfectants used were found to be potentially harmful to steel drills, causing corrosion zones that worsened after each decontamination cycle, while the zirconia drills did not show any structural damage, and the depth marks were preserved and remained clearly visible. No damage was observed for the steel and zirconia drills when they were only subjected to autoclave sterilization cycles. The results of the present study provide practical and valuable information that can help conserve the cutting efficiency of the drills by preventing metal release and overheating of the bone, both of which can increase the chances of implant failure [28].

Identifying factors and mechanisms with regards to implant failures should not be limited to the implants, but should also include the host and the drills. Drills are one of the main components of an implant procedure and play an important role in the success of an implant procedure [29,30]. Therefore, it is of primary importance to identify critical factors and develop appropriate therapies and prevention strategies. It is extremely useful to know the histopathology (macroscopic and microscopic aspects of the disease), the pathogenesis (source of the disease), and the physiopathology (mechanism of the disease) of the complications of implant failures, as well as changes in the structure of the bone drills during the processes of decontamination, cleaning, and sterilization.

From the results observed during this study, it is clear that the disinfectants used in clinical practice are potentially harmful to steel drills by contributing to corrosion of their surfaces and the loss of cutting efficiency.

5. Conclusions

The present study demonstrates that repeated immersions of steel drills in disinfecting chemical agents result in corrosion on the surface of steel drills. Conversely, these chemicals do not have any effect on zirconia ceramic drills, proving their inertness and structural stability, even in the harshest environment. Autoclave sterilization cycles have no effect on any of the drills. Cleansing, sterilization, and maintenance of the drills are crucially important for patients' health and protection, but also for the drills' long-term durability and performance. It can be concluded that zirconia ceramic drills offer a surface that is not affected by disinfecting liquids. The fact that zirconia is immune to corrosion attack eliminates the possibility of the release of microparticles and ions in the peri-implant tissue during osteotomy, thus minimizing the chance of aseptic osteolysis [31].

Author Contributions: Conceptualization, A.S.; data curation, A.S.; formal analysis, S.N. and S.G.; investigation, A.S.; methodology, A.S.; project administration, A.S.; software, F.L. and P.S.; supervision, P.S.; F.I.; validation, A.S., S.N., F.I., and S.G.; visualization, P.S. and F.L.; writing—original draft, A.S.; writing—review and editing, S.N.

References

1. Scarano, A.; Piattelli, A.; Quaranta, A.; Lorusso, F. Bone Response to Two Dental Implants with Different Sandblasted/Acid-Etched Implant Surfaces: A Histological and Histomorphometrical Study in Rabbits. *BioMed Res. Int.* **2017**, *2017*, 8724951. [CrossRef] [PubMed]
2. Eriksson, A.; Albrektsson, T. Temperature threshold levels for heat-induced bone tissue injury: A vital-microscopic study in the rabbit. *J. Prosthet. Dent.* **1983**, *50*, 101–107. [CrossRef]
3. Scarano, A.; Carinci, F.; Lorusso, F.; Festa, F.; Bevilacqua, L.; Santos de Oliveira, P.; Maglione, M. Ultrasonic vs Drill Implant Site Preparation: Post-Operative Pain Measurement through VAS, Swelling and Crestal Bone Remodeling: A Randomized Clinical Study. *Materials* **2018**, *11*, 2516. [CrossRef] [PubMed]
4. Eriksson, R.; Adell, R. Temperatures during drilling for the placement of implants using the osseointegration technique. *J. Oral Maxillofac. Surg.* **1986**, *44*, 4–7. [CrossRef]
5. Scarano, A.; Di Carlo, F.; Piattelli, A. Effect of sterilization and cleansing on implantology drills: Zirconia vs steel. *Ital. Oral Surg.* **2008**, *3*, 61–72.
6. Hochscheidt, C.J.; Shimizu, R.H.; Andrighetto, A.R.; Pierezan, R.; Thomé, G.; Salatti, R. Comparative Analysis of Cutting Efficiency and Surface Maintenance between Different Types of Implant Drills: An In Vitro Study. *Implant Dent.* **2017**, *26*, 723–729. [CrossRef] [PubMed]
7. Hein, C.; Inceoglu, S.; Juma, D.; Zuckerman, L. Heat Generation during Bone Drilling: A Comparison between Industrial and Orthopaedic Drill Bits. *J. Orthop. Trauma* **2017**, *31*, e55–e59. [CrossRef] [PubMed]
8. Louropoulou, A.; Slot, D.E.; Van der Weijden, F.A. Titanium surface alterations following the use of different mechanical instruments: A systematic review. *Clin. Oral Implant. Res.* **2012**, *23*, 643–658. [CrossRef]
9. Noumbissi, S.; Scarano, A.; Gupta, S. A Literature Review Study on Atomic Ions Dissolution of Titanium and Its Alloys in Implant Dentistry. *Materials* **2019**, *12*, 368. [CrossRef]
10. Dubruille, J.H.; Viguier, E.; Le Naour, G.; Dubruille, M.T.; Auriol, M.; Le Charpentier, Y. Evaluation of combinations of titanium, zirconia, and alumina implants with 2 bone fillers in the dog. *Int. J. Oral Maxillofac. Implant.* **1999**, *14*, 271–277.
11. Scarano, A.; Di Carlo, F.; Quaranta, M.; Piattelli, A. Bone Response to Zirconia Ceramic Implants: An Experimental Study in Rabbits. *J. Oral Implant.* **2003**, *29*, 8–12. [CrossRef]
12. Jackson, M.C. Restoration of posterior implants using a new ceramic material. *J. Dent. Technol.* **1999**, *16*, 19–22. [PubMed]
13. Spinelli, M.; Maccauro, G.; Graci, C.; Cittadini, A.; Magnani, G.; Sangiorgi, S.; Del Bravo, V.; Manicone, P.; Raffaelli, L.; Muratori, F.; et al. Zirconia Toughened Alumina (ZTA) Powders: Ultrastructural and Histological Analysis. *Int. J. Immunopathol. Pharmacol.* **2011**, *24*, 153–156. [CrossRef] [PubMed]
14. Lin, W.; Niu, B.; Yi, J.; Deng, Z.; Song, J.; Chen, Q. Toxicity and Metal Corrosion of Glutaraldehyde-Didecyldimethylammonium Bromide as a Disinfectant Agent. *BioMed Res. Int.* **2018**, *2018*, 9814209. [CrossRef] [PubMed]
15. Urayama, S.; Kozarek, R.A.; Sumida, S.; Raltz, S.; Merriam, L.; Pethigal, P. Mycobacteria and glutaraldehyde: Is high-level disinfection of endoscopes possible? *Gastrointest. Endosc.* **1996**, *43*, 451–456. [CrossRef]
16. Chenjiao, W.; HongYan, Z.; Qing, G.; Xiaoqi, Z.; Liying, G.; Ying, F. In-Use Evaluation of Peracetic Acid for High-Level Disinfection of Endoscopes. *Gastroenterol. Nurs.* **2016**, *39*, 116–120. [PubMed]

17. Omidbakhsh, N.; Sattar, S.A. Broad-spectrum microbicidal activity, toxicologic assessment, and materials compatibility of a new generation of accelerated hydrogen peroxide-based environmental surface disinfectant. *Am. J. Infect. Control* **2006**, *34*, 251–257. [CrossRef]
18. Scarano, A.; Carinci, F.; Quaranta, A.; Di Iorio, D.; Assenza, B.; Piattelli, A. Effects of Bur Wear during Implant Site Preparation: An in Vitro Study. *Int. J. Immunopathol. Pharmacol.* **2007**, *20*, 23–26. [CrossRef]
19. Bagg, J.; Smith, A.J.; Hurrell, D.; McHugh, S.; Irvine, G. Pre-sterilisation cleaning of re-usable instruments in general dental practice. *Br. Dent. J.* **2007**, *202*, E22. [CrossRef]
20. Laheij, A.M.G.A.; Kistler, J.O.; Belibasakis, G.N.; Välimaa, H.; de Soet, J.J.; European Oral Microbiology Workshop (EOMW) 2011. Healthcare-associated viral and bacterial infections in dentistry. *J. Oral Microbiol.* **2012**, *4*. [CrossRef]
21. Bourgeois, D.; Dussart, C.; Saliasi, I.; Laforest, L.; Tramini, P.; Carrouel, F. Observance of Sterilization Protocol Guideline Procedures of Critical Instruments for Preventing Iatrogenic Transmission of Creutzfeldt-Jakob Disease in Dental Practice in France, 2017. *Int. J. Environ. Res. Public Health* **2018**, *15*, 853. [CrossRef] [PubMed]
22. Douet, J.Y.; Lacroux, C.; Aron, N.; Head, M.W.; Lugan, S.; Tillier, C.; Huor, A.; Cassard, H.; Arnold, M.; Beringue, V.; et al. Distribution and Quantitative Estimates of Variant Creutzfeldt-Jakob Disease Prions in Tissues of Clinical and Asymptomatic Patients. *Emerg. Infect. Dis.* **2017**, *23*, 946–956. [CrossRef] [PubMed]
23. Scarano, A.; Assenza, B.; Di Iorio, D.; Quaranta, A. Effect of sterilization and cleansing on implantology drills. *Ital. Oral Surg.* **2008**, *2*, 4–13.
24. Ministero della Sanità. *Norme di Protezione dal Contagio Professionale da HIV Nelle Strutture Sanitarie e Assistenziali Pubbliche e Private*; Ministero della Sanità: Rome, Italy, 1990.
25. Spaulding, E.H. Chemical disinfection and antisepsis in the hospital. *J. Hosp. Res.* **1972**, *9*, 5–31.
26. Tehemar, S.H. Factors affecting heat generation during implant site preparation: A review of biologic observations and future considerations. *Int. J. Oral Maxillofac. Implant.* **1999**, *14*, 127–136.
27. Rutala, W.A.; Weber, D.J. Disinfection, sterilization, and antisepsis: An overview. *Am. J. Infect. Control* **2016**, *44*, e1–e6. [CrossRef] [PubMed]
28. Scarano, A.; Piattelli, A.; Assenza, B.; Carinci, F.; Di Donato, L.; Romani, G.L.; Merla, A. Infrared thermographic evaluation of temperature modifications induced during implant site preparation with cylindrical versus conical drills. *Clin. Implant Dent. Relat. Res.* **2011**, *13*, 319–323. [CrossRef] [PubMed]
29. Sridhar, S.; Wilson, T.G.; Valderrama, P.; Watkins-Curry, P.; Chan, J.Y.; Rodrigues, D.C. In Vitro Evaluation of Titanium Exfoliation during Simulated Surgical Insertion of Dental Implants. *J. Oral Implant.* **2016**, *42*, 34–40. [CrossRef]
30. Scarano, A.; Piattelli, A.; Polimeni, A.; Di Iorio, D.; Carinci, F. Bacterial Adhesion on Commercially Pure Titanium and Anatase-Coated Titanium Healing Screws: An In Vivo Human Study. *J. Periodontol.* **2010**, *81*, 1466–1471. [CrossRef]
31. Scarano, A.; Cholakis, A.; Piattelli, A. Histologic Evaluation of Sinus Grafting Materials after Peri-implantitis–Induced Failure: A Case Series. *Int. J. Oral Maxillofac. Implant.* **2017**, *32*, e36–e75. [CrossRef]

8

Comparative Study of the use of Different Sizes of an Ergonomic Instrument Handle for Laparoscopic Surgery

Juan A. Sánchez-Margallo [1,*], Alfonso González González [2], Lorenzo García Moruno [3], J. Carlos Gómez-Blanco [1], J. Blas Pagador [1] and Francisco M. Sánchez-Margallo [4]

1 Bioengineering and Health Technologies Unit, Jesús Usón Minimally Invasive Surgery Centre, 10071 Cáceres, Spain; jcgomez@ccmijesususon.com (J.C.G.-B.); jbpagador@ccmijesususon.com (J.B.P.)
2 Department of Mechanical, Energy, and Materials Engineering, University of Extremadura, 06800 Mérida, Spain; agg@unex.es
3 Department of Graphical Expression, University of Extremadura, 06800 Mérida, Spain; lgmoruno@unex.es
4 Scientific Direction, Jesús Usón Minimally Invasive Surgery Centre, 10071 Cáceres, Spain; msanchez@ccmijesususon.com
* Correspondence: jasanchez@ccmijesususon.com

Abstract: Previous studies have shown that the handle design of laparoscopic instruments is crucial to surgical performance and surgeon's ergonomics. In this study, four different sizes of an ergonomic laparoscopic handle design were tested in a blind and randomized fashion with twelve surgeons. They performed three laparoscopic tasks in order to analyze the influence of handle size. Execution time, wrist posture, and finger and palm pressure were evaluated during the performance of each task. The results show a significant reduction in the time required to complete the eye-manual coordination task using the appropriate handle. The incorrectly sized handle resulted in a rise in palm pressure and a reduction in the force exerted by the thumb during the transfer task. In the hand-eye coordination task, the use of the right handle size led to an increase in middle finger pressure. In general, surgeons had an ergonomically adequate wrist flexion in all tasks and an acceptable radio-ulnar deviation during the transfer task using the ergonomic instrument handle. Surgeons found it comfortable the use of the ergonomic handle. Therefore, the use of an appropriately sized instrument handle allows surgeons to improve ergonomics and surgical performance during the laparoscopic practice.

Keywords: laparoscopy; instrument handle; ergonomics; hand pressure; wrist posture; parametric design

---

1. Introduction

Laparoscopic surgery has become a standard procedure instead of open approach for many surgical interventions and it is widely used in health services around the world. This rising interest in laparoscopy is based on several benefits, such as better surgical outcomes for patients and resource optimization for healthcare services [1]. Furthermore, this surgical technique has constantly evolved over the past few years, mainly due to training efforts of surgeons [2–4] and technological advances of surgical equipment [5]. However, there are some important technical limitations that should be addressed in order to increase both performance and wellbeing of surgeons: reduced freedom of movements due to the fixed location of the surgical ports, the need for high precision through long instruments, loss of tactile feedback (no direct touch of intracorporeal anatomical structures), and the use of bidimensional vision instead of real stereoscopic (3D) vision. The combination of these features of laparoscopy makes it difficult for surgeons to achieve hand-eye coordination, depth perception and performance of certain intracorporeal maneuvers, resulting in prolonged forced postures and the consequent impairment of surgeons' performance and precision and the potential onset of musculoskeletal disorders [6]. In order to overcome some of these problems, ergonomic criteria should be applied to both patients and surgeons [7,8]. In this respect, an important field of application of ergonomics for surgeons is the improvement of surgical equipment and tools, as well as its adaptation to the surgeon's needs. The design of ergonomically better surgical tools would reduce the surgeon's muscle fatigue and other associated diseases [9], with the potential improvement of the surgical performance [7]. This results in enhanced patient safety and surgical results.

In view of the above, an ergonomic laparoscopic instrument handle has been designed and developed in previous studies [10,11]. This new surgical tool follows the design criteria for universal objects named "Design for All" criteria [12]. These criteria were included in the Universal Design guide that enumerates the seven principles of a universal design [13]. One of these principles is to facilitate "flexibility in use" so that most people could use the designed products [14,15]. In this regard, hand tools must meet these design criteria in order to overcome obstacles such as age, gender, psychomotor skills or laterality.

An important challenge to be dealt with is to ensure a consistent tool design, both in shape and dimensions, for a specific functionality [16]. Stoklasek et al. demonstrated the onset of pain and discomfort after long use of hand tools with a poor ergonomic design that eventually led to fingers' numbness and, in some cases, paresthesia [17]. Additionally, anthropometric dimensions of hand tools is another fundamental design aspect. Hand size is a critical factor for precision tools, specifically in laparoscopic instruments [18]. Surgeons with small or large hands often have problems gripping laparoscopic tools, mainly because of the size or shape of the instrument handle. For this reason, they sometimes have to grip these instrument handles in a different way to that the designers intended [18]. It is important to note that laparoscopic surgical tools are commonly sold in a standard size [19–21].

Specifically, the opening and closing mechanisms of surgical instruments present complications for surgeons with large and small hands. Surgeons with small hands often have difficulties in using instruments with a bigger size than the ideal one, mainly for instruments with a power grip [16]. For this reason, several studies have focused on addressing this problem by analyzing the opening and closing system of laparoscopic instruments [22], force applied during its use [23], hand and fingers kinematics [24,25], and EMG activity during the laparoscopic practice [26–28]. Changes in the handle design of laparoscopic instruments have been shown to affect localized muscle fatigue, mainly in the muscle groups of the surgeons' forearms [6,29–31].

Therefore, the objective of this work is to carry out a blind study to analyze the effects of different sizes of the ergonomic design of a laparoscopic handle on the surgeon's ergonomics and surgical performance. This will be done by comparing the use of a handle that is the appropriate size for the surgeon's hand with one that is the wrong size. The study will be carried out during the performance of various basic training tasks for laparoscopic surgery.

2. Materials and Methods

2.1. Description of the New Hhandle Design

Figure 1 shows a functional prototype of the patented laparoscopic instrument handle (EP10382362) used to carry out this study. This intellectual property resulted from the ERGOLAP project (Obtaining Criteria for Ergonomic Design of Laparoscopic Surgery Instruments. DPI2007-65902-C03-03) developed by the University of Extremadura (UEX), Jesús Usón Minimally Invasive Surgery Centre (JUMISC) and Institute of Biomechanics of Valencia (IBV). This novel instrument handle design is mainly characterized by a power grip that keeps the precision of movements. The parameters of the laparoscopic instrument handle design in relation to the anthropometry of the surgeon's hand are described in [10,11]. This design provides the surgeon with a neutral posture of the wrist thanks to the wide contact surface between the palm and the handle, promoting the reduction in fatigue and possible associated musculoskeletal disorders.

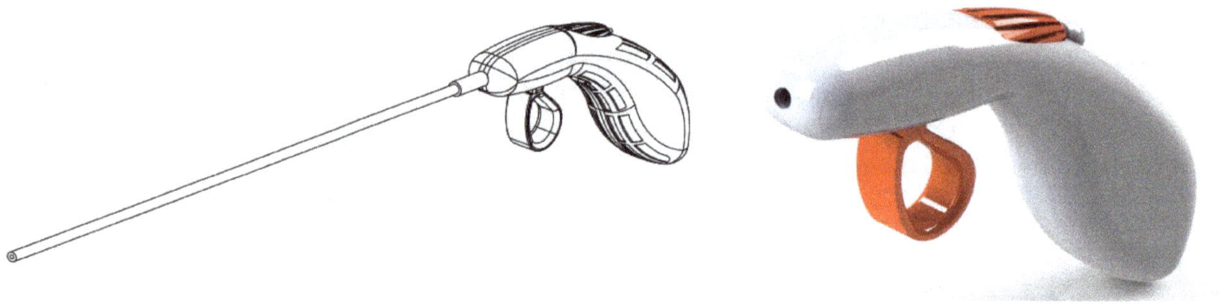

Figure 1. Design of the laparoscopic instrument handle (patent EP2471473A1) developed in the ERGOLAP project.

Additionally, the parametric 3D CAD design allowed us to easily scale the model to fit different hand sizes in an ergonomic way using the Palm Length Measured (PLM) [11]. Therefore, four different sizes (XS, S, M and L) (Figure 2) were 3D printed for this study following the specifications defined in previous studies [10,11].

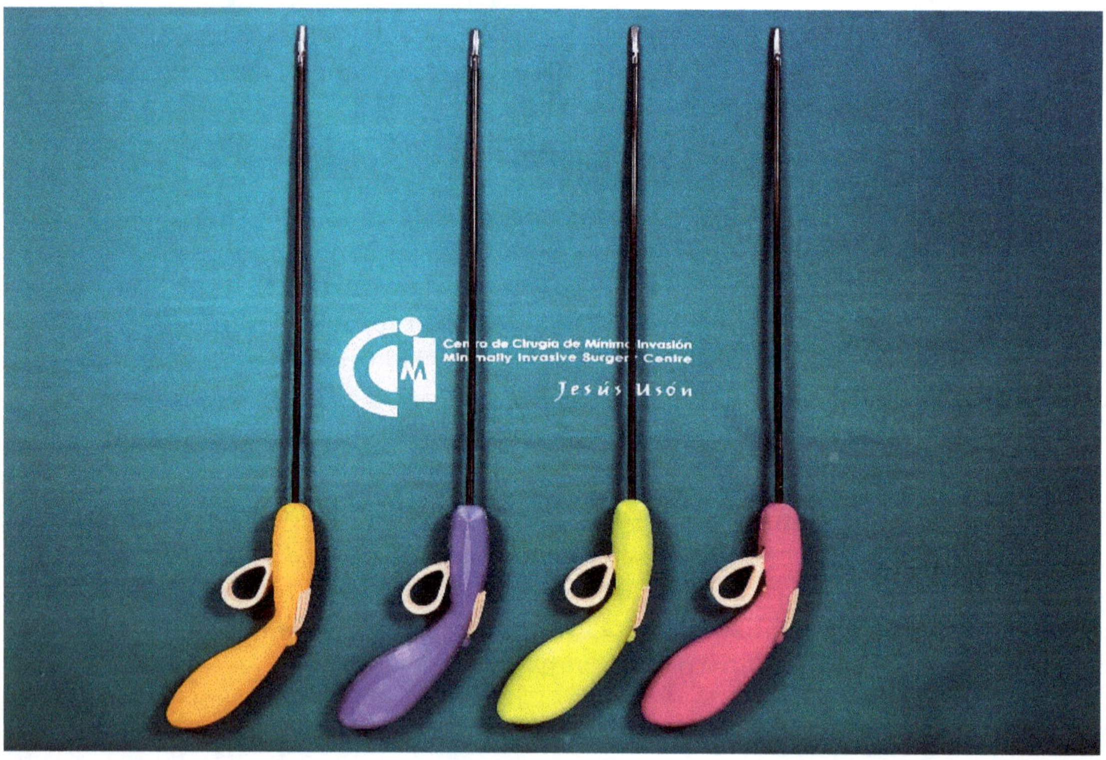

Figure 2. Prototypes of the handles for laparoscopic instruments developed. The sizes of the handles, from left to right, are XS, S, M and L.

2.2. Development of the Prototypes

As described above, the four instrument handles were 3D printed with PLA using a Prusa Original MK3 MMUS2.5 (Prusa Research s.r.o., Prague, Czech Republic), together with the triggers to control the opening and closing of the instrument tip and the wheels to rotate it. In order to obtain fully functional prototypes, these components were mounted on the internal mechanism of a standard laparoscopic forceps. This allows surgeons to test these new handle designs during the execution of conventional laparoscopic tasks.

2.3. *Participants*

Twelve surgeons participated in this study. Two surgeons were left-handed. All participants performed the tasks using the new design of the instrument handle with their dominant hand and a conventional laparoscopic instrument with their non-dominant hand. Four participants were novice surgeons (<10 laparoscopic procedures performed), 5 had an intermediate level of experience in laparoscopic surgery (between 10 and 100 laparoscopic procedures) and 3 were experienced surgeons (>100 laparoscopic procedures).

2.4. *Tasks*

At the beginning of the study, the size category (XS, S, M and L) of each participant's hand was identified using a template. Each task was performed using both an instrument handle with the correct size for the surgeon and a handle with a difference of two sizes (wrong size) in a blind and randomized fashion. The type of laparoscopic instrument used with both the left and right hands to perform the activities was grasping forceps. For this study, participants were asked to perform three different basic laparoscopic tasks on a physical simulator (SIMULAP®; CCMIJU, Cáceres, Spain) with a 10-mm, 30-degree rigid laparoscope (Karl Storz GmbH & Co. KG, Tuttlingen, Germany) as the vision system (Figure 3). The height of the table and monitor were adapted to the comfort needs of each participant and the laparoscopic camera was fixed to prevent movements during the execution of the tasks. Surgeons were given a brief explanation of how to operate the controls on the new instrument handle (trigger and wheel). Since the study was randomized, participants received no training period with the instrument in order to prevent them from being familiar with a specific handle size and thus avoid possible bias.

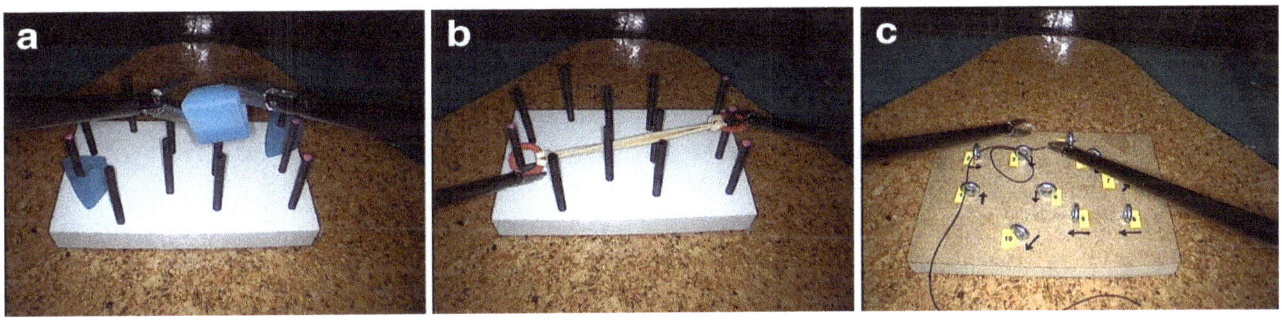

Figure 3. Tasks: (**a**) Hand-eye coordination, (**b**) coordinated traction and (**c**) transfer task (labyrinth).

2.4.1. Hand-Eye Coordination

To perform this task, participants were asked to grasp three colored objects from one side of the pegboard with their closest hand, transfer the object mid-air to their opposite hand, and place the object on a peg on the other side of the pegboard (Figure 3a). Once all three objects had been transferred, the process was reversed.

2.4.2. Coordinated Traction

This task required the placement of an elastic band from a peg placed on one side of the pegboard to three other pegs on the other side, sequentially (Figure 3b). The starting peg was on the opposite side of the participant's dominant hand.

2.4.3. Transfer Task (Labyrinth)

Participants were asked to transfer a straight needle through a circuit of rings, distributed at different angles (Figure 3c). The needle was driven through the rings using the dominant hand and with the support of the non-dominant hand. The order of the rings and orientation of the needle driving were indicated with numbers and arrows on the pegboard, respectively.

2.5. Assessment

The execution time was recorded for each trial. In addition, ergonomic aspects of using the new instrument handle design during the execution of each task, such as wrist posture and pressure exerted on the instrument handle, were analyzed (Figure 4).

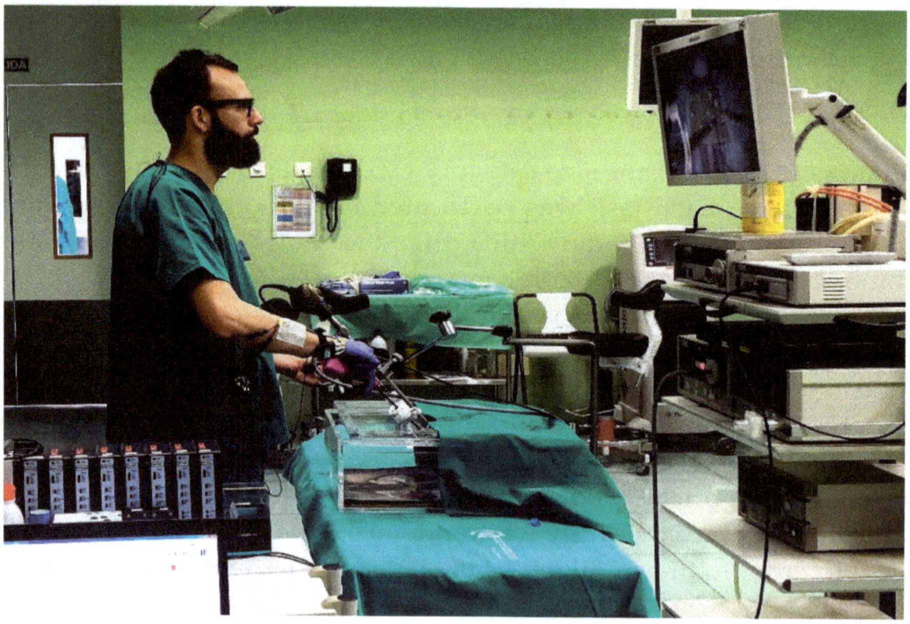

Figure 4. Setup of the study. A surgeon is performing the transfer task using an instrument handle with a size L.

2.5.1. Hand Pressure

To measure the fingers and hand pressure while using the instrument handle, the FingerTPS™ (Pressure Profile Systems, Inc., Hawthorne, CA, USA) wearable and wireless system was employed. In this study, a set of five sensors to record the pressure exerted by the surgeon's distal phalanges of the thumb and index, middle and ring fingers, as well as the palm, were used. The system was calibrated for each participant.

2.5.2. Wrist Posture

The flexion-extension and radio-ulnar deviation of the wrist were recorded using a dual-axis electrogoniometer (Biopac Systems, Inc., Goleta, CA, USA) attached to the surgeon's hand and forearm using medical adhesive tape. In order to measure both axes simultaneously, two DA100C amplifiers (Biopac Systems, Inc.) were used. This device was calibrated at the beginning of the study. The risk level of the wrist posture was determined by means of a modified version of the RULA (Rapid Upper Limb Assessment) method as described in [32]. Risk values were defined according to the wrist angle, with wrist flexion-extension and radio-ulnar deviation angles between −15° and 15° being considered ergonomically acceptable.

2.5.3. Subjective Assessment

At the end of each task, the participants were asked to complete a questionnaire to evaluate, using a visual scale from 1 to 10, the comfort of performing the task with each instrument handle used.

2.6. Statistical Analysis

For statistical analysis, the Wilcoxon signed rank test was used to compare the surgeons' performance and ergonomic data of both study groups (right and wrong instrument handle size).

All statistical analyses were carried out using R version 3.6.1 (R Foundation for Statistical Computing, Vienna, Austria). The results are shown as mean and standard deviation. For all tests, $p < 0.05$ was considered statistically significant.

3. Results

3.1. Execution Time

The surgeons required significantly less time to complete the hand-eye coordination task using the adequate size of instrument handle (Figure 5). The execution time was similar for the other tasks, regardless of the type of instrument handle used.

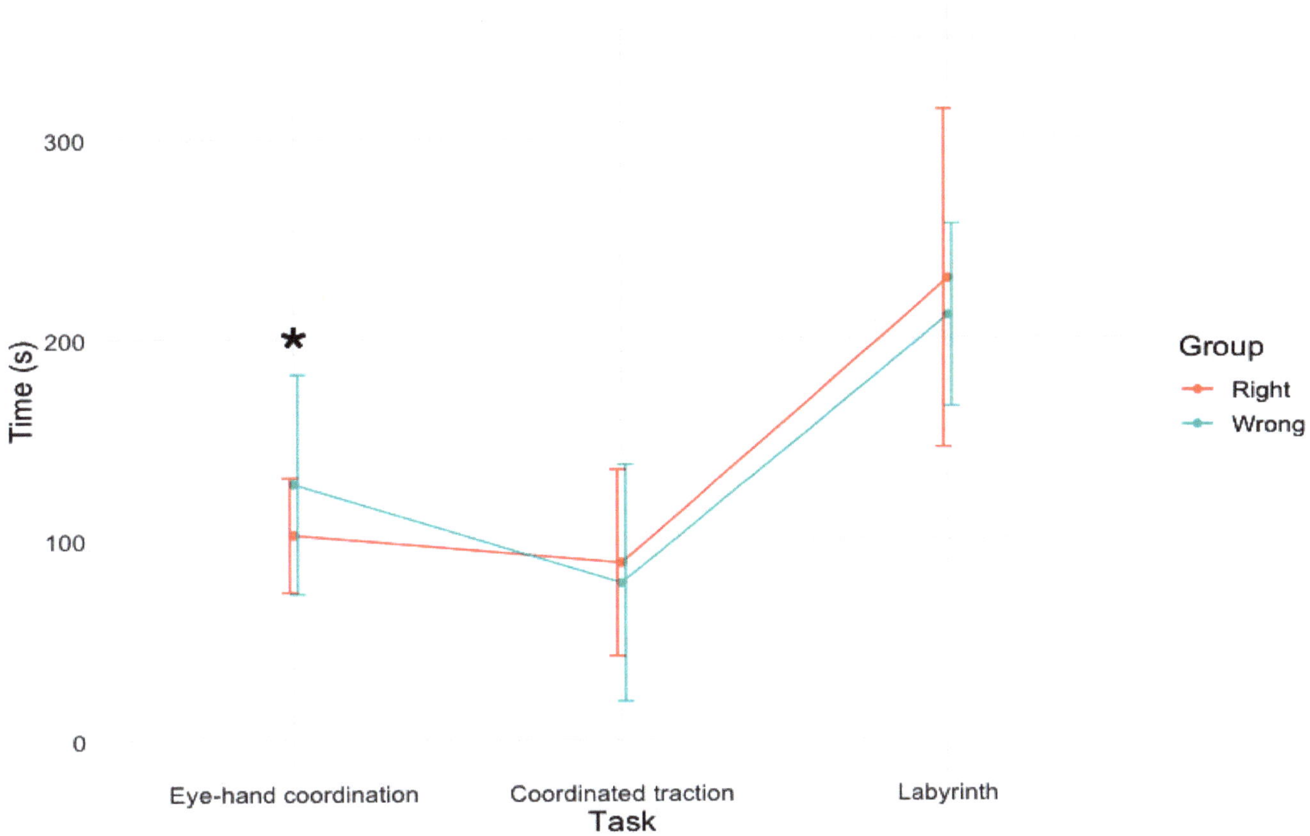

Figure 5. Execution time of the three laparoscopic tasks using the right and wrong instrument handle size. * $p < 0.05$.

3.2. Hand Pressure

There was a remarkable increase in palmar pressure on the wrong size instrument handle for the coordinated traction and transfer tasks compared to the right size handle, being statistically significant for the latter task (Figure 6). Using the right size of instrument handle led surgeons to apply more pressure with the thumb and middle fingers during the transfer and hand-eye coordination tasks, respectively, when compared to the use of the wrong size handle.

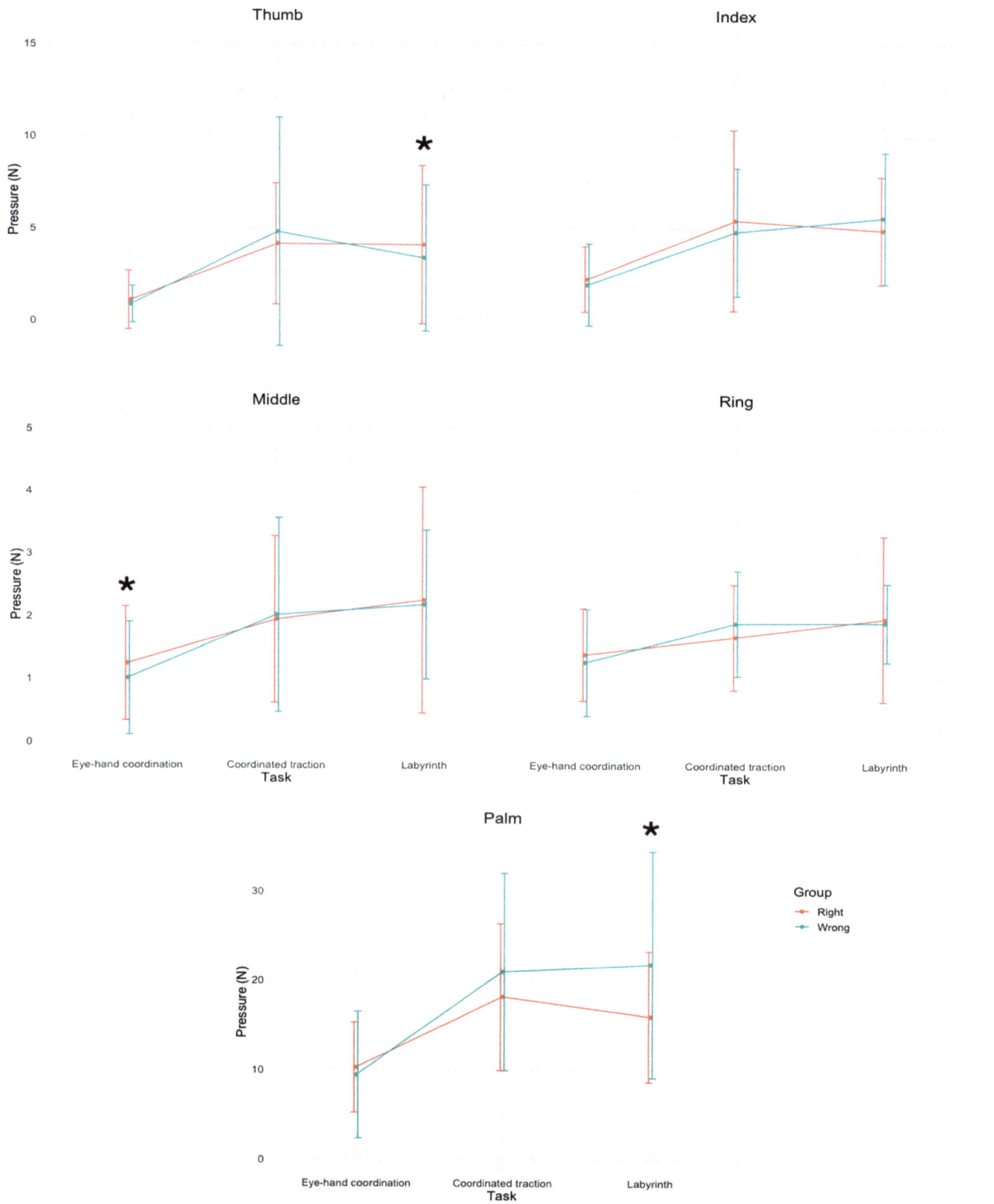

Figure 6. Pressure exerted by the surgeons' fingers (thumb, index, middle and ring fingers) and palm during the laparoscopic tasks using the right and wrong instrument handle size. The range of pressure values (y axis) has been adapted to each data set. * $p < 0.05$.

3.3. *Wrist Posture*

No statistically significant differences in wrist posture with each instrument handle were shown for any of the laparoscopic tasks (Figures 7 and 8). Regarding the wrist radio-ulnar deviation, the surgeons only obtained an ergonomically acceptable wrist posture, according to the criteria of RULA method, during the transfer task and for both sizes of instrument handle. In the case of wrist flexion-extension, both groups of handles led to an adequate posture of the wrist for all the tasks.

3.4. *Subjective Assessment*

The results from the questionnaires show that there were no statistically significant differences in the comfort of using the two different sizes of instrument handle for the three performed tasks (Figure 9).

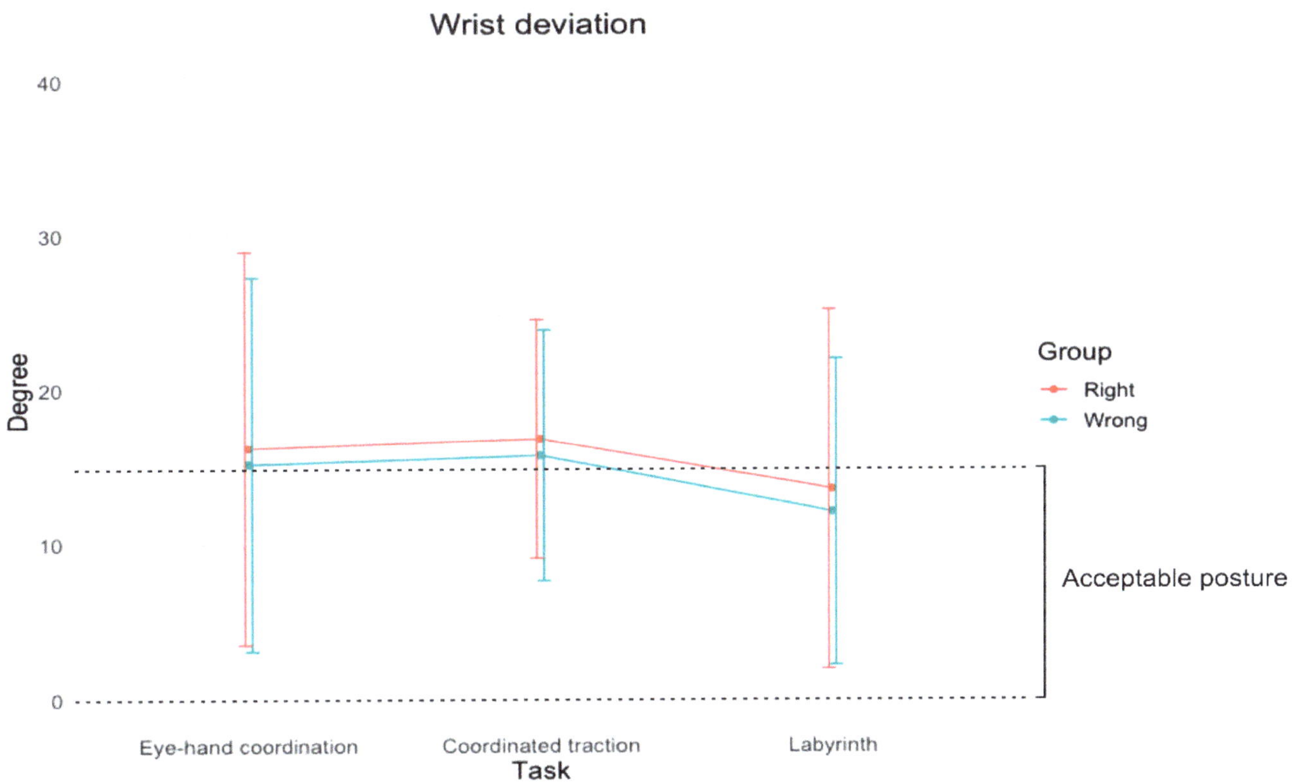

Figure 7. Radio-ulnar deviation of the surgeons' wrist during the laparoscopic tasks using the right and wrong size of instrument handle. The graph indicates the acceptable posture of the wrist according to RULA method.

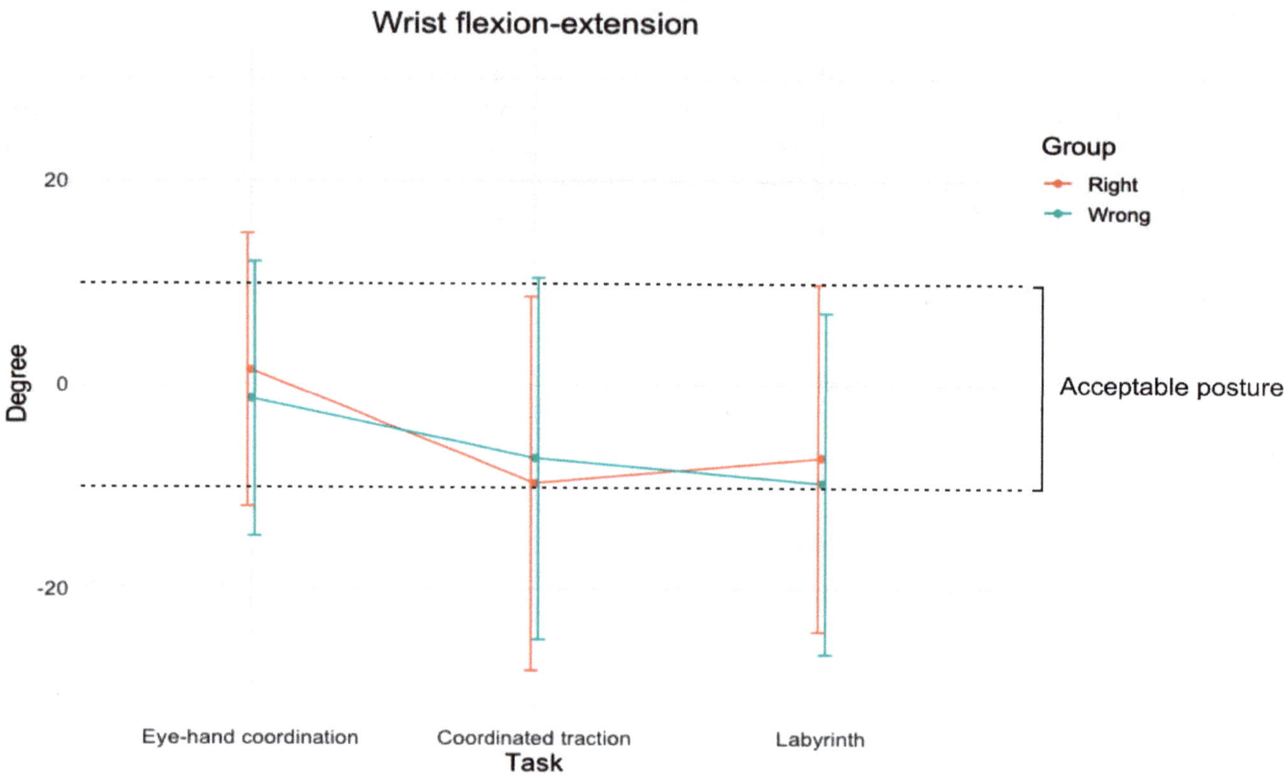

Figure 8. Flexion-extension of the surgeons' wrist during the laparoscopic tasks using the right and wrong size of instrument handle. The graph indicates the acceptable posture of the wrist according to RULA method.

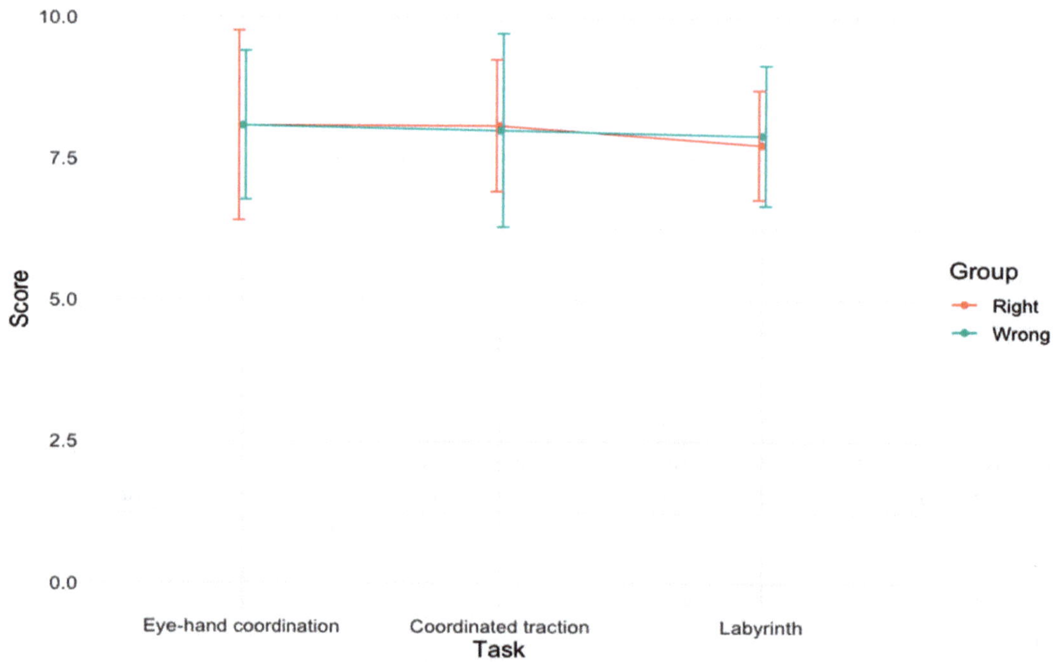

Figure 9. Results of the surgeons' evaluation regarding the comfort of performing each task using the two types of instrument handles.

4. Discussion

There are several studies in the scientific literature that confirm the need to improve the comfort and ergonomic criteria of instruments for laparoscopic surgery. The instrument handle is an essential part of laparoscopic instruments, whose inappropriate design can have a detrimental effect on the surgeon's efficiency and wellbeing [33]. The rate of work-related musculoskeletal disorders in laparoscopy are from 73% to 100%, with poor instrument handle design being one of the main risk factors [34,35]. In a survey by Santos-Carreras et al., they assessed the acceptance of different surgical instrument handle designs and they reported that conventional laparoscopic instrument handles such as the axial handle scored lowest in terms of comfort [36]. Other studies also indicated that axial handles require significantly more muscle activity than the other common types of instrument handle [37]. In this study, we have analyzed the relationship between the surgeons' ergonomics and performance and different sizes of a novel laparoscopic instrument handle design [11]. The results verify that the use of different instrument handle sizes has consequences on the surgeon's grip pressure and surgical skills.

It seems that the use of an adequate size of instrument handle helps hand-eye coordination and bimanual dexterity in the development of laparoscopic tasks, reducing the execution time, as shown by the results of this study. Tung et al. also presented an innovative laparoscopic handle design with a pistol grip attempting to address some of the ergonomic limitations in laparoscopic surgery [38]. Although the validation of this handle design was mainly subjective, they reported significantly shorter execution times in performing cutting and peg transfer tasks when compared to a conventional laparoscopic tool. However, execution time may not be a very meaningful assessment parameter in the case of the coordinated traction task. This task requires participants to exert a high degree of traction with the instruments and, therefore, to firmly the instrument handle. Due to the metal material of the rings, they sometimes slipped off the instrument tip, thus increasing the time required to complete the task, despite the surgeon's skills.

Regarding the pressure exerted by the surgeon's fingers and palm using the instrument handle, the palm exerted the highest amount of pressure on the handle when compared to the rest of the anatomical sites analyzed. This result was also reported by Rossi et al. using a power grip configuration [39]. In the case of the fingers, the thumb and index finger applied a greater amount of pressure than the middle and ring fingers. This may be because of the primary use of the thumb to control the wheel to rotate the instrument tip and the index finger to operate the trigger that opens and closes it. It should be noted that the use of an inappropriate handle size, especially in more complex tasks such as the transfer task (labyrinth), led to a significant increase in the pressure on the palm. It seems that this substantial increase in palmar pressure was accompanied by a reduction in the pressure exerted by the thumb when controlling the instrument wheel. Therefore, instead of distributing the force exerted by the fingers and the palm in a more balanced way, in this case it was mainly focused on the surgeon's palmar area. In a power grip configuration, like the one we have in our design, the handle should be held by the partially bent fingers and the palm, exerting a counter pressure with the thumb lying near the plane of the palm. Excessive strain and repetitive hand actions associated with power gripping contribute to trauma and localized fatigue [39].

The instrument handle design presented in this study allowed for an ergonomically acceptable wrist flexion-extension posture during the laparoscopic practice. This posture was also maintained for all the different handle sizes evaluated in the study. Other studies, using commercially available instruments [40] and prototypes of instrument handles [41,42], also reported that a pistol handle configuration provides an ergonomically adequate wrist flexion, providing a significantly better wrist posture than using a conventional laparoscopic tool. The results of the presented study are consistent with those presented in a previous study in which we evaluated another ergonomic power grip handle for a handheld robotic laparoscopic instrument [43]. The ergonomic analysis showed that, after training, the use of the robotic instrument resulted in an ergonomically acceptable flexion–extension of the wrist, in contrast to the posture acquired by using the conventional needle holder with axial handle. In addition, in another study we analyzed the surgeon's wrist flexion-extension posture when handling conventional instruments for laparoscopic surgery, including axial, curved, and ringed handles [44]. The results showed that, for all instruments, most surgeons have ergonomically unfavorable angles of wrist flexion, which were prone to possible musculoskeletal disorders. One of the first ergonomic studies of laparoscopic instrument handles by Matern et al. also warned of ergonomic deficiencies in wrist flexion when using ring handles and excessive radial deviation in axial handles [45]. In the case of the wrist radio-ulnar deviation, we observed the most notable improvements using the ergonomic instrument handle during the execution of the transfer task. These results reinforce the ergonomic benefits to the surgeon of using the presented handle design for laparoscopic practice.

The general design of the handle has been positively evaluated by the participants of this study with regard to the comfort of use, without showing significant differences between the groups of handle sizes. Perhaps in this study we have been conservative and a difference of only two sizes is not enough to appreciate noticeable changes in the use of the presented instrument handle design. For future studies, we will seek to compare designs with larger size differences, which could be also a very common situation in surgical practice, mainly between female and male surgeons.

This study presents some limitations of which we are aware of. Although there are other studies in the same field with a similar or smaller number of subjects [37,40], the number of participants in this study is restricted. In further studies, we will increase the study population in order to obtain more representative results and allow comparison by experience levels in laparoscopic surgery. The skills acquired by experienced surgeons in handling laparoscopic instruments may be an influential factor in their ergonomics when using different sizes of instrument handles. On the other hand, in this study we only analyzed the instrument handles with laparoscopic grasping forceps. Future work will be carried out on the use of this handle design for other laparoscopic instruments, such as a needle holder, and thus analyze the experience of surgeons in more complex tasks as intracorporeal suturing.

5. Conclusions

The results of this study show that the ergonomic design of the instrument handle improves the surgeon's ergonomics and comfort during laparoscopic practice, promoting a more neutral operating wrist posture. The use of an adequate size of the instrument handle allows for improved surgical performance, surgeons required less time to complete the eye-hand coordination task than using the incorrect size, and ergonomics by reducing the contact pressure on the surgeon's palm during the transfer task.

Author Contributions: Conceptualization, J.A.S.-M., A.G.G., L.G.M., J.B.P., J.C.G.-B., F.M.S.-M.; methodology, J.A.S.-M., A.G.G., L.G.M., J.B.P., J.C.G.-B., F.M.S.-M.; software, A.G.G., J.C.G.-B., J.A.S.-M.; validation, J.A.S.-M.; formal analysis, J.A.S.-M.; investigation, J.A.S.-M., A.G.G., J.C.G.-B.; resources, F.M.S.-M. and L.G.M.; data curation, J.A.S.-M., J.B.P., A.G.G.; writing—original draft preparation, J.A.S.-M., J.B.P., A.G.G.; writing—review and editing, F.M.S.-M. and L.G.M.; visualization, J.A.S.-M.; supervision, F.M.S.-M. and L.G.M.; project administration, F.M.S.-M. and L.G.M.; funding acquisition, F.M.S.-M., A.G.G. and L.G.M. All authors have read and agreed to the published version of the manuscript.

Acknowledgments: The authors wish to acknowledge the support of this research work to the VI Regional Research Plan and to the Regional Government of Extremadura and the European Regional Development Fund (ERDF) linked to the financial of the research groups Manufacturing Engineering (GR18029), Jesús Usón Minimally Invasive Surgery Centre (GR18199) and INNOVA (GR18176). The authors appreciate the excellent willingness to cooperate of the surgeons who participated in the study.

References

1. Tozzi, F.; Berardi, G.; Vierstraete, M.; Kasai, M.; de Carvalho, L.A.; Vivarelli, M.; Troisi, R.I. Laparoscopic versus open approach for Formal right and left hepatectomy: A propensity score matching analysis. *World J. Surg.* **2018**, *42*, 2627–2634. [CrossRef]
2. Sánchez-Margallo, F.M.; Pérez-Duarte, F.J.; Azevedo, A.M.; Sánchez-Margallo, J.A.; Sánchez-Hurtado, M.A.; Díaz-Güemes, I. An Analysis of Skills Acquisition During a Training Program for Experienced Laparoscopists in Laparoendoscopic Single-Site Surgery. *Surg. Innov.* **2014**, *21*, 320–326.

3. Sánchez-Peralta, L.F.; Sánchez-Margallo, F.M.; Moyano-Cuevas, J.L.; Pagador, J.B.; Enciso, S.; Gómez-Aguilera, E.J.; Usón-Gargallo, J. Learning curves of basic laparoscopic psychomotor skills in SINERGIA VR simulator. *Int. J. Comput. Assist. Radiol. Surg.* **2012**, *7*, 881–889.
4. Sánchez-Margallo, J.A.; Sánchez-Margallo, F.M.; Pagador, J.B.; Gómez, E.J.; Sánchez-González, P.; Usón, J.; Moreno, J. Video-based assistance system for training in minimally invasive surgery. *Minim. Invasive Ther. Allied Technol.* **2011**, *20*, 197–205. [CrossRef]
5. Büchel, D.; Mårvik, R.; Hallabrin, B.; Matern, U. Ergonomics of disposable handles for minimally invasive surgery. *Surg. Endosc.* **2010**, *24*, 992–1004. [CrossRef]
6. Berguer, R.; Gerber, S.; Kilpatrick, G.; Remler, M.; Beckley, D. A comparison of forearm and thumb muscle electromyographic responses to the use of laparoscopic instruments with either a finger grasp or a palm grasp. *Ergonomics* **1999**, *42*, 1634–1645. [CrossRef]
7. Park, A.; Lee, G.; Seagull, F.J.; Meenaghan, N.; Dexter, D. Patients benefit while surgeons suffer: an impending epidemic. *J. Am. Coll. Surg.* **2010**, *210*, 306–313. [CrossRef]
8. Manasnayakorn, S.; Cuschieri, A.; Hanna, G. Ideal manipulation angle and instrument length in hand-assisted laparoscopic surgery. *Surg. Endosc.* **2008**, *22*, 924–929. [CrossRef]
9. Sari, V.; Nieboer, T.E.; Vierhout, M.E.; Stegeman, D.F.; Kluivers, K.B. The operation room as a hostile environment for surgeons: physical complaints during and after laparoscopy. *Minim Invasive Ther. Allied Technol.* **2010**, *19*, 105–109. [CrossRef]
10. González, A.G.; Salgado, D.R.; Moruno, L.G. Optimisation of a laparoscopic tool handle dimension based on ergonomic analysis. *Int. J. Ind. Ergonom.* **2015**, *48*, 16–24. [CrossRef]
11. González, A.G.; Salgado, D.R.; García Moruno, L.; Sánchez Ríos, A. An ergonomic customized-tool handle design for precision tools using additive manufacturing: a case study. *Appl. Sci.* **2018**, *8*, 1200. [CrossRef]
12. Mace, R. Universal design: Barrier free environments for everyone. *Des. West* **1985**, *33*, 147–152.
13. Mace, R.L.; Ostroff, E.; Connell, B.R.; Jones, M.; Mueller, J.; Mullick, A.; Sanford, J.; Steinfeld, E.; Follette Story, M.; Vanderheiden, G. *The Principles of Universal Design*; NC State University: Raleigh, ND, USA, 1997.
14. Story, M.F.; Mueller, J.L.; Mace, R.L. *The Universal Design File: Designing for People of all Ages and Abilities*; NC State University: Raleigh, ND, USA, 1998.
15. Clarkson, P.J.; Coleman, R. History of Inclusive Design in the UK. *Appl. Ergon.* **2015**, *46*, 235–247. [CrossRef] [PubMed]
16. Berguer, R.; Hreljac, A. The relationship between hand size and difficulty using surgical instruments: a survey of 726 laparoscopic surgeons. *Surg. Endosc.* **2004**, *18*, 508–512. [CrossRef] [PubMed]
17. Stoklasek, P.; Mizera, A.; Manas, M.; Manas, D. Improvement of handle grip using reverse engineering, CAE and Rapid Prototyping. In Proceedings of the MATEC Web of Conferences 20th International Conference on Circuits, Systems, Communications and Computers (CSCC 2016), Corfu Island, Greece, 14–17 July 2016.
18. Sutton, E.; Irvin, M.; Zeigler, C.; Lee, G.; Park, A. The ergonomics of women in surgery. *Surg. Endosc.* **2014**, *28*, 1051–1055. [CrossRef] [PubMed]
19. Kong, Y.K.; Lowe, B.; Lee, S.J.; Krieg, E. Evaluation of handle design characteristics in a maximum screwdriving torque task. *Ergonomics* **2007**, *50*, 1404–1418. [CrossRef] [PubMed]
20. Harih, G.; Dolšak, B. Tool-handle design based on a digital human hand model. *Int. J. Ind. Ergonom.* **2013**, *43*, 288–295. [CrossRef]
21. Harih, G.; Dolšak, B. Comparison of subjective comfort ratings between anatomically shaped and cylindrical handles. *Appl. Ergon.* **2014**, *45*, 943–954. [CrossRef]
22. Maithel, S.; Villegas, L.; Stylopoulos, N.; Dawson, S.; Jones, D. Simulated laparoscopy using a head-mounted display vs traditional video monitor: an assessment of performance and muscle fatigue. *Surg. Endosc.* **2005**, *19*, 406–411. [CrossRef]
23. Horeman, T.; Dankelman, J.; Jansen, F.W.; van den Dobbelsteen, J.J. Assessment of laparoscopic skills based on force and motion parameters. *IEEE Trans. Biomed. Eng.* **2013**, *61*, 805–813. [CrossRef]
24. Pérez-Duarte, F.J.; Lucas-Hernández, M.; Matos-Azevedo, A.M.; Sánchez-Margallo, J.A.; Díaz-Güemes, I.; Sánchez-Margallo, F.M. Objective analysis of surgeons' ergonomy during laparoendoscopic single-site surgery through the use of surface electromyography and a motion capture data glove. *Surg. Endosc.* **2014**, *28*, 1314–1320. [CrossRef]
25. Loukas, C.; Georgiou, E. Multivariate autoregressive modeling of hand kinematics for laparoscopic skills assessment of surgical trainees. *IEEE Trans. Biomed. Eng.* **2011**, *58*, 3289–3297. [CrossRef]

26. Pérez-Duarte, F.J.; Sánchez-Margallo, F.M.; Martín-Portugués, I.; Sánchez-Hurtado, M.A.; Lucas-Hernández, M.; Sánchez-Margallo, J.A.; Usón-Gargallo, J. Ergonomic Analysis of Muscle Activity in the Forearm and Back Muscles During Laparoscopic Surgery. *Surg. Laparosc. Endosc. Percutan. Tech.* **2013**, *23*, 203–207. [CrossRef]
27. Szeto, G.P.; Poon, J.T.; Law, W.L. A comparison of surgeon's postural muscle activity during robotic-assisted and laparoscopic rectal surgery. *J. Robot. Surg.* **2013**, *7*, 305–308. [CrossRef]
28. Dufaug, A.; Barthod, C.; Goujon, L.; Forestier, N. Ergonomic surgical practice analysed through sEMG monitoring of muscular activity. In Proceedings of the 2016 IEEE 18th International Conference on e-Health Networking, Applications and Services (Healthcom), Munich, Germany, 14–17 September 2016; pp. 1–6.
29. Quick, N.; Gillette, J.; Shapiro, R.; Adrales, G.; Gerlach, D.; Park, A. The effect of using laparoscopic instruments on muscle activation patterns during minimally invasive surgical training procedures. *Surg. Endosc.* **2003**, *17*, 462–465. [CrossRef]
30. Emam, T.; Frank, T.; Hanna, G.; Cuschieri, A. Influence of handle design on the surgeon's upper limb movements, muscle recruitment, and fatigue during endoscopic suturing. *Surg. Endosc.* **2001**, *15*, 667–672. [CrossRef]
31. Emam, T.; Hanna, G.; Cuschieri, A. Ergonomic principles of task alignment, visual display, and direction of execution of laparoscopic bowel suturing. *Surg. Endosc.* **2002**, *16*, 267–271. [CrossRef]
32. Sánchez-Margallo, F.M.; Sánchez-Margallo, J.A. Assessment of Postural Ergonomics and Surgical Performance in Laparoendoscopic Single-Site Surgery Using a Handheld Robotic Device. *Surg. Innov.* **2018**, *25*, 208–217. [CrossRef]
33. Li, Z.; Wang, G.; Tan, J.; Sun, X.; Lin, H.; Zhu, S. Building a framework for ergonomic research on laparoscopic instrument handles. *Int. J. Surg.* **2016**, *30*, 74–82. [CrossRef]
34. Catanzarite, T.; Tan-Kim, J.; Whitcomb, E.L.; Menefee, S. Ergonomics in Surgery: A. Review. *Female Pelvic. Med. Reconstr. Surg.* **2018**, *24*, 1–12. [CrossRef]
35. Lucas-Hernández, M.; Pagador, J.B.; Pérez-Duarte, F.J.; Castelló, P.; Sánchez-Margallo, F.M. Ergonomics problems due to the use and design of dissector and needle holder: A survey in minimally invasive surgery. *Surg. Laparosc. Endosc. Percutan. Tech.* **2014**, *24*, e170–e177. [CrossRef] [PubMed]
36. Santos-Carreras, L.; Hagen, M.; Gassert, R.; Bleuler, H. Survey on Surgical Instrument Handle Design. *Surg. Innov.* **2012**, *19*, 50–59. [CrossRef] [PubMed]
37. Matern, U.; Kuttler, G.; Giebmeyer, C.; Waller, P.; Faist, M. Ergonomic aspects of five different types of laparoscopic instrument handles under dynamic conditions with respect to specific laparoscopic tasks: An electromyographic-based study. *Surg. Endosc.* **2004**, *18*, 1231–1241. [CrossRef] [PubMed]
38. Tung, K.D.; Shorti, R.M.; Downey, E.C.; Bloswick, D.S.; Merryweather, A.S. The effect of ergonomic laparoscopic tool handle design on performance and efficiency. *Surg. Endosc.* **2015**, *29*, 2500–2505. [CrossRef] [PubMed]
39. Rossi, J.; Berton, E.; Grélot, L.; Barla, C.; Vigouroux, L. Characterisation of forces exerted by the entire hand during the power grip: effect of the handle diameter. *Ergonomics* **2012**, *55*, 682–692. [CrossRef]
40. Yu, D.; Lowndes, B.; Morrow, M.; Kaufman, K.; Bingener, J.; Hallbeck, S. Impact of novel shift handle laparoscopic tool on wrist ergonomics and task performance. *Surg. Endosc.* **2016**, *30*, 3480–3490. [CrossRef]
41. Sancibrian, R.; Gutierrez-Diez, M.C.; Torre-Ferrero, C.; Benito-Gonzalez, M.A.; Redondo-Figuero, C.; Manuel-Palazuelos, J.C. Design and evaluation of a new ergonomic handle for instruments in minimally invasive surgery. *J. Surg. Res.* **2014**, *188*, 88–99. [CrossRef]
42. Van Veelen, M.A.; Meijer, D.W.; Uijttewaal, I.; Goossens, R.H.M.; Snijders, C.J.; Kazemiere, G. Improvement of the laparoscopic needle holder based on new ergonomic guidelines. *Surg. Endosc.* **2003**, *17*, 699–703. [CrossRef]
43. Sánchez-Margallo, J.A.; Sánchez-Margallo, F.M. Initial experience using a robotic-driven laparoscopic needle holder with ergonomic handle: assessment of surgeons' task performance and ergonomics. *Int. J. Comput. Assist. Radiol. Surg.* **2017**, *12*, 2069–2077. [CrossRef]
44. Sánchez-Margallo, F.M.; Sánchez-Margallo, J.A.; Pagador, J.B.; Moyano, J.L.; Moreno, J.; Usón, J. Ergonomic Assessment of Hand Movements in Laparoscopic Surgery Using the CyberGlove. In *Computational Biomechanics for Medicine*; Miller, K., Nielsen, P.M.F., Eds.; Springer: New York, NY, USA, 2010; pp. 121–128.
45. Matern, U.; Waller, P. Instruments for minimally invasive surgery: Principles of ergonomic handles. *Surg. Endosc.* **1999**, *13*, 174–182. [CrossRef]

9

3D Soft-Tissue Prediction Methodologies for Orthognathic Surgery

Elena Carlotta Olivetti [1], Sara Nicotera [1], Federica Marcolin [1,*], Enrico Vezzetti [1], Jacqueline P. A. Sotong [2], Emanuele Zavattero [2] and Guglielmo Ramieri [2]

[1] Department of Management and Production Engineering, Politecnico di Torino, corso Duca degli Abruzzi 24, 10129 Torino, Italy; elena.olivetti@polito.it (E.C.O.); sara.nicotera@studenti.polito.it (S.N.); enrico.vezzetti@polito.it (E.V.)

[2] Department of Maxillofacial unit, Città della Salute e della Scienza HOSPITAL, 10129 Torino, Italy; slim_js2000@yahoo.fr (J.P.A.S.); emanuele.zavattero@gmail.com (E.Z.); guglielmo.ramieri@unito.it (G.R.)

* Correspondence: federica.marcolin@polito.it

Abstract: Three-dimensional technologies have had a wide diffusion in several fields of application throughout the last decades; medicine is no exception and the interest in their introduction in clinical applications has grown with the refinement of such technologies. We focus on the application of 3D methodologies in maxillofacial surgery, where they can give concrete support in surgical planning and in the prediction of involuntary facial soft-tissue changes after planned bony repositioning. The purpose of this literature review is to offer a panorama of the existing prediction methods and software with a comparison of their reliability and to propose a series of still pending issues. Various software are available for surgical planning and for the prediction of tissue displacements, but their reliability is still an unknown variable in respect of the accuracy needed by surgeons. Maxilim, Dolphin and other common planning software provide a realistic result, but with some inaccuracies in specific areas of the face; it also is not totally clear how the prediction is obtained by the software and what is the theoretical model they are based on.

Keywords: orthognathic surgery; 3D face analysis; surgical planning; soft tissue prediction; prediction methods

1. Introduction

Patients presenting dentofacial deformities are commonly subject to combined orthodontic and surgical treatment such as Le Fort I osteotomy (LFI), bilateral sagittal split osteotomy (BSSO), intraoral ramus vertical osteotomy (IVRO), sagittal split ramus osteotomy (SSRO), bimaxillary surgery and genioplasty. These interventions have been commonly planned with two-dimensional methodologies; today, the last challenge is the three-dimensional (3D) surgery planning. The refining of 3D graphics and imaging tools gives the chance to explore surgical planning and prediction of the effects of different clinical approaches; these techniques are based on images acquired with computed tomography (CT), cone bean computed tomography (CBCT) and multi-slice computed tomography (MSCT), which provide volumetric images of facial anatomical structure. Additionally, the surface of the face can be scanned and mapped to underline the effect of changes in facial appearance using 3D laser technology [1] that gives a great contribution to surgeons to decide on the type of surgeries as well as on the magnitude and direction of surgical movements to correct facial dysmorphology. Moreover, a deep interest in the prediction of soft-tissue response to hard tissue movements has been growing and two-dimensional conventional methodologies seem to be insufficient for this aim as they do not take into account the third dimension.

Indeed, the possibility to know the soft-tissue response to surgical operations helps surgeons to plan surgical movements and it gives surgeons more information about the need of orthodontic decompensation. Furthermore, the purpose of these interventions is not only to correct the facial dysmorphology from a functional point of view, but also to obtain an aesthetic enhancement of patients' facial aspect. Therefore, an accurate treatment planning is very important to obtain a good aesthetic and occlusal result [2]. For the aforementioned reasons, having a preview of the soft-tissue arrangement is extremely important. In future, this opportunity could bring to have a surgical planning methodology able to best match patients' aesthetic expectations, additionally to the functional corrective aspect.

Several methods have been considered to forecast soft tissue responses; the most common are the mass-spring model (MSM), finite element model (FEM) and mass tensor model (MTM). Most of the software packages currently adopted in clinical practice are based on these models. Generally, those softwares seem to reach an acceptable overall accuracy, but with inaccuracies for specific areas of the face, for example around the lips.

Studies have been conducted to develop 2D prevision models based on the ratio between facial and bony movements, particularly focusing on face sub regions [3]; by comparing predictive models constructed on this ratio and patients' post-operative conditions, it is stated that traditional approaches show limits in forecasting the outcome of large and complex movements. Moreover, a large number of variables must be selected [4].

Although there are several studies on the soft tissue changes after maxillary osteotomies, few of them report a systematic analysis.

The target of this systematic review is to gather information on the existing prediction methods and software of soft tissue displacements after dysmorphism corrective surgery, and to draw conclusions on the accuracy and reliability of these software in the preview of surgical outcome. Additionally, some problems related to the level of accuracy needed by surgeons, to the predictive imprecision reported in the studies and to the magnitude of the acceptable error are presented.

This work is structured as follows. The section Material and Methods describes the methods that have been adopted for the literature review. The section Results includes the clinical details of patients involved and the details of the articles considered; the articles have been divided in subsections according to the software used by the authors. Finally, the section Discussion and Conclusions discusses the current prediction methods and concludes the work.

2. Materials and Methods

The research of this systematic review is based on the Population Intervention Control Outcome Study design (PICOS) format (Table 1). PubMed and Scopus are the databases adopted for our research. The considered keywords are: orthognathic surgery, facial dysmorphism, surgical planning, 3D, 3D face analysis, soft tissue, BSSO, bilateral sagittal split osteotomy, Le Fort I, prediction methods.

The research has been set on different combinations of keywords; at first, we focused generically on the orthognathic surgery, then the type of interventions has been specified: BSSO, IVRO, SSRO and LFI. Finally, the research has been limited to soft tissue simulation and prediction.

All the articles found were assessed by three authors and classified in: prospective study (PS), retrospective study (RS), case series study (CS).

Single cases reports have been excluded from our analysis because they have been considered not clinically significant.

Articles published before 2000 have not been considered.

The following data have been recorded for each eligible study: first author and year of publication, journal, study design, sample size, gender, mean age, diagnosis, imaging technology, typologies of surgery, software used for the prediction, soft and hard tissue landmarks considered, time interval from surgery to post-surgical imaging, results and conclusions of the authors.

Table 1. PICOS (Population Intervention Control Outcome Study) criteria for the systematic review.

Population	Patients with angle class II, III dentoskeletal deformities, indicated for a maxillary osteotomy to correct the malocclusion
Intervention	Le Fort I osteotomy, bimaxillary osteotomy, BSSO (bilateral sagittal split osteotomy), IVRO (intraoral ramus vertical osteotomy), SSRO (sagittal split ramus osteotomy), genioplasty
Comparison	3D orthognathic surgery planning and prediction method
Outcome	Soft tissue post-operative change, prediction and accuracy of the technique
Study design	Clinical trials, retrospective and prospective studies (CT, RS and PS, respectively) with the aim of assessing the methodologies of soft and hard tissue prediction.

3. Results

Different responses have been obtained varying the insertion order of the keywords. After having combined the outcomes and removed the duplicates, the remaining articles have been evaluated on the basis of their relevance to the topic. In the end, 24 articles to be deepened and a number of interesting articles to be referenced for a better comprehension of the topic have been selected.

3.1. Clinincal Details

A total of 24 articles have been compared in this work; 12 are retrospective studies, two are case studies and five are prospective studies. Remaining articles have not declared categorization. The sample of patients involved in each study vary from seven to 100 subjects. The soft tissue prediction has been assessed for Le Fort I osteotomy, BSSO, BSSRO and genioplasty in the correction of different types of facial dysmorphism.

Tables 2 and 3 report a brief summary of the referenced papers we focused on. In particular, the demographic details of the patients are summarized in Table 2. A brief overview of methodologies and results of each article is reported in Table 3.

CBCT has been used for the assessment of soft tissues changes in twelve of the twenty-four studies, with the addition of 3D photographs for one article, while cephalometric radiographs have been used in the remaining eight works, with the addition of CT and MSCT for two of them.

The timing of post-surgical imaging has been stated in all articles.

3.2. Prediction Methodologies

Several approaches have been considered to make a mathematical three-dimensional prediction of soft tissue changes after orthognathic surgery. MSM, FEM [5,6] and MTM are the most common. These have been developed into software packages which are currently used in clinical practice. The functioning of these software is generally acceptable if we consider the creation of a plausible facial outcome, but this prediction does not necessarily match with the real outcome. Moreover, studies show that the prediction accuracy decreases for specific facial areas, especially around the lip, and with the increasing complexity of the surgery (larger bony repositioning often results in a higher inaccuracy of the prediction). The studies presented in this literature review evaluate soft-tissue predictions obtained with different software packages.

Table 2. Demographic details of patients (acronyms: PS is prospective study, RS is retrospective study, CS is case series study, NA is not available/not reported).

References	Journal	Study Design	Sample Size	Male Pts.	Female Pts.	Mean Age	Diagnosis	Surgery
N. Abe et al. 2015	Int J Oral and maxillofacial surgery	RS	45	NA	NA	NA	Asymmetry, Class I, Class II	LFI, SSRO, IVRO
C.M. Resnick et al. 2016	J oral maxillofacial surgery	RS	7	2	5	18.1	Maxilla hypoplasia	A single segment LFI osteotomy
A. Bianchi et al. 2010	J oral maxillofacial surgery	NA	10	6	4	24	NA	LFI, BSSO, genioplasty
B. Khambay et al. 2015	Int J Oral and maxillofacial surgery	NA	10	NA	NA	NA	NA	LFI
M.I. Shafi et al. 2013	Int J Oral and maxillofacial surgery	NA	13	8	5	NA	NA	LFI
J. Liebregts et al. 2014	J of cranio-maxillo-facial surgery	NA	60	15	45	26	NA	LFI, BSSO
A. Marchetti et al. 2011	Int J Oral and maxillofacial surgery	NA	10	5	5	NA	NA	LFI, BSSO, genioplasty
T. Mundluru et al. 2017	Int J Oral and maxillofacial surgery	RS	13	NA	NA	NA	Asymmetry	Bimaxillary, BSSO
Ana de Lourdes sa de lira et al. 2012	J Oral Maxillofacial Surgery	CS, RS	80	19(group1) 20(group2)	21(group1) 20(group2)	22.8(group1) 22.4(group2)	Class II	group1: BSSO group2: bimaxillary
Ana de Lourdes sa de lira et al. 2012	J Oral Maxillofacial Surgery	CS, RS	76	10(group1) 26(group2)	26(group1) 14(group2)	25.4(group1) 25.6(group2)	Class III	LFI, bimaxillary
A. Terzic et al. 2013	Aesthetic Plastic Surgery	RS	13	5	8	25.2	NA	Bimaxillary (10 pts.) BSSO (3 pts.)
R.J. Peterman et al. 2016	Progress in Orthodontic	RS	14	3	11	22.5	Class III	LFI, BSSO
R. Ullah et al. 2014	British J of Oral and Maxillofacial Surgery	RS	13	5	8	23	Class III	LFI
Osvaldo Magro Filho et al. 2010	Am J Orthod Dentofacial Orthop	NA	10	NA	NA	NA	Class III	LFI, BSSO
D. Holzinger et al. 2018	J of cranio-maxillo-facial surgery	PS	16	8	8	26	Class III,II,I	NA
Chay Hui Koh et al. 2004	J Oral Maxillofacial Surgery	NA	35	14	21	22.8	Class III	Bimaxillary
O. Donatsky et al. 2009	J of cranio-maxillo-facial surgery	PS	52	21	31	20	Class III	LFI, SSRO
Z.Ö. Pektas et al. 2007	Int J Med and Robotics Comput Assist Surg	RS	11	4	7	23.5	NA	LFI, BSSO
De Riu et al. 2018	J of cranio-maxillo-facial surgery	RS	49	19	30	26.4	NA	Bimaxillary
Van Hemelen et al. 2015	J of cranio-maxillo-facial surgery	PS	66	29	37	NA	Angle class II/class III malocclusion	Bimaxillary, BSSO, LFI, genioplasty
Knoops et al. 2019	Int J Oral and maxillofacial surgery	RS	7	2	5	18	Maxillary sagittal hypoplasia	LFI maxillary advancement
Liebregts et al. 2015	J Oral Maxillofacial Surgery	PS	100	35	65	32	Nonsyndromic mandibular hypoplasia	BSSO
Nam et al. 2015	J of craniofacial surgery	PS	29	16	13	NA	NA	LFI, BSSRO, genioplasry
Nadjmi et al. 2013	Am J Orthod Dent Orthop	RS	13	2	11	NA	NA	LFI, BSSO

Table 3. Imaging technology, software used for prediction, number of landmarks for soft tissue and hard tissue, time interval from surgery to post-operative imaging and results.

Reference	Imaging Technology	Software Adopted for Prediction	Adoption of Land-Marks	Soft Tissue Land-Marks	Hard Tissue Land-Marks	Time Interval from Surgery to Post-Surgery CT	Results	Conclusions
N. Abe et al. 2015	CBCT	OrthoForecast	yes	11 on frontal image, 13 on lateral image, 3 lines	None	12 months	Mean difference in the location of points on predicted and actual postoperative <3.4 mm and <10° in considered angles	Useful, accurate, reliable software to predict soft tissue changes after surgery
C.M. Resnick et al. 2016	CBCT, 3D photographs	Dolphin 3D	yes	37	42	14 months	Mean linear prediction error of 2.91 ± 2.16 mm; mean error at nasolabial angle of 8.1° ± 5.6°. Poorest agreement at subnasale. Most accurate lateral point: maxillary buttress (mean error 3.31 ± 1.81 mm). Least accurate lateral point: lateral ala (mean error 4.54 ± 1.97 mm)	Prediction accuracy acceptable for linear changes in the midline, not for lateral points. In the midline changes at nasal base most prone to prediction error (mean error 2.84 ± 2.55 mm)
B. Khambay et al. 2015	CBCT	3dMDvul-tus	yes	10	None	6 months	85.2%–94.4% points with error <2 mm; RMS error 0.94–2.49 mm	The use of specific anatomic regions is more meaningful than full face
M.I. Shafi et al. 2013	CBCT	Maxilim	yes	NA	NA	6–12 months	Accuracy <3 mm except for upper lip region	Clinically satisfactory for assessed regions but associated with marked errors in upper lip region
J. Liebregts et al. 2014	CBCT	Maxilim	yes	11	None	12 months	Mean absolute error for whole face: 0.81 ± 0.22 mm. Accuracy for whole face, upper lip, lower lip, chin subregion: 100%, 93%, 90%, 95% respectively.	The prediction accuracy is influenced by the magnitude of maxillary/mandibular advancement, age of patient, usage of V-Y closure. Low predictability on upper/lower lip regions.
A. Marchetti et al. 2011	MSCT, cephalo-metric radio-graphs	SurgiCase_CMF	yes	NA	NA	6 months	Mean abs error: 0.50–1.15 mm; percentage of simulation with error ≤ 2 mm: 76–99%	Reliability of soft tissue preview > 91% Realistic, accurate forecast of pt's face after surgery
D. Holzinger et al. 2018	CT, cephalo-metric radio-graphs	Sotirios planning software	yes	NA	15	6 months	Mean error of 1.46 mm ± 1.53 mm	Quite accurate software; clinically satisfactory 3D soft tissue prediction
A. Bianchi et al. 2010	CBCT	SurgiCase_CMF	yes	NA	NA	6 months	Average abs error: 0.94 mm. St.dev: 0.90 mm Percentage of error <2 mm for 86.8%	Reliability results shows that the software makes a realistic preview with low X-ray exposure
T. Mundluru et al. 2017	CBCT	Maxilim	yes	NA	NA	6–12 months	Mean abs distance < 2 mm for all regions.	Prediction of soft tissue clinically acceptable; prediction error < 2 mm; under-prediction around the cheek and chin medio-laterally with opposite effect at inferior border of mandible bilaterally
O. Donatsky et al. 2009	Cephalometric radiographs	TIOPS	yes	8	8	5–6 weeks	Mean accuracy: 0.0–0.5 mm. Inaccuracies: 0.2–1.1 mm	Useful in surgical simulation, planning and prediction. High variability of predicted individual outcome for hard and soft tissue

Table 3. *Cont.*

Z.Ö. Pektas et al. 2007	Cephalometric radiographs	Dolphin imaging version 10.0	yes	7	5	12 months	Least accurate site: lower lip. Most accurate sites: tip of nose, subnasale. Mean difference < 1 mm (4 pts on 7)	Satisfactory in predicting soft tissue outcome
R.J. Peterman et al. 2016	Lateral cephalometric radiographs	Dolphin imaging version 11.0.03.37	yes	9	14	6 months	Error range: ±2 mm (X axis).	Not useful for precise treatment planning
Ana de Lourdes sa de Lira et al. 2012	Lateral cephalogram	Dolphin imaging	no	NA	NA	12 months	Surgeries more extensive than planned. Similar values between predicted and actual results for facial convexity and distance from lips to cranial base	Statistical differences do not invalidate surgical predictability because predicted modifications close to surgical results
Ana de Lourdes sa de Lira et al. 2012	Lateral cephalogram	Dolphin imaging version 11.0	no	NA	NA	12 months	Predicted surgical reduction in mandibular length and angle significantly greater than actual post-operative	Statistical differences do not invalidate surgical predictability because predicted modifications close to surgical results
R. Ullah et al. 2014	CBCT	3dMDvultus	yes	NA	NA	6–12 months	Mean abs distance between actual and predicted soft tissue < 3 mm and ranged from 0.65 mm (chin) to 1.17 (upper lip)	3D soft tissue prediction is acceptable for LFI advancement osteotomy
Osvaldo Magro Filho et al. 2010	Lateral cephalometric radiographs	Dentofacial planner plus (DFP), Dolphin imaging (DI)	no	NA	NA	6 months	No statistical differences between the two software ($p = 0.7945$)	DFP better in predicting nasolabial angle, upper/lower lips. DI better in predicting nasal tip, chin, sub mandibular area
A. Terzic et al. 2013	CT, CBCT	3dMDvultus version 2.2.0.8	yes	NA	NA	6 months	Mean difference between surfaces: −0.64 mm (surgically treated lower half). Errors >3 mm: 4% for upper half and 29.8% for lower half	Accuracy in soft tissue prediction is insufficient
Chay Hui Koh et al. 2004	Lateral cephalograms	CASSOS	yes	16	NA	6 months	Significant differences between 16 of 32 soft tissue measurements ($p < 0.05$) Under estimation of vertical position for upper/lower lips, over estimation of horizontal position of lower lip	Clinically useful prediction of soft tissue profile change in Chinese patients
De Riu et al. 2018	Frontal/lateral cephalometric radiograph, CBCT	Maxilim, Dolphin	yes	NA	NA	3–5 days	Differences among 12 of the 15 parameters were considered not significant. Significant differences reported for SNA ($p = 0.008$), SNB ($p = 0.006$), anterior facial height ($p = 0.033$). Average error: 1.98 mm (linear measures), 1.19° (angle measures)	Good degree of accuracy for most of parameters assessed. Tendency towards under-projection of jaws. 3D simulation of soft tissue currently does not allow an accurate management of facial height and chin position
Van Hemelen et al. 2015	Frontal/lateral cephalometric radiograph, CBCT	Onyx Ceph, Maxilim	yes	17 (3D) 16 (2D)	17 (3D) 16 (2D)	4 months	horizontal direction: 2.29 mm (2D) vs. 1.48 mm (3D) vertical direction: 2.07 mm (2D) vs. 1.46 mm (3D)	3D method more predictive, but more time consuming and more difficult to use.

Table 3. *Cont.*

Knoops et al. 2019	CBCT	Dolphin 3D, ProPlan CMF, PFEM	Yes (Dolphin 3D)	NA	NA	1 year	Dolphin 3D: RMS = 1.8 ± 0.3 mm ProPlan: RMS = 1.2 ± 0.4 mm PFEM: RMS = 1.3 ± 0.4 mm	Dolphin 3D: limited accuracy ProPlan/PFEM: better 3D prediction, mismatch in maxillary position (predicted/real)
Liebregts et al. 2015	CBCT	Maxilim	yes	5	5	6 months	Mean abs. err: whole face: 0.9 ± 0.3 mm upper lip: 1.2 ± 0.5 mm chin area: 0.8 ± 0.5 mm	Accurate soft tissue simulation for single surgery
Nam et al. 2015	CT	Simplant Pro	yes	NA	30	6 months	Mean differences: 0.73 mm (x axis), 1.39 mm (y axis), 0.85 mm (z axis). Accuracy: 52.8%	It is needed to improve soft tissue prediction accuracy
Nadjmi et al. 2013	CBCT, lateral cephalograms, profile photographs	Maxilim, Dolphin	yes	25	15	4 months	Error range (horizontal plane): −1.41 to 1.20 mm (Dolphin) −1.60 to 1.50 mm (Maxilim) Error range (vertical plane): −1.85 to 1.55 mm (Dolphin) −4.25 to 2.42 mm (Maxilim)	Errors with Dolphin are higher than with Maxilim, but not statistically significant ($p >$ 0.05). Both showed inaccuracies (chin, lips) for complicate surgeries

3.2.1. Works Based on Traditional (2D) Methodologies

Since a certain number of 3D software currently available for clinical practice are based on algorithm developed to work on 2D and then adapted to 3D representation of data, a section dedicated to traditional soft-tissue prediction is introduced. Moreover, since many surgeons currently rely more on traditional techniques than on three-dimensional methods, it is reasonable to focus on the limitations of this technology; 2D analysis based on lateral cephalograms is subject to errors caused by the impossibility to accurately locate points on both hard and soft tissue relying only on 2D anatomic structures [7]. Analysis performed on cephalograms reported that reasonable prediction can be made on soft-tissue landmarks positions, but with low accuracy concerning the lips and particularly in the vertical prediction of displacements [8]. Moreover, the inaccuracy increases with a higher level of complexity of intervention, which leads to errors both in hard- and soft-tissue simulation [9].

In this section, we particularly focused on study assessing the accuracy of Dolphin Imaging, but we also reported studies that took into consideration other software.

Peterman et al. worked on the quantification of the accuracy of Dolphin VTO (visual treatment objective) in predicting soft tissue changes in patients with a class III deformity and on the validation of its efficacy. In their study, authors considered fourteen patients receiving comprehensive orthodontic treatment and orthognathic surgery including both maxillary advancement and/or mandibular setback. Cephalometric tracing and analysis were performed with Dolphin Imaging software; pre- and post-operative and traced cephalometrics were superimposed using the cranial base as reference. The maxillary movements were recorded at the anterior nasal spine (ANS) and A point, while the mandibular changes were recorded at B point and pogonion (Pg) in both x and y axis. Subsequently, the pre-treatment profile pictures were superimposed to digitally-traced soft-tissue landmarks of pre-treatment cephalometric radiograph to initiate software VTO simulation (Figure 1). Finally, a prediction profile photograph generated by the software was compared to actual post-operative patient's profile photograph; coordinates of nine soft-tissue landmarks were used to quantify on each axis the differences between the predicted and the actual of patients. The results reported in this study are consistent with the prevision error calculated in previous works; Dolphin Imaging software was found to have a much larger standard deviation in the Y direction than in the X, with various degrees of accuracy in both directions for all soft tissue landmarks. The accuracy was 79% and 61% for X-axis and Y-axis respectively, with an acceptable error set at 2.00 mm. Furthermore, for these surgical cases, the least accurate prediction was the one concerning the lower lip region. In conclusion, authors affirmed that VTO program can be useful for rough movement previsions during surgical planning, but surgeons cannot rely on it for precise surgical movements (measurement range lower than 1.00 mm) [10].

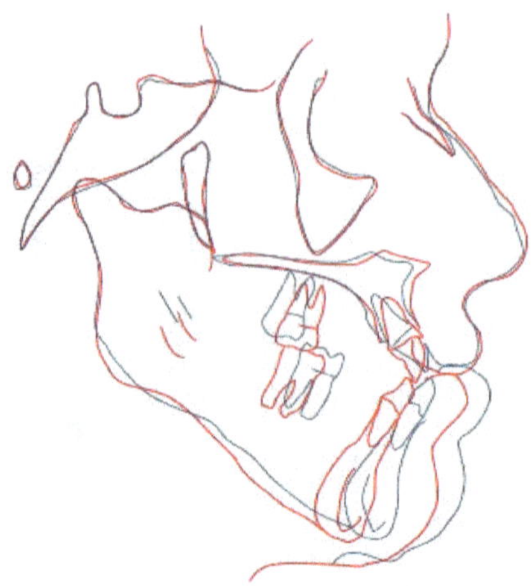

Figure 1. Super-imposition of pre- and post- and traced cephalometric tracing showing advancement of the maxilla and setback of the mandible [10].

In the study of Pektas et al., the treatment planning for each patient was constituted on the base of clinical and cephalometric evaluations, and pre-operative study models. All patients were treated with pre- and post-surgical fixed orthodontic appliances. Scanned images of cephalometric radiographs were processed using Dolphin Imaging software; the Ricketts and Steiner analysis was selected to start the digitization. To compare actual outcome and software simulation, firstly the superimposition of pre- and post-operative cephalograms was performed on the sella-nasion plane registered at sella. Landmarks located on structures not involved in the surgery were directly transposed from pre-operative to post-operative cephalogram to refine the superimposition process. The objective of an accurate superimposition of pre- and post-operative cephalograms was to construct a spreadsheet for landmarks movements to quantify changes of each point after operation; the position of points was defined in form of x and y. In accordance with the spreadsheet, a simulation of the treatment was produced, and the prediction tracings were obtained from actual post-operative changes amount. Actual post treatment tracings and prediction tracings were superimposed and differences have been measured again according to an x, y coordinate system.

The mean differences between the predicted and the actual result were less than 1 mm in four of seven soft tissue measurements; predictions turn out to be more accurate for the sagittal plane than for the vertical one. The largest errors were reported for the lower lip region, in accordance with other studies considered by authors and investigating other software [11].

Ana de Lourdes sá de Líra et al. studied the accuracy of digital prediction with respect to the actual post-operative outcome with Dolphin program. Patients with class II malocclusion were involved. Eighty Caucasian subjects treated with combined surgical and orthodontic treatment were considered. Cephalometric radiographs of pre- and post-operative were digitized; a time of at least one year from surgical to post-operative was required to rule out any effects of post-operative swelling. Digital tracings were performed with Dolphin imaging software and digital lateral cephalometric radiographs were traced at the same time to minimize the error variance; before tracing, Dolphin program was used to carry out the compensation for the effect of radiographic magnification. An x y coordinates system was constructed with the x axes corresponding to the horizontal Frankfort plane and the y-axes passing through Nasion and perpendicular to x-axes. On x-axes, vertical changes have been measured, while on y-axes authors evaluated horizontal changes. Dalberg formula was used in evaluating the reproducibility of measurements; with regard to the method error, it did not exceed 0.37° for angular measurements and 0.29 mm for linear measurements. Results of the statistical analysis were based on mean values found in each studied group. The analysis of the authors underlined that there were no significant differences between soft-tissue values at pre-operative (t1), post-operative (t2) and predicted (t3) stages. In both groups, surgeries have been more extensive than planned; facial convexity and the distance between the lips and the cranial base presented similar values between t2 and t3. The conclusion of the authors was that statistical differences in the considered measurements did not invalidate surgical prediction performed with the software, because forecasted changes were sufficiently close to of the surgical outcomes [12].

Lira et al. followed the same approach of the previous article on two groups of patients; the former underwent Le Fort I without segmental surgery, while on the latter, in addition to LFI surgery, mandibular setback was performed with an SSRO. What came out from this study was that 12 months after the operation surgical reductions in mandibular length and angle were substantially greater than indicated by predictive cephalometric tracings. The analysis of dental and skeletal mandibular changes in anteroposterior and vertical directions revealed that the effect on the profile was greater than those of the maxilla; this is probably due to the fact that the mandible is a moving structure and the upper lip leans upon the lower lip. Maxilla advancements were performed for both groups according to the planning provided by Dolphin imaging software; in group two, mandibular setback was statistically overestimated by the software planning. Nevertheless, authors concluded that statistically the differences in the considered measurements do not invalidate the surgical prediction generated with the software, because the predicted result was close to the surgical outcome. Moreover, they noticed that concerning the mandible, dentoskeletal measurements in horizontal and vertical directions showed a greater correlation to the profile than the maxillary measurements [13].

Magro-Filho et al. worked on a subjective comparison of the soft-tissue surgical simulation of two software: Dentofacial Planner Plus (Dentofacial Software, Toronto, Ontario, Canada) and Dolphin Imaging (version 9.0). Surgeries considered in the study involved retro-positioning of the mandible and advancement of the maxilla, in which linear movements were at least 4 mm for one bone segment or in the sum of both mandibular and maxillary movements, without, or least possible, postsurgical orthodontic movements. Profile predictions were made six months after the surgery; real movements, obtained from the superimposition of the cephalometries of pre- and post-operative of each subject, were used as values of the prediction. Soft-tissue images of pre-operative, real predictive images of Dentofacial Planner Plus (DFP) and Dolphin Imaging (DI) and post-operative images were compared (Figure 2). With Photoshop program (version 6.0, Adobe, San Jose, Calif), pre- and post-operative profile images were digitized and standardized; then, images were imported in DFP and DI. Movements of maxilla and mandible were made using the real values extracted from the comparison between pre- and post-operative lateral cephalograms of the surgical displacements along the vertical and horizontal directions for molars and incisors of the maxilla and for incisors of the mandible. The tip of the nose, the nasolabial angle, upper and lower lips, menton region, the base of the mandible and the complete profile were used to compare simulated and real images. A group of orthodontists, maxillofacial surgeons and general dentists evaluated the similarity among the programs simulated images and the real post-operative images with a scale ranging from "very similar" to "different". For the comparison of soft-tissue cephalometric points, to compare the two programs and to judge the criteria of similarity, chi-square test was used. From their analysis, the authors reported that for nasal tip, chin area and mandibular base DI gave better results, while for nasolabial angle, upper lip and lower lip DFP produced a more accurate prediction; authors also reported that there was no difference in the evaluation of the complete profile. Moreover, in terms of time, working with DI was longer than working with DFP. In conclusion, it was stated that in treating subjects affected by dentofacial deformities, it would be better if orthodontists and oral maxillofacial surgeons were to base on their clinical experience and to use software just as a co adjuvant. Considering the methodology of the study, there were not many differences in obtaining a two-dimensional prediction of patient's profile [14].

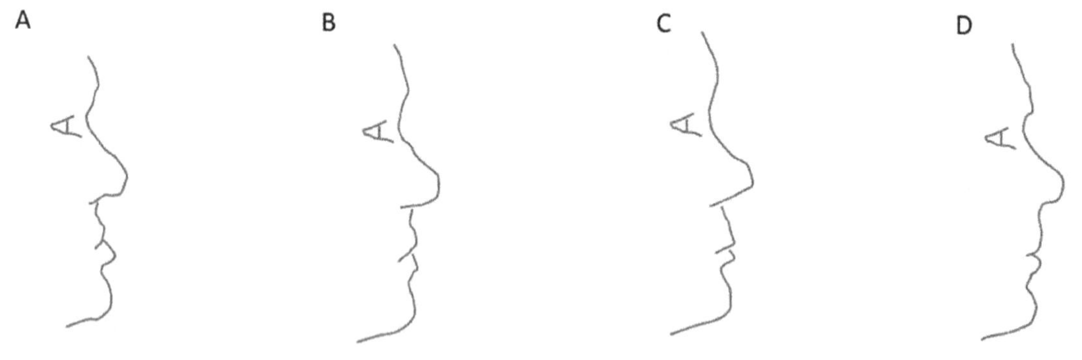

Figure 2. Profile images of a patient with Class III malocclusion, treated with orthognathic surgery: (**A**) pre-treatment; (**B**) simulation from Dentofacial Planner Plus (DFP); (**C**) simulation from Dolphin Imaging (DI); (**D**) actual post-operative photograph [14].

Other software are available for the prediction of soft tissue changes. OrthoForecast is a data-based prediction software; its database contains information of 400 patients (100 pts with asymmetry, 100 pts with skeletal class II jaw relationship and 200 pts with skeletal class III jaw relationship). All patients underwent SSRO or IVRO, with or without LFI osteotomy (respectively, 352 and 48 cases). It was evaluated by Abe et al.; the study included 15 patients with facial asymmetry, 15 with skeletal class II jaw relationship and 15 with skeletal class III jaw relationship. Patients underwent LFI osteotomy,

SSRO and IVRO. Twenty-four landmarks were chosen and digitized. Some angles were also compared between the following lines: line 1, the line connecting the bilateral mandibular angles; line 3, the line connecting the bilateral eyespots; line 2, the line connecting the bilateral oral angles. In the asymmetry group, they measured angle 1, identified by line 1 and line 3 and angle 2, identified by line 2 and line 3 on the frontal facial photograph to assess the asymmetry of the face. In the class II and class III groups, the value of angle 3, identified by the angle formed by lines connecting eyespot, upper lip, and soft tissue B-point on the lateral facial photograph was measured. Angle 3 was the reference for evaluating the convexity of the face, which was originally defined as soft-tissue convexity (Figure 3). The distances measured between landmarks on the actual and on the predicted images were analyzed, and the similarity between real and software-generated images was assessed by 39 evaluators. The mean difference measured between the positions of landmarks is less than 3.4 mm and less than 1.0° in the evaluated angles. Moreover, more than half of the evaluators stated that, in all groups, the predicted images were very 'similar' or 'similar' to the actual situation of the patients in the post-operative condition. Less than 6% of the evaluators ranked the predicted images as 'different' from the actual outcome. In conclusion, OrthoForecast is considered by the authors to be a software with high levels of accuracy, reliability and usefulness [15].

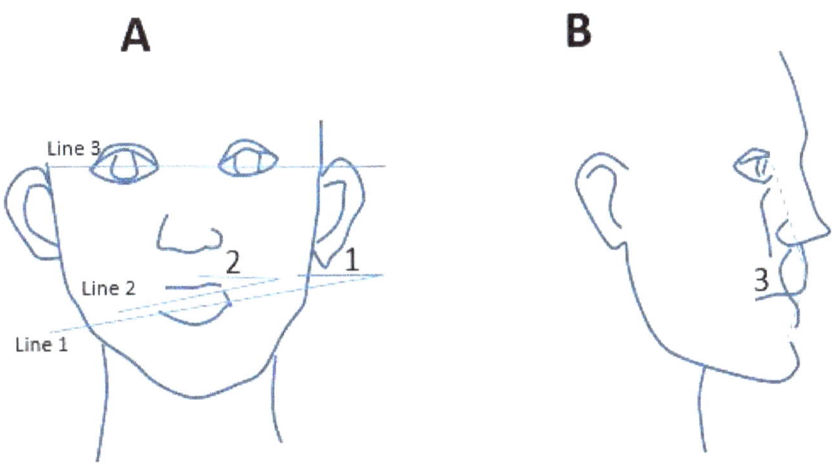

Figure 3. Construction of feature points and lines (**A**) 1, Angle between line 1 (connecting the bilateral mandibular angles) and line 3 (connecting the bilateral eyespots); 2, angle between line 2 (connecting the bilateral oral angles) and line 3; (**B**) 3, angle formed with lines connecting the eyespot point, upper lip point, and soft tissue B-point [15].

Donatsky et al. evaluated another prediction software, TIOPS. This is a computerized, cephalometric, orthognathic surgical planning system previously used in studies on hard tissue stability and accuracy. As other soft tissue prediction systems, TIOPS is based on predefined ratios of hard to soft tissue movements; its present algorithms partly rely on cephalometric observation of the post-operative situation. The study included 52 patients. Clinical photographs, study models mounted on an articulator (SAM) and standardized lateral cephalometric radiographs of the pre-operative situation were performed. Standardized lateral cephalometric radiographs were performed 5–6 weeks after surgery. The mean accuracy of the planned and predicted results of both hard and soft tissue varied from 0.0 mm to 0.5 mm from one cephalometric reference point to another. In the locus of cephalometric reference points, where it was shown that there were significant differences between planned/predicted hard and soft tissue changing in terms of position, these significant inaccuracies were moderately small and varied from 0.2 mm to 1.1 mm, with the exception of the horizontal position of the lower lip. However, the variability of the previewed hard and soft tissue individual result was evaluated to be relatively high. The study demonstrated moderately high predictability of the immediate post-surgical hard and soft tissue outcome. However, due to the significant variability of simulated individual results, it would be better to be cautious in presenting the planned and predicted hard and soft-tissue results to the individual patient in the pre-operative [16].

Finally, Chai Hui Koh et al. evaluated the accuracy of soft tissue predictions generated by the CASSOS (Computer-Assisted Simulation System for Orthognathic Surgery) software in Chinese skeletal class III patients underwent bimaxillary surgery. The digitization of pre-surgical and post-surgical lateral cephalograms of 35 patients was performed with the CASSOS program. A simulation of the surgery was performed on the pre-surgical tracing. An analysis was performed on thirty-two linear measurements on the cephalograms superimposition to assess the differences in the soft tissue profile between the post treatment results and the predicted result. It showed differences on 16 linear measurements with the most prediction errors on the upper and lower lip having a mean difference relatively small, with a greatest mean difference of 2 mm in the vertical position of stomion inferius. The authors concluded that CASSOS 2001 produced a clinically meaningful forecast of soft-tissue profile changes following bimaxillary surgery [17].

The same CASSOS software was evaluated by Jones et al. for 33 patients affected by class III skeletal deformities and underwent maxillary advancement (17 patients) or bimaxillary surgery (16 patients) [18]. The post-operative cephalograms were used to determine surgical bony movements to produce the CASSOS profile simulation. Linear differences between the predicted profile and the real outcome were measured at 12 soft tissue landmarks. The authors' conclusion was that the profile predictions obtained with CASSOS could be considered useful for both type of surgeries, even if substantial variations were found. As previously [17], the most inaccuracies were found in the lip region.

3.2.2. Works Based on Maxilim Software (3D)

In this section a collection of studies is presented considering patients' soft tissue prediction obtained with Maxilim software (Medicim—Medical Image Computing, Mechelen, Belgium). This software, based on the mass tensor model algorithm (MTM), allows surgeons to determine bony movements and to see the effect of the procedure [19]. MTM has been introduced by Cotin et al.; the geometry of the anatomical structure is discretized into a tetrahedral mesh in which the displacement vector at a generic internal point is defined as a function of vertices displacement vectors. The elastic force is written as a function of these same four vectors. The displacement for a set of mass points is set fixed and other model points will move as consequence of elastic forces due to the displacements of fixed points; finally, the new rest position of the free points is computed by integrating the Newtonian motion equation [20].

Shafi et al. [21] investigated the accuracy of Maxilim using cone-beam computed tomography (CBCT) scans in pre- and post-surgery phases (6–12 months after surgery) for 13 patients subjected to Le Fort I surgery. A 3D mesh was generated from skeletal movements (predicted model). Subsequently, the mesh generated from the post-operative of the patient and the predicted model were compared to evaluate the accuracy of the prediction. The soft tissue was divided in different areas: nose, right and left nares, right and left paranasal regions upper and lower lip and chin. The absolute distance was calculated between the meshes for each region. For each facial region, the absolute distance was calculated between the meshes.

In almost all the facial regions, the accuracy was significantly less than 3.00 mm (3.00 mm is clinically acceptable). The upper lip area was the exception; in fact, for this region, the accuracy was greater than 3.00 mm. In all cases, Maxilim produced an over prediction of the new position of the upper lip. A possible reason could be a non-linear response of the upper lip to some hard-tissue movements and, consequently, the modeling algorithm used (MTM) hardly previewed this response.

The conclusion of the authors was that the 3D soft tissue prediction for Le Fort I advancements produced by Maxilim was in general clinically satisfactory, but it was associated with marked errors around the region of the upper lip.

Liebregts et al. evaluated the accuracy of Maxilim for 3D simulation of soft tissue changes after bimaxillary osteotomy. The 3D rendered pre- and post-operative scans were matched. Segmented maxilla and mandible were aligned to the post-operative position. In order to calculate the error between the simulation and the actual post-operative condition, authors used 3D distance maps and cephalometric analysis. Concerning the facial profile, the mean absolute error between the 3D simulation and the actual post-operative facial profile was 0.81 ± 0.22 mm for the face as a whole. In this study, the accuracies of the simulation (average absolute error ≤2 mm) for the whole face and for the upper lip, lower lip and chin sub regions were 100%, 93%, 90% and 95%, respectively.

Authors affirmed that the MTM based soft tissue simulation is an accurate model for the prediction of soft tissue changes following bimaxillary surgery. The magnitude of skeletal movements influences the accuracy of the prediction; moreover, the age of the patient and the use of V–Y closure affect the precision of the predicted model. Low predictability on the upper and lower lip regions is registered once again [22].

The same authors evaluated Maxilim performances for soft-tissue simulation in 100 patients underwent BSSO for mandibular advancement [23]. As in the previous case, the accuracy of the simulation was assessed with two methods, a 3D cephalometric analysis and a 3D distance map for the entire face and for specific regions of interest. Their analysis showed that for the entire face the mean absolute 90th percentile error was less than 2 mm (clinically acceptable); the least accuracy resulted in the region of the lower lip, while the most accurate prediction involved the sub nasal region. A possible explanation suggested by authors for labial inaccuracies was the difficulty to replicate labial position during different image acquisition.

The conclusion drawn by authors on the basis of this analysis was that the soft-tissue prediction produced by Maxilim software was clinically acceptable both for the whole face and for restricted regions, but the limitation was the fact that patients considered in the study underwent a single type of surgery instead of combined operations.

In the analysis by Mundluru et al., 13 non-syndromatic adults with a midline deviation of the chin point not less than 2.0 mm underwent Le Fort I or bimaxillary osteotomies (BSSO) to correct facial asymmetry. The accuracy of an innovative concept for the soft-tissue changes prediction was evaluated. The segmentation of the 3D model was performed to identify the following regions: upper lip, lower lip, chin area, right and left paranasal regions, nose and right and left cheeks. To evaluate the prediction reliability, the surface distances between predicted and actual post-operative positions were measured. Particularly, mean (signed) and mean absolute distances were calculated on 3D meshes for each region. Through a directional analysis, the accuracy of the prediction of soft-tissue changes was evaluated. The results showed that the distances between the predicted and the actual post-operative soft tissue models were less than 2.0 mm in all regions. In details, a general tendency to the under prediction was found in the area of the cheek and of the chin (medio-laterally). An over-prediction of changes was found at the inferior border of the mandible (bilaterally) [24].

De Riu, et al. realized a retrospective study with the purpose of giving an objective quantification of accuracy of the Maxilim virtual planning method, through the comparison between planned and actual movements in jaw osteotomy. They started from the assumption that a simple superimposition of simulation and cephalometry results did not allow to define a correlation between positional error and surgical movements. Indeed, a slight positional error could be insignificant talking about large movements, but could be unacceptable dealing with small displacements. A 3D planning was performed, and virtual frontal and lateral cephalometries of pre-operative and simulated surgery were extracted; those were compared to define the predicted movements of the jaw in reference to cranial bones. All surgeries have been planned by the same surgeons using Maxilim software, with digital intermediate splints to guide osteotomies. Cephalometric analysis has been performed with Dolphin. To evaluate the accuracy, the mean linear difference between planned and actual movements was considered. Measurement of the differences between planned and actual movements were deemed accurate. As reported by authors, most of the clinical studies validating the virtual surgical planning set to 2 mm the criterion for the prediction success, with a success rate slightly lower than 100%. In this study, some significant differences with other works were found; first, differences between planned and achieved anterior facial heights were found ($p = 0.033$). This discrepancy was relevant ($p = 0.042$) in patients that did not undergo genioplasty, while it was not significant in patients who underwent this surgery (0.235). This error is probably due to the approximation of the soft tissue model, which does not allow the management of the vertical dimension. Presumably, genioplasty compensate the error on facial eight. The second error reported by authors was in the differences between actual and planned measurements for SNA (angle between Sella, Nasion and A point) and for SNB (angle between Sella, Nasion and B point), with $p = 0.008$ and $p = 0.006$ respectively. In the opinion of the authors, virtual planning inaccuracies were principally caused by the difficulty of simulate the soft tissue changes. Moreover, they concluded that virtual planning could not relieve surgeons of the necessity of monitoring jaws movements intraoperatively and of a real time supervision of planned and actual outcome, despite a high level of accuracy for most of the analyzed parameters [25].

The double blind prospective study performed by Van Hemelen et al. had the aim of providing a comparison between a traditional planning method and a 3D planning performed with Maxilim, both for hard and soft tissue [26]. In their analysis, authors considered 66 patients affected by class II or class III angle malocclusion underwent bimaxillary osteotomy (46 patients), BSSO (17) patients and LeFort I osteotomy (3 patients). Genioplasty was performed on 28 patients. For the 2D planning, clinical facial examination, lateral and frontal cephalograms were taken; 17 and 16 cephalometric landmarks were considered for 3D and for 2D respectively, to perform the validation of both 2D and 3D planning. The traditional planning was performed with Onyx Ceph Version 3.1.111 and the analyses of accuracy was performed by measuring projections on x and y axis of distances between the 16 selected points on the planned and on the actual post-operative. In the case of the 3D planning, the landmarks were defined in three dimensions and the planned and post-operative data were aligned. Distances between the 17 cephalometric points defined on planned and actual models were evaluated in depth, height and distance in the sagittal plane.

As a result of the analysis, authors reported that, for hard tissue planning, the mean differences occurring between actual and planned outcome evaluated at cephalometric points were 1.71 mm and 1.42 mm in the horizontal direction and 1.69 mm and 1.44 mm in the vertical direction, for 2D and 3D respectively. Concerning soft tissue displacements, the mean values computed in the horizontal direction were 2.29 mm for traditional planning and 1.48 for Maxilim prediction; in the vertical direction, authors noted mean values of 2.07 mm and 1.46 mm for 2D and 3D techniques respectively. These evaluations led authors to conclude that there was a statistically significant difference in the soft-tissue prediction between the two considered methods (chi-squared test and independent t-test were used to determine statistical significance, with $p < 0.005$); particularly, the 3D approach seemed to be more predictive than the traditional one. No statistically significant differences were reported for hard tissue planning.

The conclusion reached by authors was that, concerning the soft tissue prediction, the 3D planning approach here performed with Maxilim software led to a more accurate planning than the traditional method, even with disadvantages such as the cost of the software and of the CBCT scans. Moreover, a higher learning time must be considered when planning with the 3D method. In the authors' opinion, 3D planning will not replace the traditional prediction if those negative aspects are not addressed.

The study by Nadjmi et al. focused on the accuracy of soft-tissue profile changes simulated by Maxilim with respect to the accuracy obtained with Dolphin. Particularly, the goal of the comparison was to assess if the 3D prevision was more accurate than the 2D one. A "natural head distance" was defined as distance between suprasternal notch and soft tissue pogonion to replicate patients' head position. On lateral cephalogram, soft tissue and hard tissue landmarks (15 and 25 points respectively) were located; soft tissue predictions were generated with Dolphin and Maxilim. The two predictive results were superimposed with patient's post-operative profile photograph and differences in terms of linear measurements of landmarks in x and y directions were measured. All comparison steps were performed by the same operator. The movements of bony structures in the simulation must be the same as performed by the surgeon, to correctly compare the two predictions. Since this study made a comparison between 2D and 3D simulations, even if Maxilim gave in output 3D models, only profile (2D) images were considered. From the analysis of the results, the authors found that both Dolphin and Maxilim predictions were accurate, but the simulation obtained with Maxilim made possible a quantification of volumetric changes (lips aspect) and a prevision of changes in the transverse plane. Even if the study focused on the comparison of accuracies (and for this reason only the lateral prediction was considered) between the two software, authors stated that 3D simulation would be helpful in complicated surgeries thanks to the third-dimensional information [27].

3.2.3. Works Based on Other 3D Software

The work of Resnick et al. investigates the accuracy of Dolphin 3D soft tissue prediction using seven patients who had a single-segment Le Fort I osteotomy. Dolphin 3D Imaging (Dolphin Imaging and Management Solutions, Chatsworth, CA, USA) is based on a landmark photographic morphing algorithm developed for 2D prediction and adapted to 3D. The user must locate 79 landmarks, 47 on the hard tissue and 37 on the soft tissue, on the CT volume; the system generates adaptable curves between the landmarks, similarly to the tracing of a lateral cephalometry.

On the pre-operative segments LF I osteotomy was simulated by Dolphin, then hard and soft tissue landmarks were assigned, morphing curves were adjusted and finally prediction image (Tp) and post-operative image (T1) were aligned and registered for the measurement of the differences. For each patient, the error was calculated as the difference occurring between Tp and T1 at 14 points, six on the midline and eight laterally and at the nasolabial angle (Figure 4). Twelve of these points are standard anthropometric or cephalometric landmarks. Two new points were introduced for the study: lateral ala (LA), obtained from the intersection of the line tangent to endocanthion (EN) and the one tangent to subalare (SBAL), and maxillary buttress (MB), traced at the intersection of lines tangent to exocanthion (EX) and SBAL (Figure 4A).

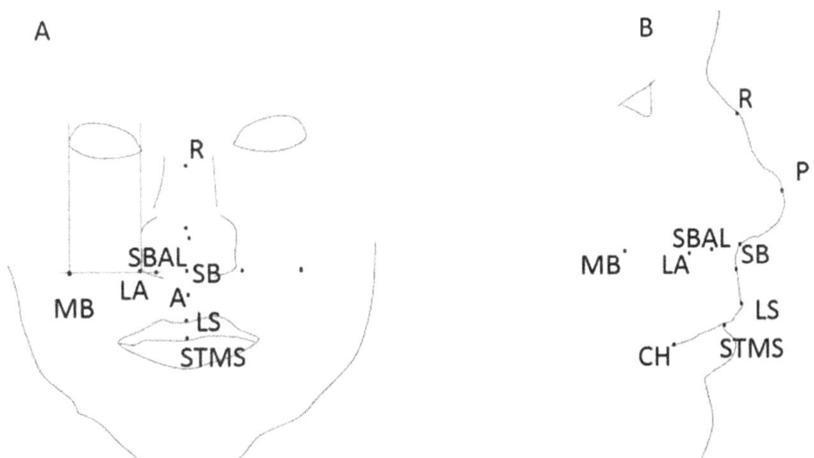

Figure 4. Points for measurement by Resnick et al. (**A**) Frontal view. The two points derived for this study are shown: lateral ala point (LA), defined as the intersection of lines tangent to endocanthion (EN) and subnasale (SBAL), and maxillary buttress (MB) point, and defined as the intersection of lines tangent to exocanthion (EX) and SBAL. (**B**) Lateral view showing all points [28].

In closing, their analysis showed that the capability to predict the soft-tissue changes in the three dimensions after LF I surgery using Dolphin software had some limitations. For linear changes, its accuracy was acceptable, while it was not acceptable for lateral points of the face. Concerning the midline, changes at nasal base were more subject to prediction errors [28].

Bianchi et al. [29] and Marchetti et al. [30] worked on SurgiCase_CMF using CBCT and MSCT respectively of 10 patients with facial deformities. In the study presented by Bianchi et al., patients underwent LFI, BSSO and genioplasty. The pre- and post-operative CT images were aligned on the top of each other. Firstly, a registration point was made, with the location of two corresponding landmarks on pre- and post-operative conditions. After the manual registration, automatic surface registration was carried out using an iterative closest point algorithm. A crucial point in surfaces registration was to indicate those that did not change after the surgery; authors used the eyes area and the forehead as fixed regions. Finally, the post-operative soft tissue surface was compared with the software virtual simulation. A comparison algorithm was used to measure the distance of every triangle corner of the post-operative surface against the preoperative one. The percentage of error was <2.0 mm for the 86.80% of patients, even if there were important errors in the top lip and chin regions. The results in the group of patients studied with CBCT (which had a reliability of 86.8%) stated that the use of SurgiCase_CMF 1.2 software combined with CBCT data allowed to achieve a realistic preview with low X-ray exposure [29].

Marchetti et al. divided virtual surgical planning in four steps (Figure 5): (1) CT data reconstruction; (2) generation of 3D models of hard and soft tissues; (3) various virtual surgical planning and simulation mode; (4) different pre-operative previews of the soft tissues. Skeletal model surgical planning and simulation were performed on the base of the 3D CT; the soft tissue model was made through a physical model. According to clinical options, the software generated a set of simulations and models of the soft tissues; in order to prevent temporomandibular functional problems, an orthodontist assessed the pre-operative plans. From the comparison of simulation and CT surgical outcomes, it was found that the prediction of soft tissue situation had a reliability greater than 91%, with a percentage of error lower than 2 mm for 76%–99%. According to the obtained results, SurgiCase_CMF was able to give a realistic and accurate preview of the face of the subjects undergoing surgery, but there were significant errors in the lip and chin regions, as in the previous studies [30].

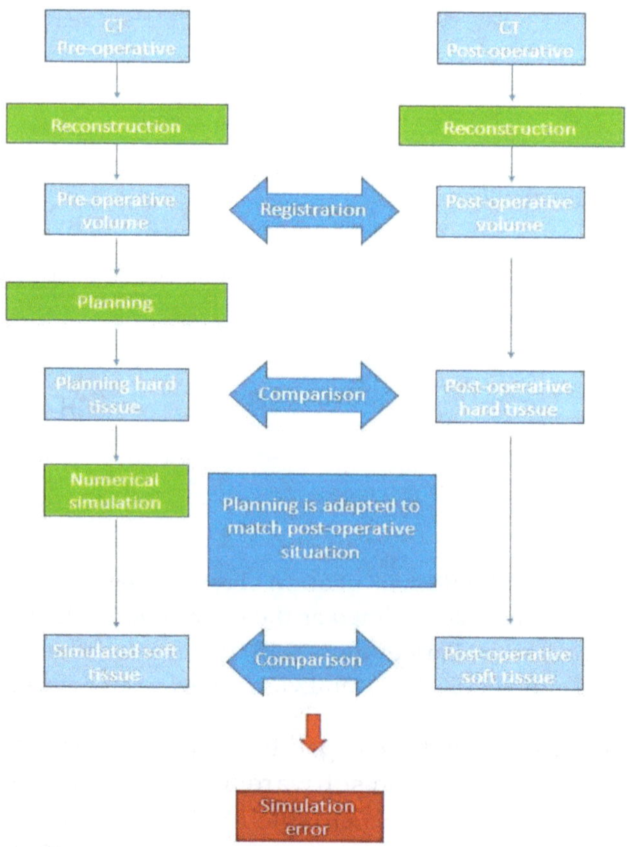

Figure 5. Virtual surgical planning proposed by Marchetti et al. [30].

3dMDvultus is a software package in which the rendering function is based on Mass Spring Model. MSM assumes a discretization of a deformable object into n mass points and a set of m connections between each n mass point. In a tetrahedral discretization, for each mesh node a point is allocated, and it is defined a linear spring for all the edges of the mesh. This linear spring follows Hook's law. This model has the advantage of being simple and computationally efficient, but the disadvantage is that the elastic behavior of the model is determined by the spring constant; the value of this constant is an approximation and it has no true bio-mechanical relevance [19].

Khambay et al. used 3dMDvultus to predict the soft tissue changes after surgery. The work included 10 patients who underwent Le Fort I osteotomy. Ten landmarks were used to measure the distances between the pre- and post- operative meshes. Moreover, the percentage of mesh points minor or equal to 2.0 mm were calculated for the full face and for specific anatomical regions. The results demonstrated that the percentage of mesh with errors minor or equal to 2.0 mm for the full face was 85.2%–94.5% and 31.3%–100% for anatomical regions. The range of root mean square (RMS) error was from 2.49 mm to 0.94 mm. The most of mean linear distances computed between the surfaces was equal or less than 0.8 mm, but it increased for the mean absolute distances. From this analysis, it was stated that the use of specific anatomical regions was more significant in clinical practice than the use of full face [31].

As in the previous article, the software considered by Terzic et al. is 3dMDvultus. Three-dimensional photographs of patients' head in natural position (lips and muscles at rest, open eyes, neutral facial expression) of pre- and post-operative were taken; CT and/or CBCT images were imported to the software platform. Pre-operative 3D photograph was fused with pre-operative CT/CBCT images. In the same manner, post-operative bony skull data was fused with pre-operatives by matching bone areas not involved in surgeries. According to actual post-surgical CT, 3D bone segments were reproduced in the pre-operative skull; the software rendering function (mass spring model) was activated. Osteotomy segments were moved to real post-operative position and the soft-tissue rendering generated the textured facial soft tissue prediction. After the fusion of 3D photographs of predicted and real post-operative soft tissue, a horizontal plane was positioned arbitrarily to divide the face in an upper part not involved in surgery, and a lower part including the overlap of simulated and real post-surgery result. Averaged distribution of absolute error showed more discrepancies between predicted and real post-operative outcome in the lower part of the face: in 29.8% of lower halves authors found errors exceeding 3.00 mm. This preliminary study concluded that the software platform had an insufficient accuracy in the forecast of 3D soft-tissue displacements [32].

Ullah et al. carried out a retrospective study in which they focused on the ability of 3dMDvultus to give a prediction of the face appearance of patients undergoing LFI maxillary advancement. The null hypothesis they started from was that the mean difference in absolute distance between the predicted surface generated by the software and the real 3D facial surface measured at eight anatomical regions did not exceed 3 mm. Pre- and post-operative CBCT for each patients were imported into 3dMDvultus and hard tissue and soft tissue were separately segmented and saved in STL (standard triangulation language) format. A template of actual surgical changes was produced using a CAD/CAM software (VRMesh, VirtualGrid, Seattle, WA, USA). Post-operative hard and soft tissue linked together were aligned to the anterior cranial base of pre-operative hard tissue of the same patient. Regions of maxilla and mandible of post-operative models were saved as STL file and imported into 3dMDvultus to generate a template of the actual maxillo-mandibular complex aligned in the same 3D space as the pre-operative image. Using the same software, a LFI osteotomy was simulated for the pre-operative hard tissue. The resulting soft-tissue prediction was exported as an STL file for the analysis. The predicted model and the real surgical result were imported as mesh in VRMesh; the differences between the two models were rendered as a color map, which showed the overall accuracy of the software. After the analysis on the overall surface, the accuracy was evaluated subdividing the mesh into anatomical regions: chin, lower lip, upper lip, nose, right and left nares, right and left paranasal areas. From the analysis of the results, the authors concluded that since the distances between software-generated surfaces and real facial surfaces were lower than 3 mm, 3dMDvultus 3D soft-tissue predictions were acceptable for clinical use in LFI osteotomy. MSM seemed to correctly predict the positions of lip and chin, while improvements should be made for nasal and paranasal regions [33].

In the prospective study by Holzinger et al., 16 patients with open bite dentofacial-dysmorphosis and underwent orthognathic surgery (surgery first) were analyzed. The surgery was planned using conventional sketches as a new software developed by the authors, SOTIRIOS planning software. A conventional pre-surgical planning was carried out using three sides X-rays and, in addition, a CT scan was performed before and 6 months after surgery. A constrained fitting approach using statistical shape modeling (SSM) technique to generate the patient-specific data was used in combination with the anatomical landmarks to compute the patient specific model. A quantitative comparison of the soft tissue prediction and post-operative data was made showing a mean error of 1.46 mm ± 1.53 mm. Authors concluded that the SOTIRIOS planning software was quite accurate and enabled the surgeon to predict the soft tissue outcome [34].

A comparison between Dolphin 3D, ProPlan CMF and an in-house probabilistic finite element (PFEM) [6] was carried out by Knoops et al. [35]. The retrospective study included seven patients who underwent LFI maxillary advancement. From CBCT taken preoperatively, 3D models of bone and soft tissue were constructed. On the base of the advancement and rotation movements measured on the post-operative images, a virtual Le Fort I osteotomy was performed and three different soft tissue predictions were realized with the three softwares. Firstly, the three predictions were compared with the pre-operative model to evaluate differences. After that, the three predictions were compared with the real post-operative outcome, to assess which was the most predictive model. As the patients involved underwent a LFI maxillary advancement, the areas of interest for the comparison with post-operative situation were the upper lip and the paranasal regions. From the outcomes analysis, it resulted that the prediction generated by Dolphin 3D was affected by a general under-prediction of paranasal displacements, while both ProPlan CMF and the PFEM model were characterized by an over-prediction of displacements involving cheilion regions. Average root mean square distances and average percentage of points less than 2 mm between real post-operative images and predictions were computed (Table 3); statistically significant differences resulted from the Friedman test. In particular, the post hoc Wilcoxon signed-rank test proved that RMS for PFEM and RMS for ProPlan had statistically significant lower values with respect to RMS for Dolphin 3D ($p = 0.016$). On the opposite, the differences between ProPlan and PFEM could not be considered statistically significant ($p = 0.219$).

The conclusions of the authors was that ProPlan CMF and PFEM gave soft-tissue predictions with significant accuracies, particularly when using the correct post-operative maxillary position; because of the limitations introduced by a landmark-based algorithm and a sparse architecture, Dolphin 3D resulted to be inaccurate when surgery involved large maxillary advancements, particularly on lateral points.

Nam et al. [36] tried to assess if a 3D virtual surgery could accurately predict the soft tissue outcome of 29 patients who underwent bimaxillary orthognatic surgery (LFI, BSSO and genioplasty) performed by the same surgeon. The predicted outcome was generated using the Simplant Pro program. All simulations were performed by the same operator. The produced simulation of the soft tissue result was superimposed on the post-operative of the patients, and 10 landmarks were designed and positioned on the two models; the simulation error was determined by measuring distances (x, y, z) between the same landmarks on predicted and real images. From this analysis, an accuracy of 52.8% resulted, disagreeing with previous study reporting accuracies around 80%. Most of the errors were found for landmarks of lower lips, mouth corner and chin area (pogonion and menton), with a general larger error in points located on the mandible. Authors suggested as a possible cause of this trend the complexity of the surgery, involving more movements in the mandible rather than in the maxilla; it could determine lower errors in the maxilla but higher inaccuracy in the mandible. Inaccuracies reported for 18 of the 30 soft-tissue landmarks were considered statistically significant ($p < 0.05$), with errors concentrated at mouth corners. Possible explanations addressed by the authors were the ethnic differences between the data used for developing the software (Caucasian population) and the data used in this study (Asian population); moreover, it was not negligible that errors up to 2 mm could be due to the positioning of soft tissue landmarks. In conclusion, authors stated that 3D software in soft tissue prediction could have great potential, but the accuracy must be improved.

Even if it is out of the scope of the present work, it is important to state that not only the surgical planning plays a crucial role in the optimal process of care of the patients. It is not negligible that maxillofacial surgery, as well as other branches of surgeries, could lead to medical complications such as venous thromboembolism, which can have fatal consequences when moving to the lung (DVT/PE) [37]. Moreover, surgeons must manage patients with rare disorders of hemostasis, which need particular care in the perioperative phase. The works by Simurda et al. [38,39], and Ghadimi et al. [40] have been referred to in order to deepen understanding of this topic.

4. Discussion and Conclusions

In this systematic review we have summarized twenty-four studies focused on the evaluation of soft-tissue prediction software for maxillofacial surgery. The treated software are commonly used in clinical procedures to have a preview of the patients' outcome after corrective surgery; the most common methodologies on which these software are based are the mass spring model, the finite element model and the mass tensor model, each of them with its advantages and disadvantages. MSM presents an easy architecture and a low memory usage but it has no real biomechanical foundations; FEM is more relevant from a biomechanical point of view, but it has a high computational cost and a rather long simulation time; MTM tries to combine the advantages of MSM and of FEM [18]. In particular, the lip region is the most difficult to predict, since lips do not rely on bony structures; moreover, it is difficult to replicate the same lip position from one acquisition to another. Due to this particularity, lips are supposed to be particularly involved in involuntary displacements caused by surgeries performed on different facial areas. The difficulty in accurately predicting the appearance of this sub region is a crucial point in the development of a prediction method, since it is particularly related to aesthetic self-perception and satisfaction of the patient. With respect to the traditional algorithms based on hard- to soft-tissue ratio, methodologies involving biomechanical models of viscoelasticity of the soft tissue to mimic its elastic deformation seems to be able to give a more realistic simulation. Despite the number of computer programs dedicated to three-dimensional prediction and surgical planning, maxillofacial practitioners often prefer to rely on conventional two-dimensional methods. This fact could be explained with the overall results given by these methodologies, which seem to be only partially relevant and/or reliable in the practice of daily clinical activity. Concerning the works based on Maxilim, Shafi et al. found that this software makes a clinically satisfactory prediction of soft tissue changes, but with an over-prediction of the position of the upper lip [21]; according to Liebregts et al., its accuracy is influenced by the magnitude of maxillary and mandibular movements, by the age of the patient and by the usage of V-Y closure, and these authors further reported a low predictability of lower and upper lips [22]. Moreover, a general tendency was reported towards an under-prediction in the area around the cheek and chin and towards an over-prediction at the mandibular inferior border [24]. It was suggested that Maxilim inaccuracy in the prediction of the lip region might be due to the modelling algorithm, i.e., mass tensor, and might indicate a non-linear response of the upper lip [21]. The study by De Riu et al., although not directly focused on soft tissue prediction, reports that inaccuracies in virtual planning are primarily due to the soft-tissue virtual model [25].

With regard to Dolphin software, Resnick et al. reported that the ability to predict 3D soft tissue changes was limited, with an accuracy that may be acceptable for linear changes but not for lateral facial points [28]. Peterman et al. reported various degrees of accuracy at each soft-tissue landmark in the horizontal and vertical axes; lower lip prediction was the least accurate. A similar result of low prediction accuracy for the lower lip region is reported by Pektas et al. [11]. Conversely, two articles affirmed that the statistical differences between Dolphin soft tissue prediction and the real outcome of the patient did not invalidate the software prediction, as it was close to real surgical results [12,13].

Dolphin 3D imaging uses a landmark-based photographic morphing algorithm that was developed for two-dimensional prediction and then adapted to three-dimensional prediction; this could be an explanation for its imprecisions. Moreover, it requires plotting 79 landmarks on the CT volume (42 for the hard tissue and 37 for the soft tissue); the localization of such a large number of points seems to require too much time for a stable usage in clinical daily practice.

Among the other considered software, SurgiCase_CMF was analyzed by Bianchi et al. [29] and Marchetti et al. [30]; they reported that the percentage of error was less than 2 mm for the majority of patients, but in both studies an important error in the areas of lips and chin was reported. Khambay et al., Terzic et al. and Ullah et al. used 3dMDvultus to predict soft tissue changes; in general, they reported that its use on specific anatomical regions was more meaningful than on the full face [31–33]. Moreover, they reported an insufficient prediction accuracy particularly for the lower part of the face with errors exceeding 3 mm [32], and for nasal and paranasal regions [33]. Surprisingly, prediction results seemed to be reliable for lips and chin.

The results reported for TIOPS showed significant inaccuracies in the predicted horizontal position of the lower lips and a relatively high variability of the predicted individual surgical outcome. The authors suggest care is needed when presenting the predicted image to patients before the operation [16,41]. The SOTIRIOS planning software and the CASSOS program were found to be quite accurate [34] and able to give a clinically useful prediction of the soft-tissue profile change [17]. OrthoForecast software resulted as being in general an accurate tool for soft-tissue prediction; indeed, more than half of the involved evaluators assessed the predicted images to be very similar or similar to the actual post-operative images [15].

As a result of this review, it seems that Dolphin, CASSOS and OrthoForecast are the most accurate software in soft-tissue prediction. However, their reliability is not sufficient when further surgery is carried out and the complexity of the operation increases; moreover, they provide only partial information on the prediction, due to the lack of the third dimension. From this viewpoint, all articles agree on the potentiality of 3D methodologies. Maxilim produced clinically meaningful results, but its inaccuracy in specific facial areas (particularly in the lip region) led to the conclusion that further steps are needed to give surgeons a tool for predicting facial movements (including involuntary movements) that significantly supports the planning of the intervention in terms of aesthetic success. The comparison between 2D and 3D methodologies shows that the first reach better results in terms of accuracy and surgeon satisfaction. Consequently, the latter are still not able to meet medical needs.

The analysis of these studies has led us to consider some issues that are still pending. Almost all of them report problems of reliability of the software or inaccuracy in specific areas; this shows that an ameliorative method would be necessary to improve prediction results. For this reason, it would be useful to clearly understand the way the existing software compute the tissue displacements. Moreover, it is important to notice that some of the considered software (Dolphin 3D) are not based purely on 3D methods, but they are an adaptation of a 2D algorithm to 3D data; the transfer of 2D data to a 3D representation may cause errors. This aspect affects both hard- and soft-tissue prediction, and it is more evident in soft tissue simulations, due to the complexity of its behavior (involuntary displacements). The tendency of surgeons to prefer conventional methods suggests that, despite the general positive opinion emerging from the studies, the reliability of automatic systems is not sufficient, since it has not significantly increased above the two-dimensional methods commonly used in clinical routine. Indeed, it seems to lack consistency between the results obtained with prediction software and practitioner satisfaction. As previously reported, if the statistical differences in the evaluated measurements do not invalidate surgical predictability software, which parameters can be used to evaluate the precision of the prediction? It may be that the evaluation of automatic output is qualitative more than quantitative. Surgeon opinion on prediction software is that, even if the soft-tissue simulation outputs are plausible with a possible result of the interventions, these do not correspond to the effective post-operative outcome; moreover, this discrepancy is even more evident when the complexity of surgery increases. Neither hard- to soft-tissue ratio-based algorithms nor those based on viscoelastic models seem to meet surgeon demand. Another aspect is that currently soft tissue prediction seems to be focused on specific intervention effects more than on involuntary displacements; presently, these displacements affect, in an unpredictable manner, the facial outcome of patients. An accurate and reliable prevision method should consider these displacements to give surgeons an effective and helpful tool.

To improve prediction, a clear technical scientific evaluation approach should be established, which seems to be lacking in certain studies. Moreover, it would be better to clarify the level of precision of the predicted outcome needed by surgeons. These aspects are also an incentive for researchers to investigate the correlation between the extent of soft tissue changes with respect to STTs (soft-tissue thickness) and BMI (body mass index).

Author Contributions: Conceptualization, F.M. and E.Z.; methodology, J.P.A.S., S.N., F.M.; software, E.C.O. and S.N.; validation, S.N., E.C.O., and J.P.A.S.; formal analysis, F.M.; investigation, S.N.; resources, J.P.A.S. and E.Z.; data curation, E.C.O. and S.N.; writing—original draft preparation, S.N., E.C.O., and J.P.A.S.; writing—review and editing, F.M. and E.Z.; visualization, F.M.; supervision, F.M., E.Z., E.V., G.R.; project administration, E.V. and G.R.; funding acquisition, E.V. and G.R.

References

1. Bruce, V. Applied Research in face Processing. In *The Oxford Handbook of Face Perception*; Oxford University Press: New York, NY, USA, 2011; pp. 131–146.
2. Eckardt, C.; Cunningham, S. How predictable is orthognathic surgery? *Eur. J. Orthod.* **2004**, *26*, 303–309. [CrossRef] [PubMed]
3. Jo, L.-J.; Weng, J.-L.; Ho, C.-T.; Lin, H.-H. Three-dimensional region-based study on the relationship between soft and hard tissue changes after orthognatic surgery in patients with prognathism. *PLoS ONE* **2018**, *13*, e0200589.
4. Suh, H.-Y.; Lee, H.-J.; Lee, Y.-S.; Eo, S.-H.; Donatelli, R.; Lee, S.-J. Predicting soft tissue changes after orthognatic surgery: The sparse partial least squares method. *Ang. Orthod.* **2019**, *89*, 910–916. [CrossRef] [PubMed]
5. Kim, D.; Chun-Yu Ho, D.; Mai, H.; Zhang, X.; Shen, S.G.F.; Shen, S.; Yuan, P.; Liu, S.; Zhang, G.; Zhou, X.; et al. A clinically validated simulation method for facial soft tissue change prediction following double jaw orthognatic surgery. *Med. Phys.* **2017**, *44*, 4252–4261. [CrossRef]
6. Knoops, P.; Borghi, A.; Ruggiero, F.; Badiali, G.; Bianchi, A.; Marchetti, C.; Rodriguez-Flores, N.; Breakey, R.; Jeelani, O.; Dunaway, D.; et al. A novel soft tissue prediction methodology for orthognatic surgery based on probabilistic finite alament modelling. *PLoS ONE* **2018**, *13*, e0197209. [CrossRef]
7. Swennen, G.; Schutyser, F.; Barth, E.; de Groeve, P.; de Mey, A. A new method of 3D cephalometery part I: The anatomic cartesian 3D reference system. *J. Craniofac. Surg.* **2006**, *17*, 314–325. [CrossRef]
8. Van Twisk, P.-H.; Tenhagen, M.; Gul, A.W.E.; Kuonstaal, M. How accurate is the soft tissue prediction of Dolphin Imaging for orthognatic surgery? *Int. Orthod.* **2019**, *17*, 488–496. [CrossRef]
9. Rustemeyer, J.; Groddeck, A.; Zwerger, S.; Bremerich, A. The accuracy of two-dimensional planning for routine orthognatic surgery. *Br. J. Oral Maxillofac. Surg.* **2010**, *48*, 271–275. [CrossRef]
10. Peterman, R.; Jiang, S.; Johe, R.; Mukherjee, P. Accuracy of Dolphin visual treatment objective (VTO) patients treated with maxillary advancement and mandibular set back. *Prog. Orthod.* **2016**, *17*, 17–19. [CrossRef]
11. Pektas, Z.; Kircelli, B.; Cilasun, U.; Uckan, S. The accuracy of computer assisted surgical planning in soft tissue prediction following orthognathic surgery. *Int. J. Med. Robot. Comput. Assist. Surg.* **2007**, *3*, 64–71. [CrossRef]
12. De Lira, A.D.L.S.; de Moura, W.L.; Artese, F.; Bittencourt, M.A.V.; Nojima, L.I. Surgical prediction of skeletal and soft tissue changes in treatment of Class II. *J. Cranio-Maxillo-Fac. Surg.* **2013**, *41*, 198–203. [CrossRef] [PubMed]
13. De Lira, A.D.L.S.; de Moura, W.L.; de Barros Vieira, J.M.; Nojima, M.G.; Nojima, L.I. Surgical prediction of skeletal and soft tissue changes in Class III treatment. *J. Oral Maxillofac. Surg.* **2012**, *70*, 290–297. [CrossRef] [PubMed]

14. Magro-Filho, O.; Magro-Hernica, N.; Queiroz, T.P.; Aranega, A.M.; Garcia, I.R., Jr. Comparative study of 2 software programs for predicting profile changes in Class III patients having double-jaw orthognathic surgery. *Am. J. Orthod. Dentofac. Orthop.* **2010**, *137*, 452.e1–452.e5. [CrossRef] [PubMed]
15. Abe, N.; Kuroda, S.; Furutani, M.; Tanaka, E. Data-based prediction of soft tissue changes after orthognathic surgery: Clinical assessment of new simulation software. *Int. J. Oral Maxillofac. Surg.* **2015**, *3*, 90–96. [CrossRef] [PubMed]
16. Donatsky, O.; Hillerup, S.; Bjorn-Jorgensen, J.; Jacobsen, P. Computerized cephalometric orthognathic surgical simulation, prediction and postoperative evaluation of precision. *Int. J. Oral Maxillofac. Surg.* **1992**, *21*, 199–203. [CrossRef]
17. Koh, C.H.; Chew, M.T. Predictability of soft tissue profile changes following bimaxillary surgery in skeletal class III chinese patients. *J. Oral Maxillofac. Surg.* **2004**, *62*, 1505–1509. [CrossRef] [PubMed]
18. Jones, R.; Khambay, B.; McHugh, S.; Ayoub, A. The validity of a computer-assisted simulation system for orthognatic surgery (CASSOS) for planning the surgical correction of class III skeletal deformities: Single jaw vs. bimaxillary surgery. *Oral Maxillofac. Surg.* **2007**, *36*, 900–908. [CrossRef]
19. Mollemans, W.; Schutyser, F.; Nadjmi, N.; Maes, F.; Suetens, P. Predicting soft tissue deformations for a maxillofacial surgery planning system: From computational strategies to a complete clinical validation. *Med. Image Anal.* **2007**, *11*, 282–301. [CrossRef]
20. Cotin, S.; Dekingette, H.; Ayache, N. A hybrid elastic model allowing real-time cutting, deformations and force-feedback for surgery training and simulation. *Vis. Comput.* **2000**, *16*, 437–452. [CrossRef]
21. Shafi, M.; Ayoub, A.; Ju, X.; Khambay, B. The accuracy of three-dimensional prediction planning for the surgical correction of facial deformities using Maxilim. *Int. J. Oral Maxillofac. Surg.* **2013**, *42*, 801–806. [CrossRef]
22. Liebregts, J.; Tong, X.; Timmermans, M.; de Konig, M.; Bergè, S.; Hoppenreijs, T.; Maal, T. Accuracy of three-dimensional soft tissue simulation in bimaxillary osteotomies. *J. Cranio-Maxillo-Fac. Surg.* **2015**, *43*, 329–335. [CrossRef] [PubMed]
23. Liebregts, J.; Timmermans, M.; de koning, M.; Bergè, S.; Maal, T. Three-dimensional facial simulation in bilateral sagittal split osteotomy: A validation study of 100 patients. *J. Oral Maxillo Fac. Surg.* **2015**, *73*, 961–970. [CrossRef] [PubMed]
24. Mundluru, T.; Almukhtar, A.; Ju, X.; Ayoub, A. The accuracy of three-dimensional prediction of soft tissue changes following the surgical correction of facial asymmetry: An innovative concept. *Int. J. Oral Maxillofac. Surg.* **2017**, *46*, 1517–1524. [CrossRef] [PubMed]
25. De Riu, G.; Virdis, P.; Meloni, S.; Lumbau, A.; Vaira, L. Accuracy of computer-assisted orthognathic surgery. *J. Cranio-Maxillofac. Surg.* **2018**, *46*, 293–298. [CrossRef]
26. Van Hemelen, G.; van Genechten, M.; Renier, L.; Desmedt, M.; Verbruggen, E.; Nadjimi, N. Three-dimensional virtual planning in orthognatic surgery enhances the accuracy of soft tissue prediction. *J. Cranio-Maxillo-Fac. Surg.* **2015**, *43*, 918–925. [CrossRef]
27. Nadjmi, N.; Tehranchi, A.; Azami, N.; Saedi, B.; Mollemans, W. Comparison of soft tissue profiles in Le Fort I osteotomy patients with Dolphin and Maxilim softwares. *Am. J. Orthod. Dentofac. Orthoprothes.* **2013**, *144*, 654–662. [CrossRef]
28. Resnick, C.; Dang, R.; Glick, S.; Padwa, B. Accuracy of three-dimensional soft tissue prediction for Le Fort I osteotomy using Dolphin 3D software: A pilot study. *Int. J. Oral Maxillofac. Surg.* **2017**, *46*, 289–295. [CrossRef]
29. Bianchi, A.; Muyldermans, L.; di Martino, M.; Lancellotti, L.; Amadori, S.; Sarti, A.; Marchetti, C. Facial Soft Tissue Esthetic Predictions: Validation in Craniomaxillofacial Surgery with Cone Beam Computed Tomography Data. *J. Oral Maxillofac. Surg.* **2010**, *68*, 1471–1479. [CrossRef]
30. Marchetti, C.; Bianchi, A.; di Martino, M.; Lancellotti, L.; Sarti, A. Validation of new soft tissue software in orthognathic surgery planning. *Int. J. Oral Maxillofac. Surg.* **2011**, *40*, 26–32. [CrossRef]
31. Khambay, B.; Ullah, R. Current methods of assessing the accuracy of three-dimensional soft tissue facial prediction: Technical and clinical considerations. *Oral Maxillofac. Surg.* **2015**, *44*, 132–138. [CrossRef]
32. Terzic, A.; Combescure, C.; Scolozzi, P. Accuracy of computational soft tissue predictions in orthognathic surgery from three-dimensional photographs 6 months after completion of surgery: A preliminary study of 13 patients. *Int. Soc. Aesthet. Plast. Surg.* **2013**, *38*, 184–191. [CrossRef] [PubMed]

33. Ullah, R.; Turner, P.; Khambay, P. Accuracy of three-dimensional soft tissue predictions in orthognathic surgery after Le Fort I advancement osteotomies. *Br. J. Oral Maxillofac. Surg.* **2014**, *53*, 153–157. [CrossRef] [PubMed]
34. Holzinger, D.; Juergens, P.; Shahim, K.; Reyes, M.; Schicho, K.; Millesi, G.; Perisanidis, C.; Zeilhofer, H.; Seemann, R. Accuracy of soft tissue prediction in surgery-first treatment concept in orthognathic surgery: A prospective study. *J. Cranio-Maxillofac. Surg.* **2018**, *46*, 1455–1460. [CrossRef] [PubMed]
35. Knoops, P.; Borghi, A.; Breakey, R.; Ong, J.; Jeelani, N.; Bruun, R.; Schievano, S.; Dunaway, D.J.; Padwa, B.L. Three-dimensional soft tissue prediction in orthognatic surgery: A clinical comparison of Dolphin, ProPlan CMF and probabilistic finite element modelling. *Int. J. Oral Maxillofac. Surg.* **2019**, *48*, 511–518. [CrossRef]
36. Nam, K.-U.; Hong, J. Is three-dimensional soft tissue prediction by software accurate? *J. Craniofac. Surg.* **2015**, *26*, e729–e733. [CrossRef]
37. Brice, W.; Indresano, A.; O'Rian, F. Venous tromboembolism in oral maxillofacial surgery: A literature review. *J. Oral Maxillo Fac. Surg.* **2011**, *69*, 840–844.
38. Simurda, T.; Kubisz, P.; Necas, L.; Stasko, J. Perioperative coagulation management in in a patient with congenital afibrinogemia during revision total hip arthroplasty. *Semin. Thromb. Emost.* **2016**, *42*, 689–692.
39. Simurda, T.; Stanciakova, L.; Stasko, J.; Dobrotova, M.; Kubisz, P. Yes or no for secondary prophilaxis in afibrinogenemia? *Blood Coagul. Fibrinolysis* **2015**, *26*, 978–980.
40. Ghadimi, K.; Levy, J.; Welsby, I. Perioperative management of the bleeding patient. *Br. J. Anaesth.* **2016**, *117*, iii18–iii30. [CrossRef]
41. Donatsky, O.; Bjorn-Jorgensen, J.; Hermund, U.; Nielsen, H.; Holmqvist-Larsen, M.; Nerder, P. Accuracy of combined maxillary and mandibular repositioning and of soft tissue prediction in relation to maxillary antero-superior repositioning combined with mandibular set-back. *J. Cranio-Maxillofac. Surg.* **2009**, *37*, 279–284. [CrossRef]

10

Laser Vision Correction for Regular Myopia and Supracor Presbyopia

Bojan Pajic [1,2,3,4], Zeljka Cvejic [2], Horace Massa [3], Brigitte Pajic-Eggspuehler [1], Mirko Resan [4] and Harald P. Studer [1,5,*]

1 Eye Clinic Orasis, Swiss Eye Research Foundation, 5734 Reinach AG, Switzerland; bpajic@datacomm.ch (B.P.); brigitte.pajic@orasis.ch (B.P.-E.)
2 Faculty of Sciences, Department of Physics, University of Novi Sad, Trg Dositeja Obradovica 4, 21000 Novi Sad, Serbia; zeljka.cvejic@df.uns.ac.rs
3 Division of Ophthalmology, Department of Clinical Neurosciences, Geneva University Hospitals, 1205 Geneva, Switzerland; horace.massa@hcuge.ch
4 Faculty of Medicine of the Military Medical Academy, University of Defense, 11000 Belgrade, Serbia; resan.mirko@gmail.com
5 OCTLab, Dept. of Ophthalmology, University of Basel, 4056 Basel, Switzerland
* Correspondence: harald.studer@gmail.com

Abstract: A study to compare femto-presbyLASIK to standard myopia femto-LASIK refractive surgical correction with a total of 45 candidates was performed. The goal was to identify a more specific set of indications for presbyopia LASIK treatments. The results showed thoroughly good uncorrected visual acuity for myopia (decimal: 1.01 ± 0.15) as well as for presbyLASIK (decimal: 0.78 ± 0.17) corrections. Astigmatism was comparable in both groups and did not change significantly from preoperative (0.98D ± 0.53 SD) to postoperative (1.01D ± 0.50 SD). Our study results suggest, that presbyLASIK treatment is as safe and effective as regular LASIK myopia correction and can hence be recommended to treat presbyopia.

Keywords: supracor; myopia; presbyopia; presbyLASIK; refractive surgery; follow-up; clinical results; lasik; excimer laser

1. Introduction

Laser Assisted In-Situ Keratomileusis (LASIK) has become the most prevalent refractive surgical procedure for myopic and hyperopic corrections (about 1.2 million procedures a year in the US)—over the last two decades. Patient satisfaction is generally found to be very high between 92 and 98 percent [1,2]. Modern excimer laser systems can restore 20/20 uncorrected visual acuity (UCVA) in myopic eyes up to—10D and hyperopic up to +6D, feature tissue saving procedures [3], provide patient-specific, wavefront and/or topography guided ablation patterns, and can treat astigmatism with elliptically shaped patterns.

The concept of multifocal PresbyLASIK is a relatively new yet attractive surgical procedure for the correction of presbyopia. It involves two steps: (1) the correction of the ametropic state for distance vision, and (2) the multifocality addition for near vision. As most commonly reported in literature, multifocality is usually implemented by combining a central corneal curvature addition for near vision correction with a paracentral corneal curvature, adjusted to correct distance vision [4–9].

The downside of multifocal LASIK treatments is that they always represent a compromise between distance—and near vision correction, as they create unwanted aberrations—especially spherical aberrations in the central pupillary region. For this reason, modern PresbyLASIK treatment algorithms are wavefront-guided to minimize unwanted aberrations. Compared to treating presbyopia with the well-established multifocal intra ocular lens (IOL) implantation, PresbyLASIK has the advantage of being less invasive because the ocular globe does not need to be opened for treatment. However, the planning of PresbyLASIK procedures is much more demanding and requires experience in the interpretation of the preoperative corneal topography, wavefront analysis and the Zernike coefficients, which all have significant impact on the surgery result. Hence, it is not enough to simply apply the common LASIK indications to PresbyLASIK as well. Presumably, the lack of specific indications—along with missing to consider refraction and wavefront analysis parameters, might well be the reason for the not all encouraging LASIK presbyopia treatment results presented in literature [10,11].

In this study we present our PresbyLASIK results and compare them to a control group of regular LASIK myopia correction cases. Further, we propose an updated set of more specific indications for the PresbyLASIK treatment.

2. Materials and Methods

Our study population included two groups of eyes, 40 eyes of 20 study patients (female: 14, male: 6, age: 30 ± 9 years) were treated with regular myopic LASIK correction, and 50 eyes of 25 study patients (female: 14, male: 11, age: 52 ± 3.8 years) were treated for presbyopia with the PresbyLASIK Supracor treatment (B&L Technolas, Munich, Germany). All surgery procedures were performed by an experienced surgeon (BP) at the Eye Clinic ORASIS between January 2014 and February 2015.

The LDV femtosecond laser (Ziemer Ophthalmology, Port, Switzerland) was used to make the LASIK flaps, whereby the hinge was superior in all cases. The flap diameter depended on the corneal curvature and was between 8.5 and 9.0 mm. The Munnerlyn formula [12] along with the B&L-Technolas proprietary transition zone algorithm was used to calculate the ablation patterns for the regular myopia corrections. In a two-step approach a 2.0 mm laser spot diameter was first used to apply the basic correction, followed by the fine-tuning step with a 1.0 mm laser spot. An eye tracker system was active during all interventions. The cyclorotation is automatically compensated which is especially important for cases where astigmatism correction was included. Whenever the angle kappa was smaller or equal 6° the laser spot was placed in the pupil center, otherwise it was placed at the point of the arithmetic mean between the pupil center and the Purkinje reflex. After the laser correction, the flap was carefully placed back onto the stromal bed, making sure no visible wrinkles are left.

The same approach as for the myopia ablation patterns is also employed to calculate the Supracor PresbyLASIK ablation patterns, however, the target refraction is chosen such that the dominant eye was at 0.0D and the follow-eye was at −0.5D. The goal of a first application phase is to obtain a perfect mono-focal correction, and only in the second phase the central cornea is steepened by the multifocal curvature addition in the 3.0 to 6.0 mm zone. Considering that such an ablation could potentially induced spherical aberration, the Supracor procedure was performed wavefront-guided for all cases.

Corneal shape was assessed one week before and then 3 months after the LASIK treatment, with the Galilei G4 tomographer (Ziemer Ophthalmic Systems, Port, Switzerland). Thereby, each individual measurement was repeated three times in a row. So, only one measurement with the median astigmatism cylinder value is selected for further data evaluation.

The statistical methods used in this study were straightforward calculations of average and standard deviation, as described in any textbook of statistics. Excel software package (Microsoft, Redmond, WA, USA) was used to import and process data, as well as, to obtain the functional dependence of the selected parameters and their visualization. Two-tailed Student *t*-test was used for calculating the parametric datas and for the nonparametric test the Wilcoxon signed rank test was used. The level of significance was set at $p < 0.05$.

3. Results

All study data were carefully analyzed and are presented in the following. Manifest refraction of the whole study population was sph: −1.99D ± 3.48 (SD), cyl: −0.80D ± 0.79 (SD) before, and sph: −0.03D ± 0.27 (SD), cyl: −0.18D ± 0.32 (SD) after the surgery. While the myopia group had a manifest refraction of sph: −3.53D ± 2.48 (SD), cyl: −0.93D ± 0.84 (SD) before, and sph: +0.05D ± 0.19 (SD), cyl: −0.09D ± 0.27 (SD) after the surgery, the presbyopia group had a manifest refraction of sph: −1.02D ± 3.78 (SD), cyl:−0.72D ± 0.75 (SD) before, and sph: −0.09D ± 0.31 (SD), cyl: −0.24D ± 0.34 (SD) after the surgery.

3.1. Uncorrected Visual Acuity

Uncorrected visual acuity (UCVA) was assessed before (decimal scale: 0.31 ± 0.24) and after the treatment (decimal scale: 0.88 ± 0.20) for the whole study population. In the myopia group UCVA was 0.19 ± 0.16 preoperatively, and 1.01 ± 0.15 postoperatively. In the presbyopia group UCVA was 0.38 ± 0.25 preoperatively, and 0.78 ± 0.17 postoperatively. A statistically significant improvement was observed in both groups ($p < 0.0001$). In 4 eyes (4.3%, two in myopia and two in presbyopia group), UCVA remained unchanged, and for two eyes (2.2%, all in the presbyopia group) UCVA was slightly worse than before the treatment. For all other eyes (93.5%), UCVA improved (see Table 1). The failure to achieve the target refraction and UCVA could be corrected with a re-treatment.

Table 1. Uncorrected visual acuity after regular myopia and Supracor presbyopia treatment.

	Average		Minimum		Maximum	
	Decimal	**Metric**	**Decimal**	**Metric**	**Decimal**	**Metric**
All eyes	0.88 ± 0.20	5.3/6	0.32	1.9/6	1.25	7.5/6
Myopia	1.01 ± 0.16	6.1/6	0.63	3.8/6	1.25	7.5/6
Supracor	0.78 ± 0.17	4.7/6	0.32	1.9/6	1.00	6/6

While the multifocal presbyopia treatments showed a small trend ($R^2 = 0.01$) towards greater corrections having a lower postoperative UCVA, this trend could not be observed ($R^2 = 1 \times 10^{-5}$) for the myopic corrections (see Figure 1).

3.2. Residual Stromal Bed and Percentage Tissue Altered

The average residual stromal bed thickness for all cases was 385 μm ± 49 (SD), with a minimum of 285 μm, and a maximum of 510 μm. The recently published and already widely accepted new criterion for LASIK safety, the percentage tissue altered (PTA) value [13] was 32.0% ± 3.0 (SD), with a minimum of 22% and a maximum of 47%.

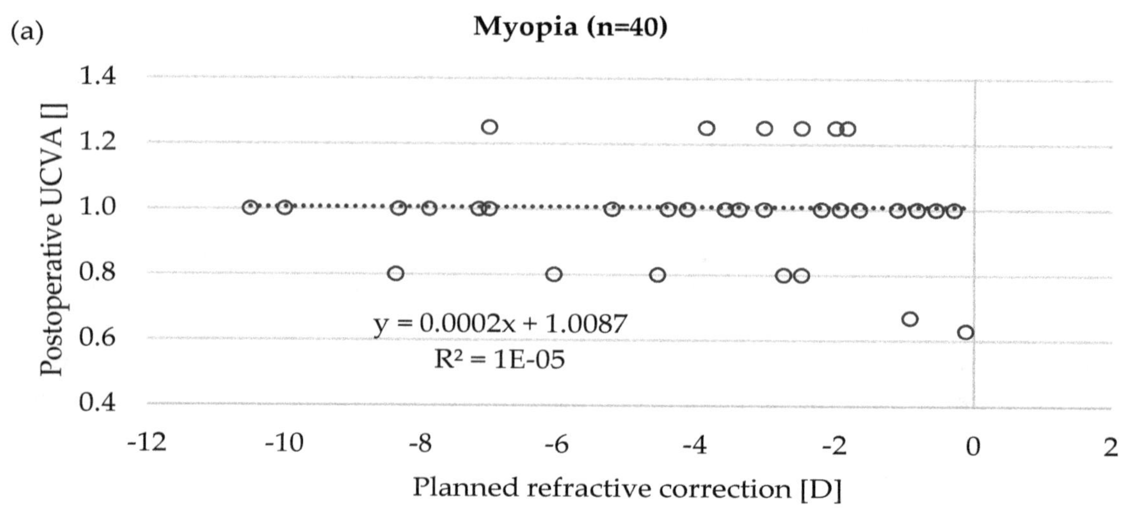

Figure 1. *Cont.*

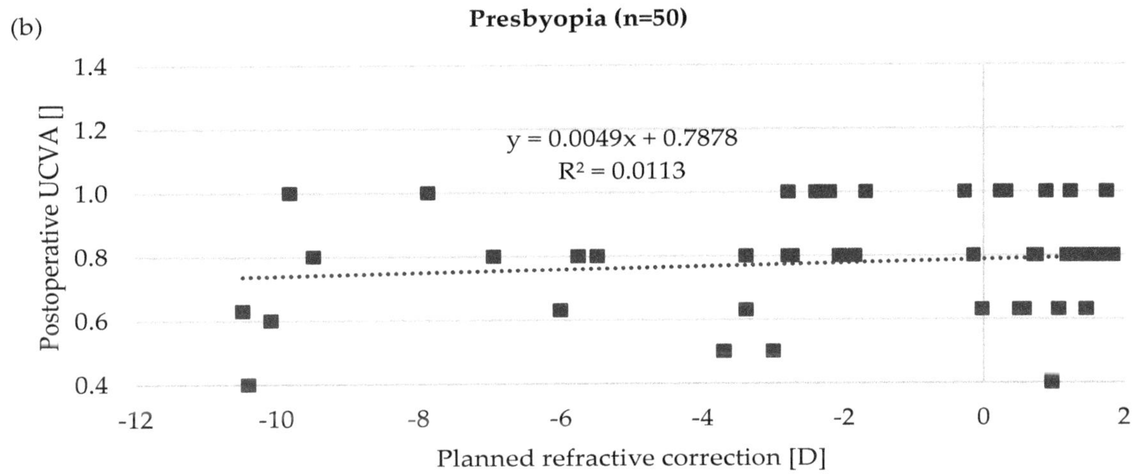

Figure 1. Trend analysis for presbyopia treatments (**b**) showed a mild correlation ($R^2 = 0.01$ with slope 0.005) that greater dioptric corrections resulted in lower uncorrected visual acuity (UCVA). No such correlation (R^2 = 1E-05 with slope < 0.001) between dioptric correction and resulting UCVA could be observed in the myopia (**a**) results, though.

3.3. *Astigmatism Change*

Corneal astigmatism, assessed with the Galilei G4, showed very little difference ($p > 0.6$), between preoperative (0.98D ± 0.53 SD) and postoperative measurements (1.01D ± 0.50 SD) over the whole study population. Likewise, the myopia group had preoperative astigmatism of 1.17D ± 0.63 (SD), which changed to postoperative astigmatism of 0.78D ± 0.74 (SD) $p > 0.02$. The presbyopia group had preoperative astigmatism of 1.02D ± 0.42 (SD), which changed to postoperative astigmatism of 0.96D ± 0.58 (SD) $p > 0.02$. Also, Figure 2 shows double-angle polar plots of pre-, and post-operative astigmatism measurements for both groups, myopia and presbyopia, and suggests only small changes in astigmatism from pre—to postoperative measurements. However, the Alpins method [14] vector analysis (including the astigmatism orientation) showed that astigmatism changed significantly, by 0.78D ± 0.74 (SD) for myopia and by 0.96D ± 0.58 (SD) for presbyopia, respectively. The intended astigmatic change (planned astigmatic LASIK ablations) was 0.94D ± 0.84 (SD) for myopia group and 0.65D ± 0.41 (SD) for presbyopia group.

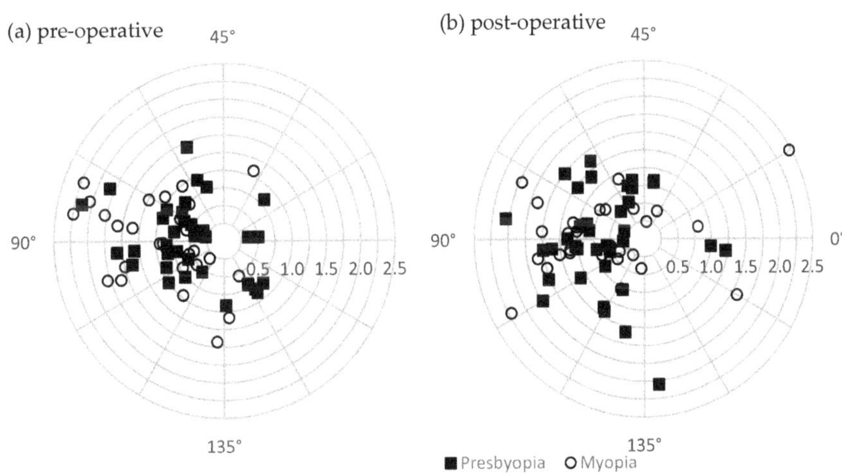

Figure 2. Double-angle polar plots comparing (**a**) pre- to (**b**) postoperative astigmatism. Myopia results are shown as circles and presbyopia results are shown as solid squares. No obvious differences between myopia and presbyopia correction were visible.

3.4. Corneal Curvature Change

The planned shape change of the anterior corneal surface was compared to the measured corneal surface average corneal curvature–AvgK (postoperative Galilei minus preoperative Galilei). In an ideally case, in Figure 3, all data points would lie on a diagonal line ($y = 1.0x + 0.0$, with an $R^2 = 1.0$). The top plot (b) in Figure 3 shows that the above graph (b) in Figure 3 shows that the presbyopia corrections showed a better match between the planned and achieved spherical correction ($y = 0.67x - 0.09$, $R^2 = 0.93$) compared to the myopia correction (see graph (a) in Figure 3) ($y = 0.45x - 1.22$, $R^2 = 0.47$).

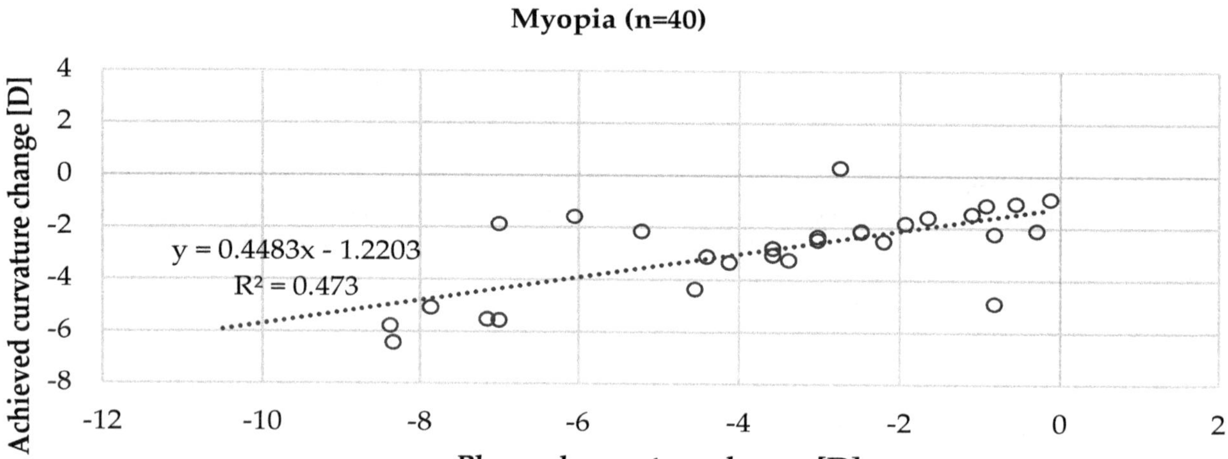

(a)

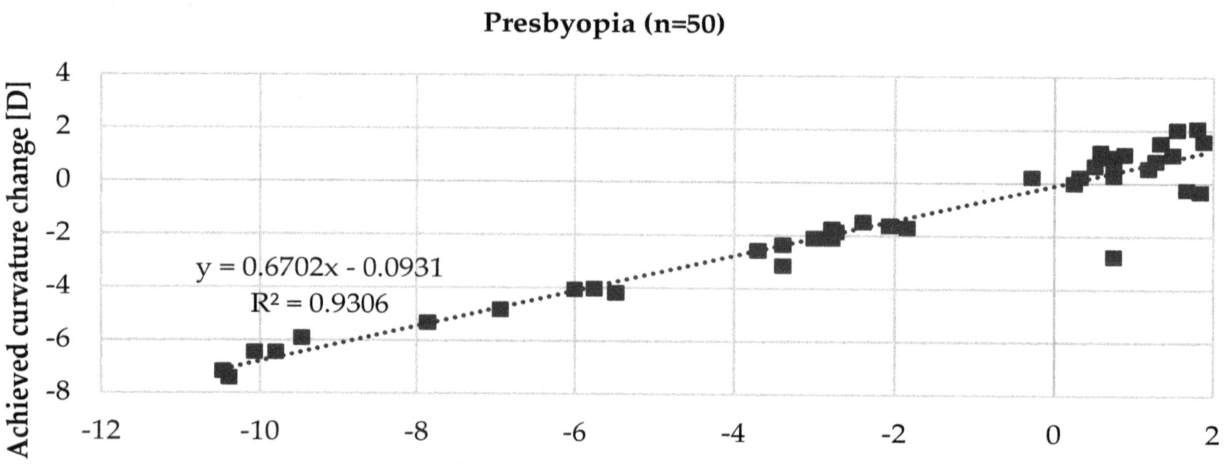

(b)

Figure 3. Comparing planned to achieved shape change of anterior corneal surface. Presbyopia treatments (**b**) showed a better match (R^2 = 0.93 and slope 0.67) than (**a**) myopia (R^2 = 0.45 and slope 0.47).

4. Discussion

In this study, femto-LASIK refractive surgical treatments were performed in two groups of study populations. While one of the groups received a standard myopia treatment, the second group was treated with a specific multifocal presbyLASIK algorithm to treat presbyopia. Study data, such as uncorrected visual acuity (UCVA), were carefully analyzed and presented as study results.

In almost all the cases (>93%), UCVA was improved after the surgery, with respect to the baseline assessment before the treatment. Thereby, the standard femto-LASIK myopia treatment showed slightly better results than the presbyLASIK treatment, where outcome UCVA was lower. This most likely arises from the fact that the subjective tolerance to eye surgical treatments including multifocal optics is greater than in monofocal treatments. Even a small deviation of 0.5D from the target value can be disturbing for the patient. Accordingly, there was a small but significant trend in recent results, where higher correction of presbyLASIK lead to lower postoperative UCVA. No similar trend was observed in the standard myopia treatment cases, where even high corrections of up to −10.5D had perfect vision with UCVA result of decimal 1.0.

The completely positive UCVA outcome was achieved, although the results suggest that astigmatism was drastically undertreated. Even though the laser was programmed with astigmatism correcting ablation patterns for all cases with treatable preoperative astigmatism, significant postoperative corneal astigmatism was observed in the topography measurements of both study groups. This observation is not supported by estimates of apparent refraction, where the cylinder of astigmatism decreased from −0.80D ± 0.79 (SD) to −0.18 D ± 0.33 (SD) ($p < 0.00001$). Thus, it could be assumed that the topography measurements were not accurate enough, but we did not have additional data to examine this in more details.

After surgical treatment, the mechanical strength of the cornea depends only on the residual stroma. It is well known that when the residual stroma is too thin to handle IOP, both its anterior and posterior surface will bulge forward as in ectasia. Nowadays, residual stroma thickness (RST) is accepted to be at least 250 μm. Conventionally, thickness less than 480 is considered abnormal, while some surgeons consider preoperative corneal thickness less than 500 μm unsuitable for LASIK. While planning the treatments, 250 μm of the RST was suggested as it accounts for 50% of 500 μm, which is the minimum corneal thickness recommended for LASIK. Also, high percentage of tissue altered (PTA) is the most common cause of ectasia after LASIK in patients with normal preoperative corneal topography. According to Santiago et al. [13], high values of PTA, especially higher than 40% is important factor in the development post-Lasik ectasia with normal preoperative corneal topography. For that reasonPTA should be taken as one of the screening parameter for refractive surgery candidates. In addition to this criterion, we have aimed at a postoperative thickness of 300 μm residual cornea stroma or more for all cases to allow re-treatment if necessary. None of the eyes in this study developed postoperative ectasia.

The observation, that postoperative central corneal curvature was steeper than planned comes from the fact that the algorithm used for the multifocality add-on causes a central steepening within the 3.0 mm zone. This is because the central zone is intended to be used for near vision. The 3.0 to 6.0 mm zone is adjusted to correct intermediate and distance vision. Both eyes thereby are treated the same way, except that the non-dominant eye is targeted at −0.5D from plano.

The results in this study suggest that the used procedure for presbyLASIK improves vision of presbyopia patients. Hence, we propose to include subjects for the presbyopia treatment older than 48 years, with a mesopic pupil of 3.5–6.5 mm diameter, and with a postoperative Kmean between 35.0D and 47.0D. The central near vision add-ons should be chosen >2.0D. We further suggest that cases where eye surgery was previously performed should not be included, especially cases where corneal refractive surgery was performed. Also, those cases with irregular corneal morphology, lens opacification, natural preoperative multifocality in the cornea, or a central corneal thickness CCT < 500 μm microns should not be included.

Author Contributions: B.P. and the team from the Orasis clinic in Switzerland conducted the clinical study and collected all the data and contributed substantially to writing the manuscript. Z.C. contributed substantially to the methodology, collecting datas and contributed substantially to writing the manuscript. H.M. performed data analyses and substantially contributed advising regarding the paper contents. B.P.-E. perform substantially data curation and contributed the study design. M.R. performed data anlysis and substantially contributed the study design. H.P.S. did the data analysis, statistical analysis and created all the plots and figures, and contributed substantially to writing the manuscript. All authors have read and agreed to the published version of the manuscript.

References

1. Tahzib, N.G.; Bootsma, S.J.; Eggink, F.A.; Nabar, V.A.; Nujits, R.M. Functional outcomes and patient satisfaction after laser in situ keratomileusis for correction of myopia. *J. Cataract Refract. Surg.* **2005**, *10*, 1943–1951. [CrossRef] [PubMed]
2. Bailey, M.D.; Mitchell, L.G.; Zadnik, K. Reasons for recommending laser in situ keratomileusis. *Optom. Vis. Sci.* **2005**, *79*, 10. [CrossRef]
3. McGhee, C.N.; Graig, J.P.; Sachdev, N.; Weed, K.H.; Brown, A.D. Functional, psychological, and satisfaction outcomes of laser in situ keratomileusis for high myopia. *J. Cataract Refract. Surg.* **2000**, *26*, 497–509. [CrossRef]
4. Alarcón, A.; Anera, R.G.; Villa, C.; Jiménez del Barco, L.; Gutierrez, R. Visual quality after monovision correction by laser in situ keratomileusis in presbyopic patients. *J. Cataract Refract. Surg.* **2011**, *37*, 1629–1635. [CrossRef] [PubMed]
5. Uthoff, D.; Pölzl, M.; Hepper, D.; Holland, D. A new method of cornea modulation with excimer laser for simultaneous correction of presbyopia and ametropia. *Graefe's Arch. Clin. Exp. Ophthalmol.* **2012**, *250*, 1649–1661. [CrossRef] [PubMed]
6. Baudu, P.; Penin, F.; Arba Mosquera, S. Uncorrected binocular performance after biaspheric ablation profile for presbyopic corneal treatment using AMARIS with the PresbyMAX module. *Am. J. Ophthalmol.* **2013**, *155*, 636–647. [CrossRef] [PubMed]
7. Jackson, W.B.; Tuan, K.M.; Mintsioulis, G. Aspheric wavefrontguided LASIK to treat hyperopic presbyopia: 12-month results with the VISX platform. *J. Refract. Surg.* **2011**, *27*, 519–529. [CrossRef] [PubMed]
8. Jung, S.W.; Kim, M.J.; Park, S.H.; Joo, C.-K. Multifocal corneal ablation for hyperopic presbyopes. *J. Refract. Surg.* **2008**, *24*, 903–910. [CrossRef] [PubMed]
9. Luger, M.H.; Ewering, T.; Arba-Mosquera, S. One-year experience in presbyopia correction with biaspheric multifocal central presbyopia laser in situ keratomileusis. *Cornea* **2013**, *32*, 644–652. [CrossRef] [PubMed]
10. Pajic, B.; Pajic-Eggspuehler, B.; Mueller, J.; Cvejic, Z.; Studer, H. A Novel Laser Refractive Surgical Treatment for Presbyopia: Optics-Based Customization for Improved Clinical Outcome. *Sensors* **2017**, *17*, 1367. [CrossRef] [PubMed]
11. Pajic, B.; Massa, H.; Eskina, E. Presbyopiekorrektur mittels Lasechirurgie. *Klin. Monatsbl. Augenheilkd.* **2017**. [CrossRef]
12. Munnerlyn, C.R.; Koons, S.J.; Marshall, J. Photorefractive keratectomy: A technique for laser refractive surgery. *J. Cataract Refract. Surg.* **1988**, *14*, 46–52. [CrossRef]
13. Santhiago, M.R.; Smadja, D.; Gomes, B.F.; Mello, G.R.; Monteiro, M.R.L.; Wilson, S.E.; Randelman, J.B. Association Between the Percentage Tissue Altered and Post-Laser In Situ Keratomileusis Ectasia in Eyes With Normal Preoperative Topography. *Am. J. Ophthalmol.* **2014**, *158*, 87–95. [CrossRef]
14. Alpins, N.A. A new method of analyzing vectors for changes in astigmatism. *J. Cataract Refract. Surg.* **1993**, *19*, 524–533. [CrossRef]

11

A New Concept Compliant Platform with Spatial Mobility and Remote Actuation

Nicola Pio Belfiore

Department of Engineering, University of Roma Tre, via della Vasca Navale 79, 00146 Rome, Italy; nicolapio.belfiore@uniroma3.it.

Abstract: This paper presents a new tendon-driven platform with spatial mobility. The system can be obtained as a monolithic structure, and its motion is based on the concept of selective compliance. The latter contributes also to optimizing the use of the material by avoiding parasitic deformations. The presented platform makes use of lumped compliance with three different kinds of elastic joints. An analysis of the platform mobility based on finite element analysis is provided together with an assembly mode analysis of the equivalent pseudo-rigid body mechanism. Surgical operations in laparoscopic environments are the natural fields of applications for this device.

Keywords: platform; spatial motion; remote actuation; cable actuation; laparoscopy; minimally-invasive surgery

---

1. Introduction

A parallel architecture offers several advantages to the designers of spatial platform mechanisms. In fact, they rely on a multi-loop topology that is certainly convenient for the stage stiffness and accuracy, whereas their forward kinematic analysis becomes more complex.

The Stewart–Gough platform, a mechanism that can be considered to be a milestone of parallel manipulators, was presented in 1965 [1]. This six-DoF (degree of freedom) system can be controlled in any combination by six motors and has the advantage of no fixed axis relative to the ground. Classical issues for parallel manipulators have been extensively studied in the literature, such as structural kinematics [2], workspace [3], singularity [4], optimal design [5], structure synthesis [6], manipulability [7], control of redundantly-actuated [8], and remotely cable-driven parallel manipulators [9]. On the other hand, more recent subjects have still not been well investigated for parallel platforms, such as connectivity and redundancy [10], topology [11], and planarity [12].

Classical parallel platforms are composed of rigid links and ordinary kinematic pairs with a geometric closure configuration. However, they could be built as compliant mechanisms [13–15], which present a series of advantageous characteristics: they are not subject to backlash and do not need lubrication; they can be also built from a unique block of material; and finally, they have generally a neutral or balance configuration from which the deformed poses can be achieved. In fact, they can reach a given configuration thanks to external forces that can be applied with a high precision to deform the elastic structure, using also a redundant driving strategy. More recently, active compliance [16,17] has been added as a further possibility in design, acting both as a series or in a parallel configuration with passive compliance.

These features make compliant mechanisms very interesting for applications where lubrication is impossible or where extreme accuracy is needed. For these reasons, a group multi-DoF compliant stages has also been developed in literature [18].

Since 1990, stiffness and conditioning maps of the workspace of parallel manipulators have been established [19], in order to prevent special types of singularities, which result in a loss of controllability. A six-DoF force sensor was designed in 1991 [20] on the base of the Stewart–Gough platform. In this layout, the fixed and mobile platforms are coupled by six spring-loaded pistons, whereas the length variations are measured by means of six linear voltage differential transformers mounted along the pistons. The Stewart–Gough inverse and forward kinematic transformations are used to calculate the forces and torques that are applied to the mobile platform. A three DoF translational compliant parallel platform was presented in 2005 [21] for nanomanipulation. Workspace, dexterity, and isotropic configurations were studied by using the pseudo rigid-body model (PRBM). A six-PSS (prismatic-spherical-spherical) nanopositioner compliant mechanism was designed [22] to be actuated by means of six multilayered piezoelectric actuators. The system is composed of one fixed plate, three two-PSS compliant mechanisms, and one end effector. The PRBM is also used in this investigation to study its kinematic analysis. A three DoF spatial translational accurate positioning compliant platform with flexible hinges and with piezoelectric actuators has been designed [23] to achieve high stiffness, a high speed of dynamic response, high kinematic accuracy, and high resolution. A six-DoF compliant parallel micro-scale manipulator with piezo-driven actuators and integrated force sensor has been designed [24] to provide real-time force information for feedback control. Kinematic and static analysis were investigated to achieve high positioning accuracy, compactness, and smooth and continuous displacements. A method for the optimal design and performance characterization of micromanipulators has been also applied to six-DOF parallel micromanipulators [25]. A three-DoF compliant platform has been studied [26] to make it able to move in three-dimensional space. The system was composed of compliant joints, actuators, and a central moving platform. The actuators consisted of three binary links, while the moving platform was an equilateral plate. The free end of each actuator and the central platform were connected by springs in such a way that the motion of the actuators was transmitted to the moving platform. Considering the applications at the micro scale and using the technology on which micro electro-mechanical systems (MEMS) are based, a compliant three-DoF plane parallel platform has been proposed [27] together with its kinetostatic optimization.

The "da Vinci" © surgical robot (by Intuitive Surgical, Inc., Sunnyvale, California, USA) is a widely-used system designed to facilitate surgical operations with a minimally-invasive approach. This robot makes use of multi-DoF end terminals as a resource to cope with different tasks, working in cooperation with robotic wrists or steerable instruments, and their characteristics have been extensively improved and refined throughout the years. For example, a 2 mm-diameter instrument equipped with a three-DoF wrist has been investigated and tested [28] for the robotic "da Vinci" platform. Moreover, new systems for measuring the end effector gripping force have also been developed by means of a torque transfer system [29]. Finally, deflection and force feedback from the "da Vinci" end effector have been provided by new types of strain gauges [30].

However, in most of the above-mentioned systems for remote manipulations that are widely adopted for minimally-invasive surgery, the wrists and end effector consist of mechanisms that have ordinary kinematic pairs, which are subject to backlash problems, and a serial kinematic structure, which is usually less robust than a parallel structure. The present paper presents a new six-DoF platform for remote manipulation that consists pf a mechanism with selective compliance (compliant mechanism) and has also a parallel structure. The device could be either part of "da Vinci" or independently driven by another positioning system. Originally, the system was conceived to work under a laparoscopic environment, and it is expected to improve its success in surgery, such as in laparoscopic sleeve gastrectomy (LSG) with cruroplasty [31], in surgical treatment of gastrointestinal stromal tumors of the duodenum [32], in colovesical fistula surgery with a minimally-invasive approach [33], in endoluminal loco-regional resection by transanal endoscopic microsurgery (TEM) [34–36], and also in low rectal anterior resection (LAR) [37].

2. Description of the New Concept Platform

In several applications, the position of a mobile platform in space has to be controlled by using remote means, such as cables. Usually, the conventional mechanisms that are able to implement such a feature are rather complicated because the platform has six degrees of freedom (DoF), and moreover, they are subject to backlash and parasitic deformations. This problem is quite general, but in this paper, a specific implementation suitable for surgical applications will be presented.

A new tendon-driven compliant mechanism is herein proposed, as a possible solution to the above-mentioned problem. The full mobility of the platform in space and, in particular, its raising motion is possible because of a new elastic joint, which combines the action of an elastic curved beam and of a portion of the conjugate surfaces. The invention consists basically of a wire-operated selective compliance mobile platform like the one represented in Figure 1. The mechanism base (k) is intended to be mounted on the end of a flexible tubular duct for endoscopic, surgical, therapeutic, or diagnostic uses.

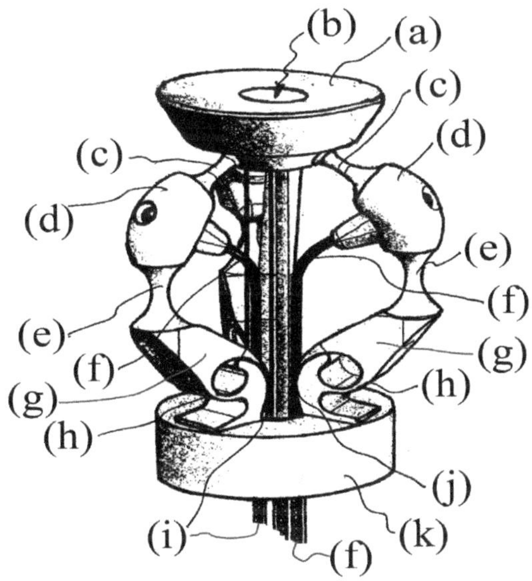

Figure 1. A view of the compliant platform and of all its elements: platform (**a**); plaform hole (**b**); type *S* elastic joints (**c**); type-U elastic joints (**e**); upper (**d**) and lower (**g**) links; upper (**f**) and lower cables (**i**); conjugate surface flexure hinge (CSFH) hinges (**h**); base link (**k**).

The platform (a) is designed for supporting surgical means, normally used during endoluminal operations, such as vision systems, forceps, scissors, cannulae, electrotomes, and so on. However, the system could be used for precision applications or in adverse environments, e.g., for operations in the aerospace environment. The base (k) and the platform (a) are connected through a plurality of legs, which provide mobility in space to the mobile surface (a), and are operated by actuating wires (i) and (f), running inside the tubular duct, to control and operate the platform remotely.

Since the mechanical structure of the mechanism is based on selective compliance and, particularly, on lumped compliance, there is a neutral configuration that is assumed when no external force is acting on the structure.

2.1. Deduction of the Pseudo-Rigid Body Equivalent Mechanism

A compliant mechanism can be generally modeled as its equivalent so-called pseudo-rigid body mechanism (PRBM). The PRBM is a mechanism with only ordinary kinematic pairs, which presents approximately the same motion as the original compliant mechanism in the neighborhood of the neutral configuration. For this purpose, each elastic joint is replaced by an ordinary kinematic pair, which can offer mobility that is compatible with the selective compliance characteristics of that elastic joint. Figure 2 shows the original compliant mechanism (Figure 2a) and its corresponding spatial PRBM (Figure 2b).

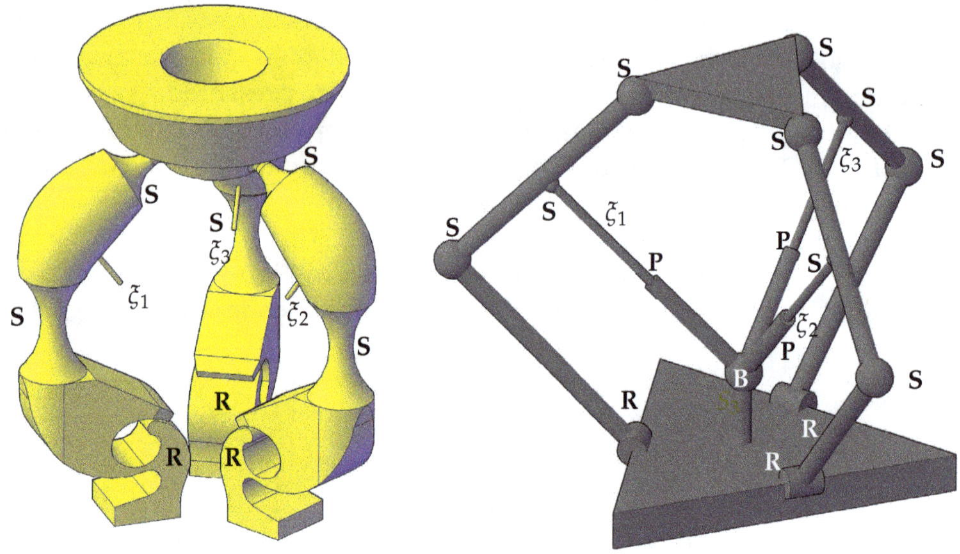

(a) (b)

Figure 2. The compliant platform (**a**) and its corresponding pseudo-rigid body mechanism (**b**), with the equivalent revolute joints R, spherical joints S, prismatic pairs P, a triple spherical joint S_3, and the cable directions ξ_1, ξ_2, and ξ_3.

With reference to Figures 1 and 2, the elastic joints can be distinguished according to the following characteristics.

- A Type (e) elastic joint is delimited by a toroidal surface obtained by revolving a circular arc around a vertical axis γ_E. As a consequence, the neck cross-sectional area is normal to γ_E and is positioned in correspondence to the symmetry middle plane of the joint surface. The relative motion between the two connected pseudo-rigid parts has at least two degrees of freedom (DoF), namely those due to the bending along two orthogonal planes passing through γ_E. Furthermore, one more DoF could be added depending on whether the neck section allows the two opposite end sections to rotate significantly, one with respect to the other, about γ_E. For Type (e) joints, the choice of the diameter of the neck section is decisive for assuming whether the amount of torsional rotation might play a significant role. If so, Type (e) can be replaced by a three-DoF spherical S joint, otherwise a two DoF (Hooke's) universal U will be used. In the latter case, the flexure works approximately as a Cardan joint whose center is placed at the center of elastic weights of the elastic joint itself.
- A Type (c) elastic joint is also delimited by a portion of a toroidal surface obtained by the rotation of a circular arc around an axis of revolution $\gamma_C \neq \gamma_E$. For this type of joint, the rotations about γ_C are considered to be always non-negligible. In fact, they are provided with an even more reduced middle cross-section that gives rise to possible torsion rotations about γ_c. Therefore, the joints (c) substantially have the function of spherical elastic joints, the equivalent center of the spherical kinematic pair being placed at the center of elastic weights of the joint itself. For this reasons, Type (c) joints will be replaced by spherical joints S.
- Type (h) elastic joints belong to the class of the conjugate surface flexure hinge (CSFH). This kind of flexure has been patented (see Section 7) and extensively studied for several aspects: their theoretical behavior [38,39], design [40,41], dynamic simulation [42], fabrication [43–45], and applications [46–51]. Type (h) CSFH hinges selectively provide rotations around the CSFH axis

with a very good accuracy, because of the presence of a portion of conjugate surfaces. Therefore, they are replaced by classical revolute joints R.

- Type (f) cables are the three moving elements for Type (d) upper links out of a total of six cables that are used to operate the six-DoF platform. For example, a simultaneous pull command on the three Type (f) cables will move the platform downward. The cables may be arranged in such a way so as to be aligned in the three directions ξ_1, ξ_2, and ξ_3, as illustrated in Figure 2a.
- Type (i) cables are the moving elements for Type (g) links. These three cables provide motion for the three CSFH hinges, and so, they regulate the orientation of Type (g) links. For example, a cable pull will induce a rotation that tends to raise the link upward.

Three linear actuators SPS are added to the system and positioned as in Figure 2b in order to replace the three actuated cables directed along the ξ_1, ξ_2, and ξ_3 directions. The three linear actuators are identified in the figure as the ones that are incident to the triple spherical joint S_3 positioned at Point B. This replacement is justified by the fact that the three cables are directed along lines that pass through the center $B$of the triple spherical joint S_3. This point is positioned in the middle of the fixed platform, in correspondence to a level that does not interfere with the CSFH hinges.

Finally, it is worth noting that the identification of a PRBM that adequately corresponds to the proposed compliant structure represents the first necessary step to further analyze the new systems, such as workspace and kinematic analysis, kinematic synthesis, and kinetostatic behavior.

2.2. Topological Analysis

Considering an equivalent mechanism PRBM with rigid bodies and classical U, S, and R pairs, three legs guarantee six degrees of freedom to the platform. In fact, the PRBM presents $\ell = 8$ rigid links and $m = 9$ kinematic pairs. In case Type (e) joints are replaced by U joints, the structure will be composed of three Type (h) revolute joints R with degree of constraint $c_i = 5$ in space, three Type (e) U joints with $c_i = 4$, and six S joints with $c_i = 3$. Therefore, according to the general topological Grubler's formula, the PRBM has:

$$F = \lambda(\ell - 1) - \sum_{i=1}^{m} c_i = 6(8-1) - 3\cdot 5 - 3\cdot 3 - 3\cdot 4 = 6 \tag{1}$$

overall degrees of freedom (DoF), where $\lambda = 6$ is the mobility number for general spatial motion.

As mentioned above, torsion cannot always be excluded on U elastic Type (e) joints, depending on the minimum diameter of the normal cross-section, which would make them practically equivalent to S joints. In this case, Grubler's formula would yield $F = 9$ DoFs for the platform, but it must be remarked that three of such DoFs would be uniquely dedicated to providing idle rotations to the upper Type (d) links. In this case, any Link (d) would be connected to the remaining parts of the structure by means of two S type pairs, and so, rotations about an axis passing through the centers of the two spherical joints would be possible. These rotations are naturally counterbalanced by internal elastic reactions that would drive the system back toward the minimum of the potential elastic energy. Alternatively, they could make it easier to achieve an optimal attitude of Type (f) cables that pull down Type (d) links. For these reasons, a different manipulator could be obtained, as an alternative, where Type (e) links are replaced by Type (c) links, with no problems for mobility.

According to the result obtained by using Equation (1) and considering that each leg is supposed to be controlled by two cables, a three-legged platform will be the one that has a number of independent actuators that is equal to the number of DoF and therefore will be considered as an optimal choice for the compliant structure. In fact, according to the principle of selective compliance, any elastic element where compliance is concentrated presents a peculiar geometry that is intended for a specific deformation, for example a prescribed flexion or torsion axis, and all the deformations different from the prescribed ones are considered to be as parasitic deformations, because they do not contribute to the desired motion, but only increase the stress level in the elastic material. For this reason, a satisfying geometry of a compliant mechanism is the one that minimizes the parasitic deformations.

2.3. Direct Position Analysis

Thanks to the construction of the PRBM depicted in Figure 2b, it is possible to identify some fundamental characteristics of the platform, as they have been introduced in the literature. For example, it is clear that this platform is not a fully-parallel platform, because two DoF are needed for each leg. With reference to Figure 3a, the ith leg (with $i = 1, \dots, 0$) will be composed of the pseudo rigid links C_iA_i and A_iP_i, which respectively correspond to Type (g) and Type (d) links of the original compliant structure.

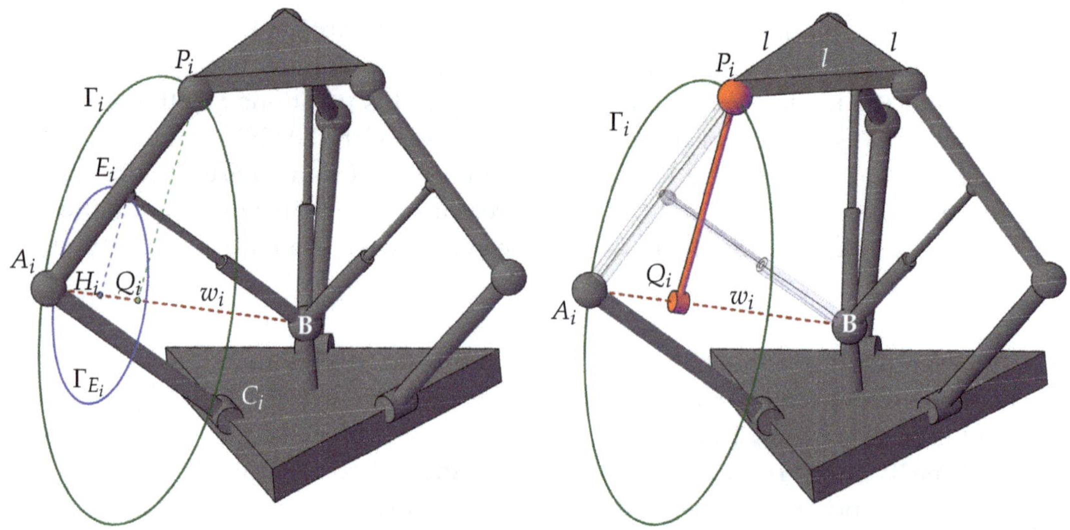

(a) (b)

Figure 3. (**a**) The circles Γ_{E_i} and Γ_i as loci of points E_i and P_i, respectively, for the ith leg; (**b**) the virtual bar Q_iP_i rotating along the axis w_i parallel to the line A_iB.

For the generic ith leg, one DoF is firstly required to define the angular position of Type (g) link C_iA_i. An angle α_i can be introduced to measure the rotation of (C_iA_i) with respect to its position in the undeformed configuration of the CSFH joint. Since the latter corresponds to a revolute joint with a known rotation axis, the angle α_i uniquely identifies the position of the center A_i of the spherical pair. Secondly, another DoF is needed to assess the position of the upper Type (d) A_iP_i link of the ith leg. Indeed, an assigned pull command on the Type (f) cable has the effect of bringing points E_i and B closer to each other. This effect could be similarly obtained by introducing in the PRBM a virtual linear actuator being active along the line BE_i. Any contraction of the linear actuator BE_i corresponds to a pull command of the (f) rope, while an extension of the linear actuator would represent a reduction of the cable tension. Since mobility is granted by the elasticity of the structure, its overall configuration will depend on the whole set of tensions that are assigned to the six cables. Furthermore, it is worth noticing that positive tensions (push) are not considered here, and therefore, the maximum elongation of the three virtual linear actuators will depend on the whole balance between the tensions that are applied to the cables and the structural elasticity. For the linear actuator BE_i, the pulled distance d_i can be introduced as the shortening of the original length $|BE_i|$ with respect to the distance between points B and E_i in the undeformed structure configuration.

Once the input parameters α_i and d_i have been assigned, the chain BA_iE_i behaves as a rigid structure, which may rotate about the axis w_i passing through points A_i and B (see Figure 3b). Therefore, point E_i describes a circle Γ_{E_i} laying on a plane π_{H_i} that is orthogonal to w_i and whose center H_i is on line w_i. Since A_iP_i can be regarded as a rigid link, point P_i is also forced to lay on a circle Γ_i that lays on a plane π_{Q_i} parallel to π_{H_i}. The center Q_i of Γ_i is on the line w_i.

Considering the three loci Γ_i (with $i = 1, \ldots, 3$) of the possible positions of the points P_i, it is clear that three points of the upper platform, coincident with P_1, P_2, and P_3, will belong to the three circles Γ_1, Γ_2, and Γ_3, respectively. However, exactly the same constraint could be imposed by introducing a virtual link Q_iP_i, represented in Figure 3b, that rotates about the w_i axis. Therefore, three new links Q_iP_i, with $i = 1, \ldots, 3$, can be used to get rid of the three whole chains made of links C_iA_i, A_iP_i, and the linear actuators BE_i. After this substitution, a new three-legged structure is obtained, as depicted in Figure 4.

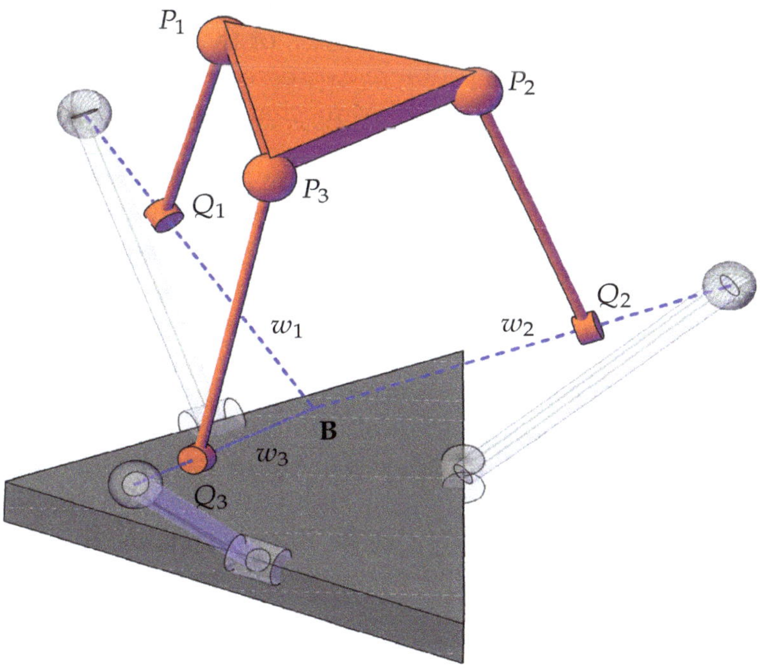

Figure 4. The reduced parallel structure: points Q_i, axes w_i and points P_i.

The new mechanism will have a null DoF because the whole set of input positions has already been assigned. In fact, after assigning a value to the three angles α_i and to the three displacements d_i, the axes w_i, the lengths $|Q_iP_i|$, and the positions of points Q_i can be uniquely identified. The resulting structure consists of a mobile platform that is connected to the base via three links only arranged in a parallel configuration, each one having one revolute R and one spherical S joint at its ends incident to the base and the platform, respectively. This structure has received the attention of several eminent scholars in the field and has been extensively studied [52–54]. From the geometric and kinematic point of view, the study of the possible assembly modes of this zero-DoF structure gives the same solution as for problem of finding the assembly modes of a six-DoF, so called 6-3-type fully-parallel mechanism, belonging to the class of Stewart platform mechanisms, once six elongation values are assigned to the six linear actuators along its legs.

Innocenti and Parenti Castelli solved the direct position analysis in 1990 [55] and found results that were coherent with Hunt's works [2]. According to this method (see also [56]), three closed-loop vector equations:

$$
\begin{aligned}
\overrightarrow{P_1P_2} &= -\overrightarrow{Q_1P_1} - \overrightarrow{P_2Q_2} - \overrightarrow{Q_2Q_1} \\
\overrightarrow{P_2P_3} &= -\overrightarrow{Q_2P_2} - \overrightarrow{P_3Q_3} - \overrightarrow{Q_3Q_2} \\
\overrightarrow{P_3P_1} &= -\overrightarrow{Q_3P_3} - \overrightarrow{P_1Q_1} - \overrightarrow{Q_3Q_1}
\end{aligned} \tag{2}
$$

can be written, where $\overrightarrow{P_1P_2}$, $\overrightarrow{P_2P_3}$, and $\overrightarrow{P_3P_1}$ are the edges of the upper platform.

For the sake of the present investigation $\overrightarrow{P_1P_2}$, $\overrightarrow{P_2P_3}$, and $\overrightarrow{P_3P_1}$ have constant modules because of the symmetry of the upper platform. Therefore, given the constant length l of the upper platform edges, Equation (2) can be rewritten as:

$$\overrightarrow{P_1P_2} \cdot \overrightarrow{P_1P_2} = l^2, \qquad \overrightarrow{P_2P_3} \cdot \overrightarrow{P_2P_3} = l^2, \qquad \overrightarrow{P_3P_1} \cdot \overrightarrow{P_3P_1} = l^2 \tag{3}$$

from which three scalar conditions are obtained where the three unknown are the rotation angles θ_i (with $i = 1, \ldots, 3$) of the virtual bars Q_iP_i around the axes w_i.

It is now essential to remind that once the three rotations α_i of the CSFHs and the three displacements d_i of the Type (f) cables have been assigned, the zero-DoF structure illustrated in Figure 4 is completely configured because the positions of the points A_i, H_i, and Q_i can be easily calculated. Therefore, the solutions of the problem expressed by the set of Equation (3) are also the solution of the assembly configuration for the PRBM mechanism depicted in Figure 3a.

The system (3) consists of three second-order algebraic equations in three unknowns θ_i (with $i = 1, \ldots, 3$), where any equation contains two unknown variables only. Therefore, the solutions can be achieved by firstly eliminating one variable $\hat{\theta}$ from two equations where $\hat{\theta}$ appears, so obtaining one equation in the other two variables, and then, by eliminating one of the other two variables, say $\tilde{\theta}$, from the remaining two equations. The result is a 16th-order polynomial equation in the remaining variable θ, with 16 real and complex solutions for θ. Since for every solution θ, unique values of $\hat{\theta}$ and $\tilde{\theta}$ exist, a unique location of the upper platform is identified for each solution θ. These solutions correspond to the possible assembly configurations of the structure represented in Figure 4 and, as a consequence, of the PRBM depicted in Figure 3a, provided that the six inputs α_i and d_i have been assigned. However, for the sake of the present investigation, the only interesting solution will be the one compatible with rotations and displacements starting from the initial undeformed configuration represented in Figure 2a. This shows that the numerical approaches could be used more conveniently than the purely analytical ones, because they could converge to the actual configuration by using the undeformed pose as the starting guess. In the next section, finite element analysis (FEA) is applied to the compliant platform illustrated in Figure 2a, by assigning three different sets of input displacements.

3. Numerical Simulation of the Platform Pose

The peculiar geometry illustrated in Figure 1 is the result of a preliminary study that led to the definition of the patented structure. Three equal legs were positioned in a parallel configuration, each leg being actuated by two cables, and so, the whole structure was a tendon-driven mechanism. The geometry of each leg was chosen in such a way that the lower and upper cables induced a raising and lowering motion, respectively. The attachment points were also selected in order not to induce cable jamming. Further optimization of the attachment points and of the angles of the pseudo-rigid links will be the object of future investigations. Considering the nomenclature introduced in Figure 1, any moving cable (i) acts on a CSFH turning pair, relevantly operates the bending of the CSFH Type (h) flexure, and actually drives the rotations of Type (g) links. Cables (f) will have the effect of pulling the platform down because they are attached to the upper links. More in general, a configuration of the platform (a) will be defined by the whole set of forces applied to all the wires, since it depends on the interaction between the applied forces and the elasticity of joints.

Finite element analysis is a convenient way to assess the deformation of the whole structure for assigned values of the cable displacements. More specifically, FEA provided evidence that the adoption of the proposed platform can be a promising approach to find an efficient way for remote handling in several contexts.

Finite Element Analysis

Finite element analyses were conducted to evaluate the static behavior of the parallel platform. Three cases were considered depending on three different sets of input parameters and using $E = 1.1 \cdot 10^9$ Pa as the material Young's modulus.

Three cases will be studied:

I pull on Type (f) cables and null tension on Type (i) cables;
II pull on Type (i) cables and null tension on Type (f) cables;
III asymmetric pull: pull on one Type (f) cable and pull on two Type (i) cables;

The fixed reference frame (x, y, z) and the unit vectors $(\vec{u}_x, \vec{u}_y, \vec{u}_z)$ attached to the mobile platform were positioned as in Figure 5a. This figure also shows the input displacement d_1. Rotations θ_x, θ_y, and θ_z were assumed to be about $\vec{u}_x$, $\vec{u}_y$, and $\vec{u}_z$, respectively.

In the first case, a displacement was imposed on each one of the Type (f) cables, equal to $d_1 = d_2 = d_3 = 0.5$ mm, and null tensions on Type (i) cables, giving rise to null rotation angles $\alpha_1 = \alpha_2 = \alpha_3 = 0$ of the three CSFH hinges. The deformed configuration is reported in Figure 5b, showing a platform displacement along the z-axis in the negative direction. No other significant displacements or rotations were registered.

The second case corresponded to $\alpha_1 = \alpha_2 = \alpha_3 = 20°$ with $d_1 = d_2 = d_3 = 0$ mm. The deformed configuration is reported in Figure 6a, showing a platform displacement along the z-axis in the positive direction. Analogous to the previous case, no other significant displacements or rotations were registered.

The third case corresponded to a general actuation scheme with $\alpha_1 = 0°, \alpha_2 = 5°, \alpha_3 = 20°$, $d_1 = 1$ mm, $d_2 = d_3 = 0$ mm. The deformed configuration is reported in Figure 6b, showing a platform displacement with components along the $x-$ and y-axes and rotations about the x- and z-axes.

The input parameters, the platform displacement, and the rotations are reported in Table 1 for the three analyzed cases.

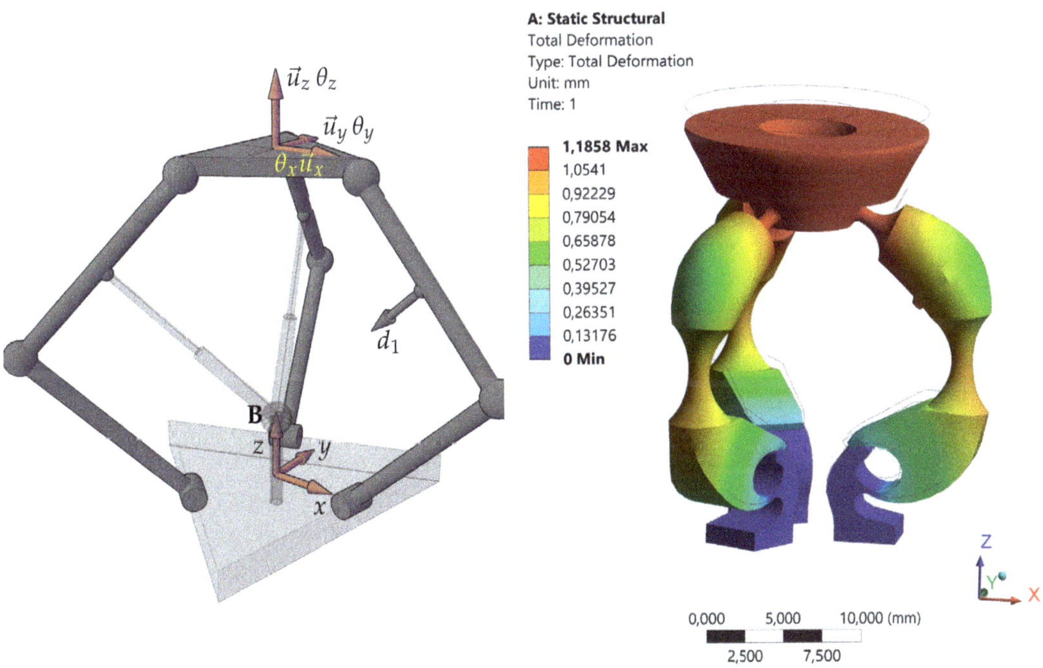

(a) (b)

Figure 5. (**a**) Reference frames and nomenclature; (**b**) platform displacement along the z-axis, negative direction (Case 1).

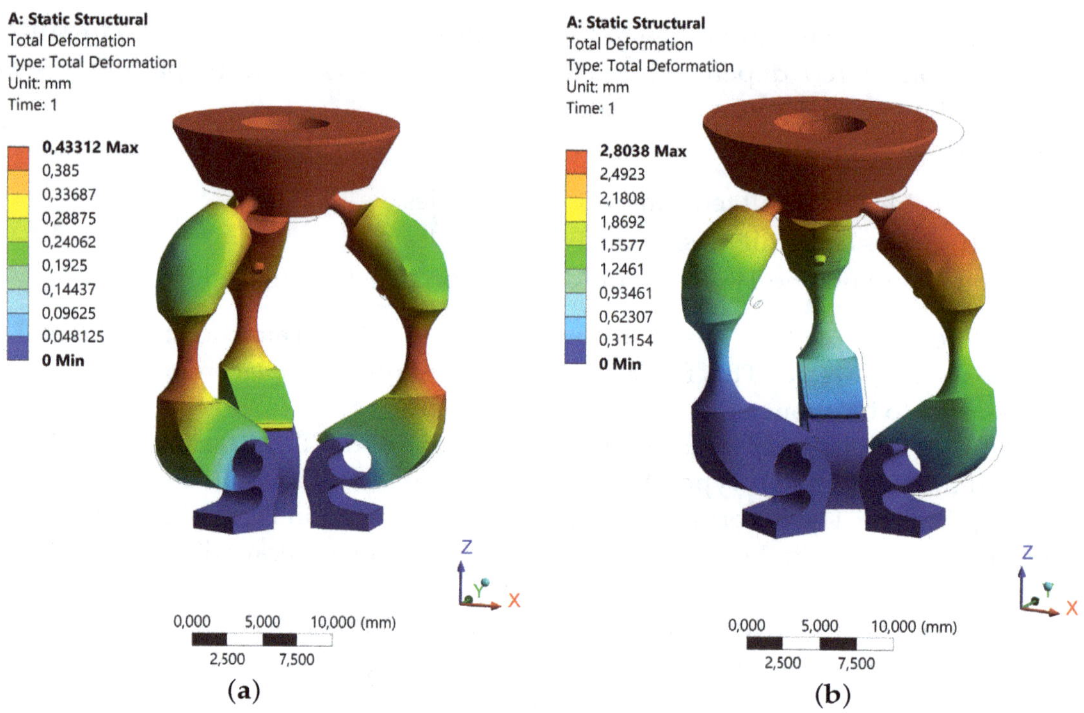

Figure 6. (**a**) Platform displacement along the *z*-axis, positive direction (Case 2); (**b**) platform pose for a generic actuation scheme (Case 3).

Table 1. Input rotations and displacements and their effect on the platform for the three analyzed cases.

Case 1		Case 2		Case 3	
Input	**Output**	**Input**	**Output**	**Input**	**Output**
$\alpha_1 = 0$	$u_x = 8 \cdot 10^{-3}$ mm	$\alpha_1 = 20°$	$u_x = -8 \cdot 10^{-3}$ mm	$\alpha_1 = 0°$	$u_x = -2.4$ mm
$\alpha_2 = 0$	$u_y = 2 \cdot 10^{-2}$ mm	$\alpha_2 = 20°$	$u_y = -1 \cdot 10^{-2}$ mm	$\alpha_2 = 5°$	$u_y = 0.1$ mm
$\alpha_3 = 0$	$u_z = -1.17$ mm	$\alpha_3 = 20°$	$u_z = 0.43$ mm	$\alpha_3 = 20°$	$u_z = -6 \cdot 10^{-2}$ mm
$d_1 = 0.5$ mm	$\theta_x = 8 \cdot 10^{-2}$ °	$d_1 = 0$ mm	$\theta_x = 2 \cdot 10^{-2}$ °	$d_1 = 1$ mm	$\theta_x = -1.7$ °
$d_2 = 0.5$ mm	$\theta_y = 4 \cdot 10^{-2}$ °	$d_2 = 0$ mm	$\theta_y = 2 \cdot 10^{-2}$ °	$d_2 = 0$ mm	$\theta_y = -5 \cdot 10^{-2}$ °
$d_3 = 0.5$ mm	$\theta_z = 9 \cdot 10^{-2}$ °	$d_3 = 0$ mm	$\theta_z = 8 \cdot 10^{-4}$ °	$d_3 = 0$ mm	$\theta_z = 1.1$ °

4. Applications

Originally, the main activities for the invention herein presented were intended to be operated in the laparoscopic environment. Figure 7 shows a possible end-effector that could be mounted on the platform. With reference to the labels used in Figure 7, the endoluminal catheter (a) carries the base platform (b), which supports three Type (c) legs on which the mobile platform (d) is mounted. The mobile platform surface holds the surgical means (f) that can vary according to the type of required operation. Other miniaturized instruments can be mounted on the controlled platform, such as vision means (e) that allow the surgeon to observe the corporal cavity wherein the device is inserted. Moreover, a communication duct (g) was designed, allowing the surgeon to access the region to be operated. For this reason, the mobile and base platforms were also provided with an opening that connects the duct (g) with the tubular duct (a). With reference to Figure 7, it should be also noted that the surgical device was comprised of a shaped surface (f) that made it easier to act as a guiding element inside the cavity during the use of the device.

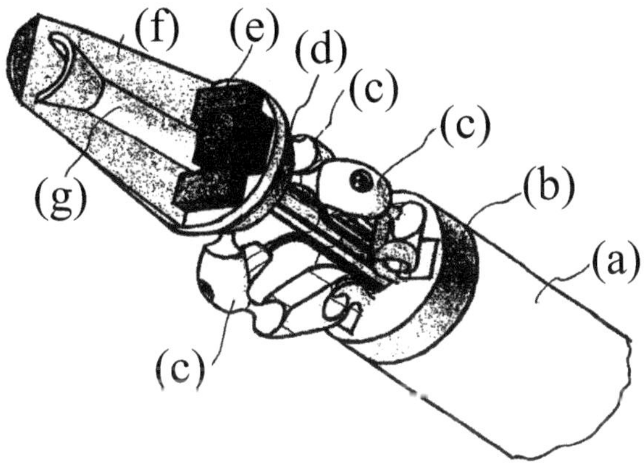

Figure 7. A view of an end-effector mounted in the platform: catheter (**a**); base link (**b**); legs (**c**); platform (**d**); on-board hardware (**e**); on-board end-effectors (**f**) and (**g**).

5. Discussion

The aim of this paper was to present a new concept high accuracy platform with spatial mobility, remotely actuated, and equipped with selective compliance joints. The system can be built on a unique material block or with a reduced number of components, which reduces the costs and time of production. It can be also built by means of 3D printing.

The platform was mounted on three arms, and it was remotely controlled by six wires. The system included a mobile plane and a connection base fixed to an endoscopic instrument. The instruments was accurate and maneuverable with continuous motion granted by the interaction between the cable tensions and the elastic energy stored in the elastic media. Based on selective compliance, the principle of design gave rise to optimal configurations where parasitic motions, friction, and wear were minimized. No lubrication was needed.

The invention is expected to drive surgical operations in laparoscopic, endogastric, or endarterial environments, but other applications are not excluded, such as in aerospace, automotive, appliances, and microelectronics. However, it is worth noting that the platform fabrication and its actual implementation for real operations deserve further refinements, and therefore, they will be treated in future contributions. Among the important subjects that still represent open problems, the following will be briefly addressed.

The first problem is the selection of an optimal material for the elastic parallel mechanism. This choice will depend on the overall size of the device and on the consequent preferred method of machining. In any case, some desired characteristics of a material that could be conveniently employed to build a compliant mechanism block were proposed in [57], among which are good performances at variable temperatures, biocompatibility, low susceptibility to creep, resistance to wear and fatigue, and the predictability of such properties. However, the most important characteristic is a high value of the ratio of the yield strength to Young's modulus. According to Table 2.1. presented in [57], there are several materials that have an acceptable ratio, among which are nylon, e-glass, Kevlar, and polyethylene.

The actual fabrication of the device will depend both on size and material. Unfortunately, the geometry is rather complicated, and so, many of the classical machining operations would be problematic.

The identification of a proper PRBM, as proposed in the present contribution, could be helpful to complete typical tasks in robotics, such as the study of the critical configurations. Furthermore, the PRBM will be useful to optimize the platform and the legs' geometry, in order to suit the required workspace, mobility, and mechanical advantage.

Finally, an efficient control algorithm would be required for each specific application.

6. Conclusions

A spatial, selective compliance, tendon-driven, and parallel platform was described and analyzed. This system was quite different from the compliant mechanisms previously presented either in the literature or the national patent institutions until today. Its mechanical structure was studied by identifying the equivalent pseudo-rigid body mechanism. The platform was also simulated with finite element analysis (FEA) by assigning different sets of cable tensions and obtaining results that matched well with the expected behavior. It is hoped that this article will offer new perspectives for general tasks of spatial body guidance and particularly in laparoscopic surgery.

7. Patents

The following patents describe the new concept platform and the related claims.

- N.P. Belfiore, M. Scaccia, F. Ianniello, M. Presta, L. Perfetti, Selective Compliance Wire Actuated Mobile Platform, particularly for Endoscopy Surgical Devices, Patent N0.2 US 8,845,520 B2, 30 September 2014.
- N.P. Belfiore, M. Scaccia, F. Ianniello, M. Presta, L. Perfetti, Selective Compliance Wire Actuated Mobile Platform, particularly for Endoscopy Surgical Devices, World Intellectual Property Organization, WO 2009/034552 A2, Int. Appl. No. PCT/IB2008/053698, Publ. Date 19 March 2009.
- N.P. Belfiore, M. Scaccia, F. Ianniello, M. Presta, Selective Compliance Hinge, US 8,191,204 B2, 5 June 2012.
- N.P. Belfiore, M. Scaccia, F. Ianniello, M. Presta, Selective Compliance Hinge, World Intellectual Property Organization, WO 2009/034551 A1, Int. Appl. No. PCT/IB2008/053697, Publ. Date 19 March 2009.

Acknowledgments: The whole staff of the "Research and Technology Transfer Area" of the University of Rome la Sapienza is gratefully acknowledged. Particular thanks go to the Manager of the "Research and Technology Transfer Area" Antonella Cammisa, the Office Manager of the "Enhancement and Technology Transfer Office" Daniele Riccioni, and the Office Manager of the "Grant Office" Alessandra Intraversato, for their counseling and support during my long stay at Sapienza University. I am also grateful to several people from my new University of Roma Tre (my list would be too long to mention all of them) for supporting and encouraging me since my arrival in October 2017.

Abbreviations

The following abbreviations are used in this manuscript:

CSFH	Conjugate surface flexure hinge
DoF	Degrees of freedom
MEMS	Micro electro-mechanical systems

References

1. Stewart, D. A Platform with Six Degrees of Freedom. *Proc. Inst. Mech. Eng.* **1965**, *180*, 371–386. [CrossRef]
2. Hunt, K.H. Structural Kinematics of in-parallel-actuated Robot-Arms. *J. Mech. Transm. Autom. Des.* **1983**, *105*, 705–712. [CrossRef]
3. Gosselin, C. Determination of the workspace of 6-DOF parallel manipulators. *J. Mech. Transm. Autom. Des.* **1990**, *112*, 331–336. [CrossRef]
4. Innocenti, C.; Parenti-Castelli, V. Singularity-free evolution from one configuration to another in serial and fully-parallel manipulators. *J. Mech. Des. Trans. ASME* **1998**, *120*, 73–79. [CrossRef]
5. Parenti-Castelli, V.; Di Gregorio, R.; Bubani, F. Workspace and optimal design of a pure translation parallel manipulator. *Meccanica* **2000**, *35*, 203–214. [CrossRef]

6. Fang, Y.; Tsai, L.W. Structure synthesis of a class of 4-DoF and 5-DoF parallel manipulators with identical limb structures. *Int. J. Robot. Res.* **2002**, *21*, 799–810. [CrossRef]
7. Merlet, J.P. Jacobian, manipulability, condition number, and accuracy of parallel robots. *J. Mech. Des. Trans. ASME* **2006**, *128*, 199–206. [CrossRef]
8. Cheng, H.; Yiu, Y.K.; Li, Z. Dynamics and Control of Redundantly Actuated Parallel Manipulators. *IEEE/ASME Trans. Mechatron.* **2003**, *8*, 483–491. [CrossRef]
9. Tang, X. An overview of the development for cable-driven parallel manipulator. *Adv. Mech. Eng.* **2014**, *2014*. [CrossRef]
10. Belfiore, N.P.; Di Benedetto, A. Connectivity and redundancy in spatial robots. *Int. J. Robot. Res.* **2000**, *19*, 1245–1261. [CrossRef]
11. Belfiore, N.P. Distributed Databases for the development of Mechanisms Topology. *Mech. Mach. Theory* **2000**, *35*, 1727–1744. [CrossRef]
12. Belfiore, N.P. Brief note on the concept of planarity for kinematic chains. *Mech. Mach. Theory* **2000**, *35*, 1745–1750. [CrossRef]
13. Howell, L.L.; Magleby, S.P.; Olsen, B.M. *Handbook of Compliant Mechanisms*; John Wiley and Sons: The Atrium Southern Gate, Terminus Road, Chichester, West Sussex, UK, 2013.
14. Howell, L.L.; Midha, A. Parametric deflection approximations for end-loaded, large-deflection beams in compliant mechanisms. *J. Mech. Des. Trans. ASME* **1995**, *117*, 156–165. [CrossRef]
15. Howell, L.L.; Midha, A. A method for the design of compliant mechanisms with small-length flexural pivots. *J. Mech. Des. Trans. ASME* **1994**, *116*, 280–290. [CrossRef]
16. Verotti, M.; Masarati, P.; Morandini, M.; Belfiore, N.P. Isotropic compliance in the Special Euclidean Group SE(3). *Mech. Mach. Theory* **2016**, *98*, 263–281. [CrossRef]
17. Verotti, M.; Belfiore, N.P. Isotropic compliance in E(3): Feasibility and workspace mapping. *J. Mech. Robot.* **2016**, *8*. [CrossRef]
18. Dunning, A.; Tolou, N.; Herder, J. Review Article: Inventory of platforms towards the design of a statically balanced six degrees of freedom compliant precision stage. *Mech. Sci.* **2011**, *2*, 157–168. [CrossRef]
19. Gosselin, C. Stiffness Mapping for Parallel Manipulators. *IEEE Trans. Robot. Autom.* **1990**, *6*, 377–382. [CrossRef]
20. Nguyen, C.C.; Antrazi, S.S.; Zhou, Z.L. Analysis and implementation of a 6 DOF Stewart platform-based force sensor for passive compliant robotic assembly. In Proceedings of the IEEE SOUTHEASTCON, Williamsburg, VA, USA, 7–10 April 1991; Volume 2, pp. 880–884.
21. Li, Y.; Xu, Q. Design and analysis of a new 3-DOF compliant parallel positioning platform for nanomanipulation. In Proceedings of the 5th IEEE Conference on Nanotechnology, Nagoya, Japan, 15 July 2005; Volume 2, pp. 133–136.
22. Wu, T.L.; Chen, J.H.; Chang, S.H. A six-dof prismatic-spherical-spherical parallel compliant nanopositioner. *IEEE Trans. Ultrason. Ferroelectr. Freq. Control* **2008**, *55*, 2544–2551.
23. Chen, Q.; Huang, Y.; Zhu, D.; Zhou, M. The design and finite element analysis of a compliant 3-DOF spatial translational ultra-precise positioning platform. In Proceedings of the IEEE International Conference on Intelligent Computing and Intelligent Systems, Xiamen, China, 29–31 October 2010; Volume 3, pp. 122–126.
24. Liang, Q.; Zhang, D.; Chi, Z.; Song, Q.; Ge, Y.; Ge, Y. Six-DOF micro-manipulator based on compliant parallel mechanism with integrated force sensor. *Robot. Comput.-Integr. Manuf.* **2011**, *27*, 124–134. [CrossRef]
25. Liu, X.J.; Wang, J.; Gao, F.; Wang, L.P. On the design of 6-DOF parallel micro-motion manipulators. In Proceedings of the IEEE International Conference on Intelligent Robots and Systems, Maui, HI, USA, 29 October–3 November 2001; Volume 1, pp. 343–348.
26. Correa, J.C.; Crane, C. Kinematic analysis of a three-degree of freedom compliant platform. *J. Mech. Des. Trans. ASME* **2013**, *135*. [CrossRef]
27. Belfiore, N.P.; Emamimeibodi, M.; Verotti, M.; Crescenzi, R.; Balucani, M.; Nenzi, P. Kinetostatic optimization of a MEMS-based compliant 3 DOF plane parallel platform. In Proceedings of the 9th International Conference on Computational Cybernetics, Tihany, Hungary, 8-10 July 2013; pp. 261–266.
28. Francis, P.; Eastwood, K.W.; Bodani, V.; Looi, T.; Drake, J. Design, Modelling and Teleoperation of a 2 mm Diameter Compliant Instrument for the da Vinci Platform. *Ann. Biomed. Eng.* **2018**, *46*, 1437–1449. [CrossRef] [PubMed]

29. Lee, C.; Park, Y.H.; Yoon, C.; Noh, S.; Lee, C.; Kim, Y.; Kim, H.C.; Kim, H.H.; Kim, S. A grip force model for the da Vinci end-effector to predict a compensation force. *Med Biol. Eng. Comput.* **2015**, *53*, 253–261. [CrossRef] [PubMed]
30. Pena, R.; Smith, M.J.; Ontiveros, N.P.; Hammond, F.L.; Wood, R.J. Printing Strain Gauges on Intuitive Surgical da Vinci Robot End Effectors. In Proceedings of the IEEE International Conference on Intelligent Robots and Systems, Madrid, Spain, 1–5 October 2018; Institute of Electrical and Electronics Engineers Inc.: Piscatawa, NJ, USA, 2018; pp. 806–812.
31. Balla, A.; Quaresima, S.; Ursi, P.; Seitaj, A.; Palmieri, L.; Badiali, D.; Paganini, A.M. Hiatoplasty with crura buttressing versus hiatoplasty alone during laparoscopic sleeve gastrectomy. *Gastroenterol. Res. Pract.* **2017**, *2017*. [CrossRef] [PubMed]
32. Popivanov, G.; Tabakov, M.; Mantese, G.; Cirocchi, R.; Piccinini, I.; D'Andrea, V.; Covarelli, P.; Boselli, C.; Barberini, F.; Tabola, R.; et al. Surgical treatment of gastrointestinal stromal tumors of the duodenum: A literature review. *Transl. Gastroenterol. Hepatol.* **2018**, *3*, 71. [CrossRef]
33. Cochetti, G.; Del Zingaro, M.; Boni, A.; Cocca, D.; Panciarola, M.; Tiezzi, A.; Gaudio, G.; Balzarini, F.; Ursi, P.; Mearini, E. Colovesical fistula: Review on conservative management, surgical techniques and minimally invasive approaches. *Giornale Chir.* **2018**, *39*, 195–207.
34. Quaresima, S.; Balla, A.; Dambrosio, G.; Bruzzone, P.; Ursi, P.; Lezoche, E.; Paganini, A.M. Endoluminal loco-regional resection by TEM after R1 endoscopic removal or recurrence of rectal tumors. *Minim. Invasive Ther. Allied Technol.* **2016**, *25*, 134–140. [CrossRef]
35. Paci, M.; Scoglio, D.; Ursi, P.; Barchetti, L.; Fabiani, B.; Ascoli, G.; Lezoche, G. Transanal Endocopic Microsurgery (TEM) in advanced rectal cancer disease treatment [Il ruolo della TEM nel trattamento dei tumori del retto extraperitoneale]. *Ann. Ital. Chir.* **2010**, *81*, 269–274.
36. Lezoche, E.; Fabiani, B.; D'Ambrosio, G.; Ursi, P.; Balla, A.; Lezoche, G.; Monteleone, F.; Paganini, A.M. Nucleotide-guided mesorectal excision combined with endoluminal locoregional resection by transanal endoscopic microsurgery in the treatment of rectal tumors: Technique and preliminary results. *Surg. Endosc.* **2013**, *27*, 4136–4141. [CrossRef]
37. Ursi, P.; Santoro, A.; Gemini, A.; Arezzo, A.; Pironi, D.; Renzi, C.; Cirocchi, R.; Di Matteo, F.; Maturo, A.; D'Andrea, V.; et al. Comparison of outcomes following intersphincteric resection vs low anterior resection for low rectal cancer: A systematic review. *G. Chir.* **2018**, *39*, 123–142.
38. Verotti, M. Effect of initial curvature in uniform flexures on position accuracy. *Mech. Mach. Theory* **2018**, *119*, 106–118. [CrossRef]
39. Verotti, M. Analysis of the center of rotation in primitive flexures: Uniform cantilever beams with constant curvature. *Mech. Mach. Theory* **2016**, *97*, 29–50. [CrossRef]
40. Sanò, P.; Verotti, M.; Bosetti, P.; Belfiore, N.P. Kinematic Synthesis of a D-Drive MEMS Device With Rigid-Body Replacement Method. *J. Mech. Des. Trans. ASME* **2018**, *140*. [CrossRef]
41. Verotti, M.; Dochshanov, A.; Belfiore, N.P. Compliance Synthesis of CSFH MEMS-Based Microgrippers. *J. Mech. Des. Trans. ASME* **2017**, *139*. [CrossRef]
42. Botta, F.; Verotti, M.; Bagolini, A.; Bellutti, P.; Belfiore, N.P. Mechanical response of four-bar linkage microgrippers with bidirectional electrostatic actuation. *Actuators* **2018**, *7*, 78. [CrossRef]
43. Veroli, A.; Buzzin, A.; Frezza, F.; de Cesare, G.; Hamidullah, M.; Giovine, E.; Verotti, M.; Belfiore, N.P. An approach to the extreme miniaturization of rotary comb drives. *Actuators* **2018**, *7*, 70. [CrossRef]
44. Bertini, S.; Verotti, M.; Bagolini, A.; Bellutti, P.; Ruta, G.; Belfiore, N.P. Scalloping and stress concentration in DRIE-manufactured comb-drives. *Actuators* **2018**, *7*, 57. [CrossRef]
45. Bagolini, A.; Ronchin, S.; Bellutti, P.; Chistè, M.; Verotti, M.; Belfiore, N.P. Fabrication of Novel MEMS Microgrippers by Deep Reactive Ion Etching with Metal Hard Mask. *J. Microelectromech. Syst.* **2017**, *26*, 926–934. [CrossRef]
46. Belfiore, N.P. Micromanipulation: A challenge for actuation. *Actuators* **2018**, *7*, 85. [CrossRef]
47. Potrich, C.; Lunelli, L.; Bagolini, A.; Bellutti, P.; Pederzolli, C.; Verotti, M.; Belfiore, N.P. Innovative silicon microgrippers for biomedical applications: Design, mechanical simulation and evaluation of protein fouling. *Actuators* **2018**, *7*,12. [CrossRef]
48. Veroli, A.; Buzzin, A.; Crescenzi, R.; Frezza, F.; de Cesare, G.; D'Andrea, V.; Mura, F.; Verotti, M.; Dochshanov, A.; Belfiore, N.P. Development of a NEMS-technology based nano gripper. *Mech. Mach. Sci.* **2018**, *49*, 601–611.

49. Di Giamberardino, P.; Bagolini, A.; Bellutti, P.; Rudas, I.J.; Verotti, M.; Botta, F.; Belfiore, N.P. New MEMS tweezers for the viscoelastic characterization of soft materials at the microscale. *Micromachines* **2017**, *9*, 15. [CrossRef]
50. Cecchi, R.; Verotti, M.; Capata, R.; Dochshanov, A.; Broggiato, G.; Crescenzi, R.; Balucani, M.; Natali, S.; Razzano, G.; Lucchese, F.; et al. Development of micro-grippers for tissue and cell manipulation with direct morphological comparison. *Micromachines* **2015**, *6*, 1710–1728. [CrossRef]
51. Belfiore, N.P.; Simeone, P. Inverse kinetostatic analysis of compliant four-bar linkages. *Mech. Mach. Theory* **2013**, *69*, 350–372. [CrossRef]
52. Tsai, L.W. *Robot Analysis: The Mechanics of Serial and Parallel Manipulators*; John Wiley and Sons: New York, NY, USA, 1999.
53. Hunt, K.H. *Kinematic Geometry of Mechanisms*; Oxford University Press: Oxford, UK, 1979.
54. Merlet, J.P. *Parallel Robots*, 2nd ed.; Springer: Dordrecht, The Netherlands, 2006.
55. Innocenti, C.; Parenti-Castelli, V. Direct position analysis of the Stewart platform mechanism. *Mech. Mach. Theory* **1990**, *25*, 611–621. [CrossRef]
56. Parenti-Castelli, V.; Di Gregorio, R. Closed-form solution of the direct kinematics of the 6-3 type Stewart Platform using one extra sensor. *Meccanica* **1996**, *31*, 705–714. [CrossRef]
57. Howell, L.L. *Compliant Mechanisms*; John Wiley and Sons, Inc.: New York, NY, USA, 2001.

12

Pressure Observer based Adaptive Dynamic Surface Control of Pneumatic Actuator with Long Transmission Lines

Deyuan Meng [1,*], Bo Lu [2], Aimin Li [1], Jiang Yin [1] and Qingyang Li [1]

1 School of Mechatronic Engineering, China University of Mining and Technology, Xuzhou 221116, China
2 National Quality Supervision and Inspection Centre of Pneumatic Products, Ningbo 315500, China
* Correspondence: tinydreams@126.com.

Featured Application: This research dedicates to develop a pressure observer based nonlinear controller for precise position control of the MRI-compatible pneumatic servo system with long transmission lines.

Abstract: In this paper, the needle insertion motion control of a magnetic resonance imaging (MRI) compatible robot, which is actuated by a pneumatic cylinder with long transmission lines, is considered and a pressure observer based adaptive dynamic surface controller is proposed. The long transmission line is assumed to be an intermediate chamber connected between the control valve and the actuator in series, and a nonlinear first order system model is constructed to characterize the pressure losses and time delay brought by it. Due to the fact that MRI-compatible pressure sensors are not commercially available, a globally stable pressure observer is employed to estimate the chamber pressure. Based on the model of the long transmission line and the pressure observer, an adaptive dynamic surface controller is further designed by using the dynamic surface control technique. Compared to the traditional backstepping design method, the proposed controller can avoid the problem of "explosion of complexity" since the repeated differentiation of virtual controls is no longer required. The stability of the closed-loop system is analytically proven by employing the Lyapunov theory. Extensive experimental results are presented to demonstrate the effectiveness and the performance robustness of the proposed controller.

Keywords: pneumatic servo system; long transmission line; pressure observer; dynamic surface control; position tracking

---

1. Introduction

The magnetic resonance imaging (MRI) technique is widely used in clinical diagnosis due to its ability to image without the use of ionizing x-rays and superior soft tissue contrast as compared to computed tomography (CT) scanning. Recently, pneumatically actuated MRI-compatible robots, which enable real-time magnetic resonance (MR) image-guided needle placement, are designed for brachytherapy and biopsy by several researchers [1–15]. To fulfill the requirements for MR compatibility of the robotic systems, pneumatic valves are commonly placed outside the scanner room in the aforementioned works. Therefore, long transmission lines between the actuators and valves are used. Since long transmission lines have a significant influence on the pressure dynamics of the pneumatic system and MRI-compatible pressure sensors are not commercially available, precise position control is one of the main technical challenges in robot development.

Indeed, considerable research effort has been devoted to addressing the issue related to long transmission lines. Richer et al. [16] suggested a formula for the time delay and amplitude attenuation between the mass flows at the outlet and inlet of the line, as well as a formula for the pressure drop along the tube. Although this approach was later employed in many other studies (Jiang et al. [14]; Richer et al. [17]), it has been proven improper for long transmission lines (>2 m) [18]. Yang et al. [8] adopted a first order transfer function with time delay to describe the 9-m transmission line dynamics. However, for some unknown reason, the authors omitted the transmission line dynamics in the subsequent controller design. Based on the discretization of a general set of equations from fluid mechanics, two similar distributed models of long pneumatic transmission lines were derived by Li et al. [19] and Krichel et al. [20]. However, this type of model is not suitable for controller design for their high order and low computational speed. Turkseven et al. [21] developed a simplified distributed model to characterize the additional dynamics brought by the long transmission lines.

As previously mentioned, direct pressure measurement is unavailable for the lack of MRI-compatible pressure sensors. However, pressure states are commonly used in controller design for precise position control of a pneumatic actuator. To solve this problem, pressure observers were used in place of a pressure sensor in many studies. Pandian et al. [22] investigated two design methods of an observer to estimate the chamber pressures in a pneumatic cylinder. While a continuous gain observer was used to estimate one of the chamber pressures with the assumption that the other one is measured in the first method, a sliding mode observer was utilized to estimate both chamber pressures in the second method. In this study, the mass flow rate was assumed to be exactly known, which is apparently too restrictive in practice. Wu et al. [23] conducted an analysis on observability and concluded that the pressure states in the pneumatic servo system are not locally observable from the measurement of the output motion within several regions in the state space. Based on the actuator pressure dynamics, various observers are developed, such as the sliding-mode observer (Bigras [24]), energy-based Lyapunov observer (Gulati et al. [25]), and adaptive nonlinear observer (Langjord et al. [26]). It should be noted that the performance of these observers relies on the accuracy of the valve model. Driver et al. [27] developed a pressure estimation algorithm by utilizing the measured actuation force and the hypothesized average air pressure in the actuator. Turkseven et al. [18] presented a pressure observation method by using the measured force and piston displacement. However, the requirement for force sensing in the MRI environment is particularly burdensome because the MRI-compatible force sensor is not available commercially and its development cost is high.

Recently, the backstepping design method has been proven to be a very effective way to develop nonlinear robust controllers for pneumatic servo systems. However, this method has the problem of "explosion of complexity" since the requirement of repeated differentiation of virtual controls. Thus, a practical implementation is difficult. To solve this problem, Swaroop et al. [28] proposed the dynamic surface control (DSC) method, in which the calculation of the virtual control variable's derivative was prevented by introducing a filter at each design step. Since then, the DSC method has been the topic of significant research efforts and a number of excellent theoretical contributions have been made. The applications of DSC can be found in many engineering fields, for example, hydraulic servo systems [29], underwater/autonomous surface vehicles [30], mobile wheeled inverted pendulum [31], pneumatic artificial muscle [32], and servo motor [33].

In this study, the needle insertion motion control of the MRI compatible robot developed in our lab is considered. The robot is actuated by a pneumatic cylinder with long transmission lines. The focus of this paper is dealing with the issue of long transmission lines and realizing a high accuracy control of a pneumatic actuator with a pressure observer. Therefore, the long transmission line is assumed to be an intermediate chamber connected between the control valve and the actuator in series, and a pressure observer based adaptive dynamic surface control is proposed. The main contributions are: (1) The long transmission line dynamic is approximated as a nonlinear first order system, which can estimate the pressure losses and time delay through the long transmission line precisely in real time. (2) A pressure observer, which is proven to be globally stable, is developed to estimate the chamber pressure in a pneumatic actuator with a long transmission line. (3) In contrast to most of the existing nonlinear robust controllers synthesized by the backstepping method, by using the dynamic surface control

(DSC) technique, the proposed controller can cope with the problem of "explosion of complexity", since the repeated differentiation of virtual controls is no longer required. The rest of this paper is organized as follows: Section 2 presents the dynamic models and problem statement; Section 3 gives the design and stability proof of the pressure observer based adaptive dynamic surface controller; Section 4 presents the experimental results to demonstrate the performance of the proposed controller; and Section 5 draws the conclusions.

2. Dynamic Models and Problem Formulation

As shown in Figure 1, a 5-DOF (degree of freedom) MRI compatible robot for abdominal and thoracic punctures was built in our laboratory. The robot's mechanism design was developed such that all motions were decoupled and actuated by pneumatic cylinders. With the help of the robot, the physician could manipulate the needle remotely without moving the patient out of the MRI scanners. A schematic of the pneumatic servo system driving the needle insertion motion is depicted in Figure 2. The pneumatic cylinder (customized product from XMC Corp., Ningbo, China), which had a 150 mm stroke and 10 mm diameter bore, was made of nonmagnetic material to ensure MRI compatibility. While Chamber A was controlled by a proportional directional control valve (FESTO MPYE-5-M5-010-B), a tank was used to maintain the pressure of Chamber B at a specified constant level for safety reasons. The control valve was connected to the cylinder via a 10 m transmission line since it had to be placed away from the MRI scanner. A pressure observer was needed to estimate the pressure of Chamber A, since direct measurement was expensive for the lack of MRI-compatible pressure sensors. The main purpose of this paper was to find a way to deal with the issue of the long transmission line and realize high accuracy control of a pneumatic cylinder with pressure observation. For the purpose of comparison, the pressures at the two ends of the long transmission line, as well as the supply pressure were measured by three pressure sensors (FESTO SDET-22T-D10-G14-I-M12). The piston position was obtained with an optical position sensor (Micronor MR328). The controller was programmed in Simulink on a dSPACE DS1103 control system with a 1 ms sampling period.

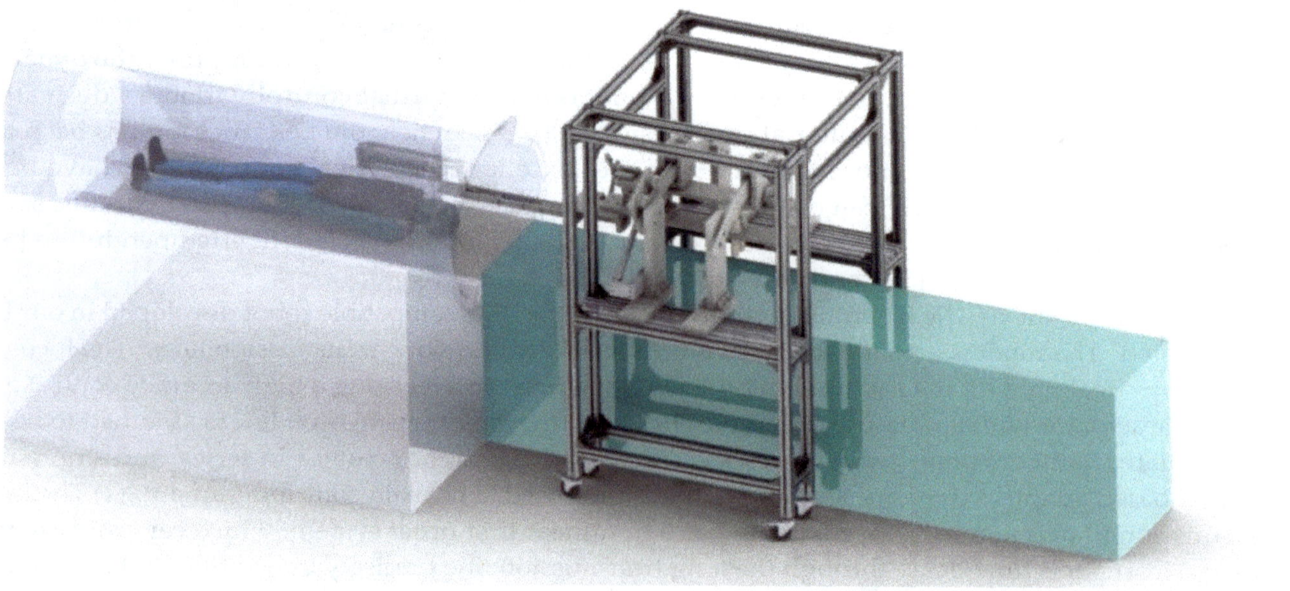

Figure 1. Virtual prototype of a 5-DOF (degree of freedom) magnetic resonance imaging (MRI) compatible robot for abdominal and thoracic punctures.

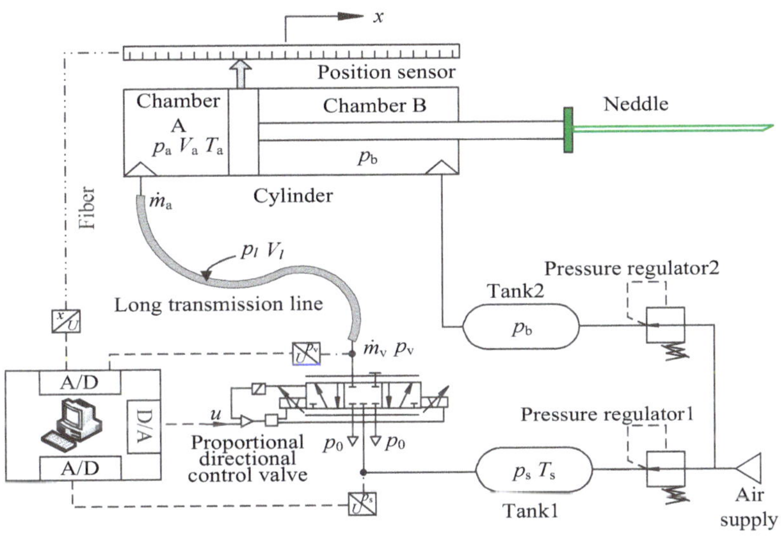

Figure 2. Schematic of the pneumatic servo system used to drive the needle insertion motion.

As shown in [34], the motion of the piston–rod–needle assembly can be expressed as:

$$m\ddot{x} = p_a A_a - p_b A_b - p_0 A_r - b\dot{x} - F_f S_f(\dot{x}) - d_f, \tag{1}$$

where x, $\dot{x}$, and $\ddot{x}$ are the piston position, velocity, and acceleration, respectively, m is the normal mass of the piston–rod–needle assembly, p_a and p_b denotes the absolute pressures of actuator chambers, p_0 is the ambience pressure, A_a and A_b are the cross section areas of piston chambers, A_r is the cross section area of the rod, b is the total load and cylinder viscous friction coefficient, F_f is the unknown friction coefficient, $S_f(\dot{x})$ is a continuous function, which is always chosen as $S_f(\dot{x}) = \frac{2}{\pi}\arctan(900\dot{x})$, $F_f S_f(\dot{x})$ is utilized as the smooth approximation for the usual static discontinuous Coulomb friction force, and d_f represents the unmodeled dynamics and external disturbances.

With the assumption that the discharging and charging processes are both isothermal, the pressure dynamic in the actuator chamber can be modeled as [16,35]:

$$\dot{p}_a = \frac{RT_s}{V_a}\dot{m}_a - \frac{A_a p_a}{V_a}\dot{x}, \quad V_a = V_{a0} + A_a(\frac{L_c}{2} + x), \tag{2}$$

where R is the gas constant, T_s is the ambient temperature, V_a is the volume of the cylinder chamber A, $\dot{m}_a$ is the mass flow entering or exiting the chamber A, V_{a0} is the dead volume of the cylinder chamber A, and L_c is stroke of the actuator. $\dot{m}_a$ can be calculated by [16]:

$$\dot{m}_a = (p_l - p_a)\frac{p_v A_l D_l}{32RT_s L_l \mu}, \tag{3}$$

where p_l is the average air pressure in the transmission line, p_v is the measured air pressure at the work port of the control valve, L_l, A_l, and D_l denote the length, cross section area, and inner diameter of the transmission line, respectively, and μ is the dynamic viscosity of air.

As shown in Figure 2, the long transmission line is assumed to be an intermediate chamber connected between the control valve and the actuator in series, thus, the following equation is formulated to represent the pressure dynamic of the line [16,35]:

$$\dot{p}_l = \frac{RT_s}{V_l}(\dot{m}_v - \dot{m}_a), \tag{4}$$

where V_l is the volume of the transmission line, and $\dot{m}_v$ is the mass flow rate through the valve, which can be calculated by [35]:

$$\dot{m}_v = A(u)K_q(p_u, p_d, T_u) = \begin{cases} A(u)C_d C_1 \frac{p_u}{\sqrt{T_u}}, & \frac{p_d}{p_u} \le p_r, \\ A(u)C_d C_1 \frac{p_u}{\sqrt{T_u}} \sqrt{1 - \left(\frac{\frac{p_d}{p_u} - p_r}{1 - p_r}\right)^2}, & \frac{p_d}{p_u} > p_r \end{cases}, \tag{5}$$

where $A(u)$ is the effective valve orifice area, u is the control valve's control input, C_d is the discharge coefficient, C_1 is a constant with a value of 0.0404, p_u and p_d are the upstream pressure and the downstream pressure, respectively, T_u is the upstream temperature of air, and p_r is the critical pressure ratio. Therefore, $\dot{m}_v = A(u)K_q(p_s, p_v, T_s)$ when the line is charging, and $\dot{m}_v = A(u)K_q(p_v, p_0, T_s)$ when the line is discharging.

Choose the state vectors $x = [x_1, x_2, x_3, x_4]^T$ as $x_1 = x$, $x_2 = \dot{x}$, $x_3 = p_a$ and $x_4 = p_l$, thus the system dynamics can be expressed in a state-space form as:

$$\begin{cases} \dot{x}_1 = x_2 \\ m\dot{x}_2 = A_a x_3 - A_b p_b - p_0 A_r - b x_2 - A_f S_f(x_2) - d_f \\ \dot{x}_3 = \frac{RT_s}{V_a}\dot{m}_a - \frac{A_a x_2}{V_a} x_3 \\ \dot{x}_4 = \frac{RT_s}{V_l}(\dot{m}_v - \dot{m}_a) \end{cases}. \tag{6}$$

The control objective is to synthesize a control input u for the system Equation (6) such that x tracks the desired trajectory x_d with a guaranteed transient and final tracking accuracy. Instead of using the pressure sensor, a globally stable pressure observer is developed to estimate the pressure in chamber A. The parametric uncertainties due to unknown b and A_f and unknown external disturbances will be explicitly considered in this paper.

Assumption 1: *The desired trajectory x_d is at least second-order differentiable, and x_d, $\dot{x}_d$, and $\ddot{x}_d$ are bounded. Then, there exists a compact set* $\Omega_0 = \left\{ \left[x_d, \dot{x}_d, \ddot{x}_d\right]^T : x_d^2 + \dot{x}_d^2 + \ddot{x}_d^2 \le B_0 \right\}$ *such that* $\left[x_d, \dot{x}_d, \ddot{x}_d\right]^T \in \Omega_0$, *where B_0 is a positive constant.*

Assumption 2: *The extent of parametric uncertainties and external disturbances can be predicted and given by* $b_{min} \le b \le b_{max}$, $F_{fmin} \le F_f \le F_{fmax}$, *and* $d_{min} \le d_f \le d_{max}$.

3. Controller Design

3.1. Pressure Observer

The following observer is proposed to estimate the pressure of the actuator chamber A and the average air pressure in the transmission line:

$$\begin{cases} \dot{\hat{p}}_a = \frac{RT_s}{V_a}\hat{\dot{m}}_a - \frac{A_a \dot{x}}{V_a}\hat{p}_a \\ \dot{\hat{p}}_l = \frac{RT_s}{V_l}(\hat{\dot{m}}_v - \hat{\dot{m}}_a) \end{cases}, \tag{7}$$

where $\hat{p}_a$ and $\hat{p}_l$ represent the estimates of p_a and p_l, $\hat{\dot{m}}_a$ and $\hat{\dot{m}}_v$ denote the estimated mass flow rates according to Equation (3) and Equation (5) based on $\hat{p}_a$ and $\hat{p}_l$. It should be noted that the proposed observers are closed loop because of the relationship between the estimated mass flow rates and the estimated pressures. Proof of the convergence between the actual pressures and the estimated ones will be given later.

To verify the convergence between the actual pressures and the estimated pressures, the following Lyapunov function candidate was considered:

$$V_o = V_{o1} + V_{o2}, V_{o1} = \frac{1}{2}(\widetilde{p}_a V_a)^2, V_{o2} = \frac{1}{2}(\widetilde{p}_l V_l)^2, \tag{8}$$

where $\widetilde{p}_a = p_a - \hat{p}_a$, and $\widetilde{p}_l = p_l - \hat{p}_l$.

The time derivative of V_{o1} is:

$$\begin{aligned} \dot{V}_{o1} &= (p_a V_a - \hat{p}_a V_a)(\dot{p}_a V_a + p_a \dot{V}_a - \dot{\hat{p}}_a V_a - \hat{p}_a \dot{V}_a) \\ &= RT_s V_a (p_a - \hat{p}_a)(\dot{m}_a - \hat{\dot{m}}_a) \end{aligned} \tag{9}$$

According the Equation (3), one can obtain:

1. $p_a > \hat{p}_a$ implies that $\dot{m}_a < \hat{\dot{m}}_a$, yielding $(p_a - \hat{p}_a)(\dot{m}_a - \hat{\dot{m}}_a) < 0$.
2. $p_a < \hat{p}_a$ implies that $\dot{m}_a > \hat{\dot{m}}_a$, yielding $(p_a - \hat{p}_a)(\dot{m}_a - \hat{\dot{m}}_a) < 0$.
3. $p_a = \hat{p}_a$ implies that $\dot{m}_a < \hat{\dot{m}}_a$, yielding $(p_a - \hat{p}_a)(\dot{m}_a - \hat{\dot{m}}_a) = 0$.

Therefore, $\dot{V}_{o1}$ is negative semi-definite.

The time derivative of V_{o2} is:

$$\begin{aligned} \dot{V}_{o2} &= (p_l V_l - \hat{p}_l V_l)(\dot{p}_l V_l - \dot{\hat{p}}_l V_l) \\ &= RT_s V_l (p_l - \hat{p}_l)(\dot{m}_v - \hat{\dot{m}}_v) - RT_s V_l (p_l - \hat{p}_l)(\dot{m}_a - \hat{\dot{m}}_a) \end{aligned} \tag{10}$$

According the Equation (3), one can obtain:

1. $p_l > \hat{p}_l$ implies that $\dot{m}_a > \hat{\dot{m}}_a$, yielding $(p_l - \hat{p}_l)(\dot{m}_a - \hat{\dot{m}}_a) > 0$.
2. $p_l < \hat{p}_l$ implies that $\dot{m}_a < \hat{\dot{m}}_a$, yielding $(p_l - \hat{p}_l)(\dot{m}_a - \hat{\dot{m}}_a) > 0$.
3. $p_l = \hat{p}_l$ implies that $\dot{m}_a = \hat{\dot{m}}_a$, yielding $(p_l - \hat{p}_l)(\dot{m}_a - \hat{\dot{m}}_a) = 0$.

For the mass flow rate relationship given by Equation (5), it has proven in [25] that the term $(p_l - \hat{p}_l)(\dot{m}_v - \hat{\dot{m}}_v)$ is always non-positive. Thus, $\dot{V}_{o2}$ and V_o are negative semi-definite, one can conclude that the proposed pressure observers are globally Lyapunov stable with regard to the errors in the estimated pressures.

3.2. Adaptive Dynamic Surface Controller

Step 1: Differentiate the trajectory tracking error $e_1 = x_1 - x_d$ with respect to time leads to:

$$\dot{e}_1 = x_2 - \dot{x}_d. \tag{11}$$

Consider x_2 as the first virtual control input, the virtual control law is designed as follows:

$$\overline{x}_{2d} = \dot{x}_d - k_1 e_1, \qquad k_1 > 0, \tag{12}$$

where k_1 is a positive control gain. Following the dynamic surface control theory [28], the signal $\overline{x}_{2d}$ is fed to a low pass filter to obtain a new one x_{2d} for the next design step:

$$\tau_1 \dot{x}_{2d} + x_{2d} = \overline{x}_{2d}, \qquad x_{2d}(0) = \overline{x}_{2d}(0), \qquad \tau_1 > 0, \tag{13}$$

where τ_1 is the filter parameter.

Step 2: Define the first surface error as $s_1 = x_2 - x_{2d}$, its time derivative can be derived as:

$$\dot{s}_1 = \dot{x}_2 - \dot{x}_{2d} = \overline{A}_a x_3 - \frac{1}{m}\left[p_b A_b + p_0 A_r + b x_2 + F_f S_f(\dot{x}) + d_f\right] - \frac{1}{\tau_1}(\overline{x}_{2d} - x_{2d}), \tag{14}$$

where $\overline{A}_\mathrm{a} = A_\mathrm{a}/m$.

Define $\widetilde{x_3} = x_3 - \hat{x}_3$, and let $\varsigma = \hat{x}_3$ be the second virtual control input, the virtual control law is designed as follows:

$$\overline{\varsigma}_\mathrm{d} = \frac{1}{\overline{A}_\mathrm{a}}\left\{\frac{1}{m}\left[p_\mathrm{b}A_\mathrm{b} + p_0A_\mathrm{r} + \hat{b}x_2 + \hat{F}_\mathrm{f}S_\mathrm{f}(\dot{x}) + \hat{d}_\mathrm{f}\right] + \frac{1}{\tau_1}(\overline{x}_{2\mathrm{d}} - x_{2\mathrm{d}}) - k_2s_1 - \frac{h_1^2}{4\eta_1}s_1\right\}, \tag{15}$$

where $k_2 > 0$ is a positive control gain, $\eta_1 > 0$ is a controller parameter, and h_1 is a known function that will be determined later, $\hat{b}$, $\hat{F}_\mathrm{f}$,and $\hat{d}_\mathrm{f}$ are the estimates of b, F_f, and d_f, respectively. $\hat{b}$, $\hat{F}_\mathrm{f}$, and $\hat{d}_\mathrm{f}$ are updated by:

$$\dot{\hat{b}} = \mathrm{Proj}_{\hat{b}}(-\frac{\gamma_1}{m}x_2s_1), \tag{16}$$

$$\dot{\hat{F}}_\mathrm{f} = \mathrm{Proj}_{\hat{F}_\mathrm{f}}(-\frac{\gamma_2}{m}S_\mathrm{f}(x_2)s_1), \tag{17}$$

$$\dot{\hat{d}}_\mathrm{f} = \mathrm{Proj}_{\hat{d}_\mathrm{f}}(-\frac{\gamma_3}{m}s_1), \tag{18}$$

where $\gamma_1 > 0$, $\gamma_2 > 0$,and $\gamma_3 > 0$ are the observer gains, and the projection mapping is defined as:

$$\mathrm{Proj}_{\hat{\xi}}(\cdot) = \begin{cases} 0, & \text{if} \quad \hat{\xi} = \xi_{\max} \quad \text{and} \quad \cdot > 0 \\ 0, & \text{if} \quad \hat{\xi} = \xi_{\min} \quad \text{and} \quad \cdot < 0 \\ \cdot, & \text{otherwise} \end{cases}, \tag{19}$$

where ξ is a symbol that can be replaced by b, F_f, and d_f.

Similarly, the signal $\overline{\varsigma}_\mathrm{d}$ is fed to a low pass filter to obtain a new one ς_d for the next design step:

$$\tau_2\dot{\varsigma}_\mathrm{d} + \varsigma_\mathrm{d} = \overline{\varsigma}_\mathrm{d}, \varsigma_\mathrm{d}(0) = \overline{\varsigma}_\mathrm{d}(0),\ \tau_2 > 0, \tag{20}$$

where τ_2 is the filter parameter.

Step 3: Define the second surface error as $s_2 = \varsigma - \varsigma_\mathrm{d}$, its time derivative can be derived as:

$$\begin{aligned} \dot{s}_2 &= \dot{\varsigma} - \dot{\varsigma}_\mathrm{d} = \dot{\hat{x}}_3 - \dot{\varsigma}_\mathrm{d} = \tfrac{RT_\mathrm{s}}{V_\mathrm{a}}\hat{\dot{m}}_\mathrm{a} - \tfrac{A_\mathrm{a}x_2}{V_\mathrm{a}}\hat{x}_3 - \tfrac{1}{\tau_2}(\overline{\varsigma}_\mathrm{d} - \varsigma_\mathrm{d}) \\ &= -\tfrac{RT_\mathrm{s}a}{V_\mathrm{a}}\hat{x}_4 + (\tfrac{RT_\mathrm{s}a}{V_\mathrm{a}} - \tfrac{A_\mathrm{a}x_2}{V_\mathrm{a}})\hat{x}_3 - \tfrac{1}{\tau_2}(\overline{\varsigma}_\mathrm{d} - \varsigma_\mathrm{d}) \end{aligned} \tag{21}$$

where $a = \frac{p_\mathrm{v}A_lD_l}{32RT_\mathrm{s}L_l\mu}$.

Let $\zeta = -\hat{x}_4$ be the third virtual control input, the virtual control law is designed as follows:

$$\overline{\zeta}_\mathrm{d} = \frac{V_\mathrm{a}}{RT_\mathrm{s}a}\left[\left(\frac{A_\mathrm{a}x_2}{V_\mathrm{a}} - \frac{RT_\mathrm{s}a}{V_\mathrm{a}}\right)\hat{x}_3 + \frac{1}{\tau_2}(\overline{\varsigma}_\mathrm{d} - \varsigma_\mathrm{d}) - k_3s_2\right], \tag{22}$$

where $k_3 > 0$ is a positive control gain. Similarly, the signal $\overline{\zeta}_\mathrm{d}$ is fed to a low pass filter to obtain a new one ζ_d for the next design step:

$$\tau_3\dot{\zeta}_\mathrm{d} + \zeta_\mathrm{d} = \overline{\zeta}_\mathrm{d}, \quad \zeta_\mathrm{d}(0) = \overline{\zeta}_\mathrm{d}(0),\ \tau_3 > 0, \tag{23}$$

where τ_3 is the filter parameter.

Step 4: Define the second surface error as $s_3 = \zeta - \zeta_\mathrm{d}$, its time derivative can be derived as:

$$\dot{s}_3 = \dot{\zeta} - \dot{\zeta}_\mathrm{d} = -\dot{\hat{x}}_4 - \dot{\zeta}_\mathrm{d} = -\frac{RT_\mathrm{s}}{V_l}(\hat{\dot{m}}_\mathrm{v} - \hat{\dot{m}}_\mathrm{a}) - \frac{1}{\tau_3}(\overline{\zeta}_\mathrm{d} - \zeta_\mathrm{d}). \tag{24}$$

Similarly, the following control law q_d for $\hat{\dot{m}}_v$ is proposed:

$$q_d = \hat{\dot{m}}_a - \frac{RT_s}{V_l}\left[\frac{1}{\tau_3}(\overline{\zeta}_d - \zeta_d) - k_4 s_3\right], \tag{25}$$

where $k_4 > 0$ is a positive control gain.

Once the q_d is calculated, the desired effective valve orifice area $A(u)$ can be calculated by:

$$A(u) = \begin{cases} \frac{q_d}{K_q(p_s, p_v, T_s)} & q_d > 0 \\ \frac{q_d}{K_q(p_v, p_0, T_s)} & q_d \leq 0 \end{cases}. \tag{26}$$

Thus, the input signal u for the proportional-directional control valve could be obtained according to the relation between the input signal and effective valve orifice area.

The proposed pressure observer based adaptive dynamic surface control is illustrated in Figure 3.

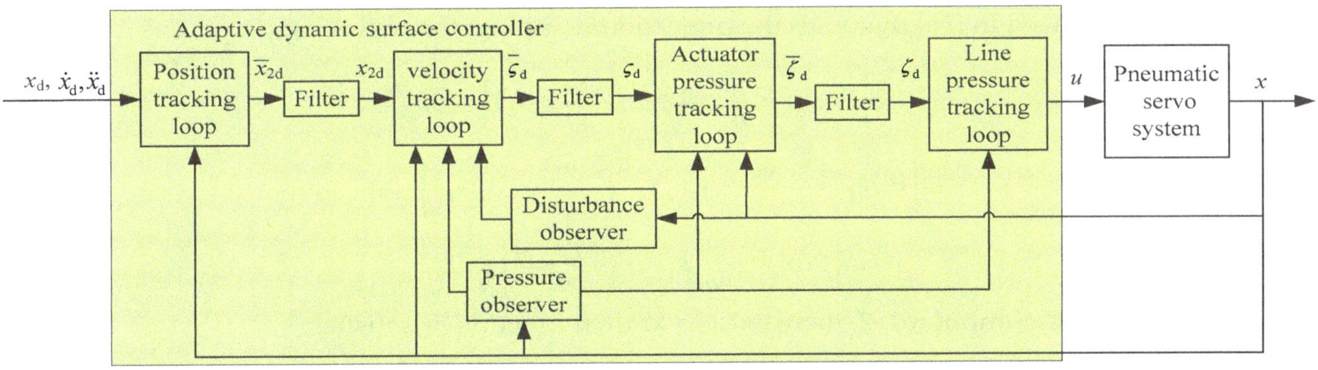

Figure 3. Block diagram of the control system.

3.3. Proof of Stability

Theorem 1. *Consider the closed loop pneumatic servo system consisting of the plant Equation (6), the nonlinear control law Equation (25), the pressure observers Equation (7), and the parameter and disturbance estimation algorithm Equations (16)–(18) under the Assumption 1–2. If there exists a set of the feedback gains and the filter constants satisfying* $\gamma = \min\left\{k_1 - 1, k_2 - \frac{1}{2} - \overline{A}_a, k_3 - \frac{\overline{A}_a}{2}, \frac{1}{\tau_1} - 1, \frac{1}{\tau_2} - \frac{1}{2} - \frac{\overline{A}_a}{2}\right\} > 0$, *then the closed loop system is uniformly and ultimately bounded.*

Proof. Consider the following Lyapunov function candidate:

$$\begin{aligned} &V_c = V_{cs} + V_{cz} + V_\theta,\ V_{cs} = \tfrac{1}{2}e_1^2 + \tfrac{1}{2}s_1^2 + \tfrac{1}{2}s_2^2 + \tfrac{1}{2}s_3^2,\ V_{cz} = \tfrac{1}{2}z_1^2 + \tfrac{1}{2}z_2^2 + \tfrac{1}{2}z_3^2, \\ &V_\theta = \tfrac{1}{2}\gamma_1^{-1}\widetilde{b}^2 + \tfrac{1}{2}\gamma_2^{-1}\widetilde{F}_f^2 + \tfrac{1}{2}\gamma_3^{-1}\widetilde{d}_f^2 \end{aligned} \tag{27}$$

where $z_1 = x_{2d} - \overline{x}_{2d}$, $z_2 = \varsigma_d - \overline{\varsigma}_d$, $z_3 = \zeta_d - \overline{\zeta}_d$. Substituting Equation (12) into Equation (11) gives:

$$\dot{e}_1 = s_1 + z_1 - k_1 e_1. \tag{28}$$

Substituting Equation (15) into Equation (14) and noting $\hat{x}_3 = s_2 + \varsigma_d = s_2 + z_2 + \overline{\varsigma}_d$ yields:

$$\dot{s}_1 = \overline{A}_a(s_2 + z_2) - \frac{1}{m}\left[\widetilde{b}x_2 + \widetilde{F}_f S_f(\dot{x}) + \widetilde{d}_f\right] + \overline{A}_a\widetilde{x}_3 - k_2 s_1 - \frac{h_1^2}{4\eta_1}s_1, \tag{29}$$

where $\widetilde{b} = b - \hat{b}$, $\widetilde{F}_f = F_f - \hat{F}_f$, $\widetilde{d}_f = d_f - \hat{d}_f$.

Substituting Equation (22) into Equation (21) and noting $\hat{x}_4 = s_3 + \zeta_d = s_3 + z_3 + \overline{\zeta}_d$ yields:

$$\dot{s}_2 = \frac{RT_s a}{V_a}(s_3 + z_3) - k_3 s_2. \tag{30}$$

Substituting Equation (25) into Equation (24) gives:

$$\dot{s}_3 = -k_4 s_3. \tag{31}$$

Therefore, the time derivative of $V_1 = V_{cs} + V_\theta$ is:

$$\begin{aligned}\dot{V}_1 = \ & -k_1e_1^2 - k_2s_1^2 - k_3s_2^2 - k_4s_3^2 + e_1s_1 + e_1z_1 + \overline{A}_a(s_1s_2 + s_1z_2) + \tfrac{RT_s a}{V_a}(s_3 + z_3) \\ & +\gamma_1^{-1}\widetilde{b}\Big[\dot{\hat{b}} - (-\tfrac{\gamma_1}{m}x_2s_1)\Big] + \gamma_2^{-1}\widetilde{F}_f\Big[\dot{\hat{F}}_f - (-\tfrac{\gamma_2}{m}S_f(x_2)s_1)\Big] + \gamma_3^{-1}\widetilde{d}_f\Big[\dot{\hat{d}}_f - (-\tfrac{\gamma_3}{m}s_1)\Big] \\ & +s_1\Big\{-\tfrac{h_1^2}{4\eta_1}s_1 - \tfrac{1}{m}\Big[\widetilde{b}x_2 + \widetilde{F}_fS_f(\dot{x}) + \widetilde{d}_f\Big] + \overline{A}_a\widetilde{x}_3\Big\}\end{aligned} \tag{32}$$

It has been proved in [36] that with the projection mapping, the following properties hold:

$$\widetilde{b}\Big[\mathrm{Proj}_{\hat{b}}(-\frac{\gamma_1}{m}x_2s_1) - (-\frac{\gamma_1}{m}x_2s_1)\Big] \le 0. \tag{33a}$$

$$\widetilde{F}_f\Big[\mathrm{Proj}_{\hat{F}_f}(-\frac{\gamma_2}{m}S_f(x_2)s_1) - (-\frac{\gamma_2}{m}S_f(x_2)s_1)\Big] \le 0. \tag{34b}$$

$$\widetilde{d}_f\Big[\mathrm{Proj}_{\hat{d}_f}(-\frac{\gamma_3}{m}s_1) - (-\frac{\gamma_3}{m}s_1)\Big] \le 0. \tag{33c}$$

According to Assumption 1–2, there exists a known function h_1 satisfies:

$$h_1(t) \ge \frac{1}{m}\Big[|b_{\max} - b_{\min}||x_2| + |F_{f\max} - F_{f\min}|\big|S_f(x_2)\big| + |d_{\max} - d_{\min}|\Big] + \overline{A}_a\big|\rho_1\big|, \tag{34}$$

where ρ_1 is the bound of $\widetilde{x}_3$ as proven in the above step. From the smoothed sliding mode control theory, the following inequality holds.

$$s_1\left\{-\frac{h_1^2}{4\eta_1}s_1 - \frac{1}{m}\Big[\widetilde{b}x_2 + \widetilde{F}_fS_f(\dot{x}) + \widetilde{d}_f\Big] + \overline{A}_a\widetilde{x}_3\right\} \le \eta_1. \tag{35}$$

Substituting Equation (34) into Equation (32) yields

$$\dot{V}_1 \le -k_1e_1^2 - k_2s_1^2 - k_3s_2^2 - k_4s_3^2 + e_1s_1 + e_1z_1 + \overline{A}_a(s_1s_2 + s_1z_2) + \frac{RT_s a}{V_a}(s_3 + z_3) + \eta_1. \tag{36}$$

The following inequalities can be obtained by using Young's inequality.

$$\begin{aligned} & e_1s_1 \le \tfrac{e_1^2}{2} + \tfrac{s_1^2}{2}, e_1z_1 \le \tfrac{e_1^2}{2} + \tfrac{z_1^2}{2}, s_1s_2 \le \tfrac{s_1^2}{2} + \tfrac{s_2^2}{2} \\ & s_1z_2 \le \tfrac{s_1^2}{2} + \tfrac{z_2^2}{2}, s_2s_3 \le \tfrac{s_2^2}{2} + \tfrac{s_3^2}{2}, s_2z_3 \le \tfrac{s_2^2}{2} + \tfrac{z_3^2}{2}\end{aligned} \tag{37}$$

Substituting Equation (37) into Equation (36) gives:

$$\begin{aligned}\dot{V}_1 \le \ & -(k_1 - 1)e_1^2 - (k_2 - \tfrac{1}{2} - \overline{A}_a)s_1^2 - (k_3 - \tfrac{\overline{A}_a}{2} - \tfrac{RT_s a}{V_a})s_2^2 - (k_4 - \tfrac{RT_s a}{2V_a})s_3^2 + \\ & \tfrac{1}{2}z_1^2 + \tfrac{\overline{A}_a}{2}z_2^2 + \tfrac{RT_s a}{2V_a}z_3^2 + \eta_1\end{aligned} \tag{38}$$

Following the similar analysis as done in [28], the following inequalities hold.

$$\dot{z}_1 + \frac{z_1}{\tau_1} \le \left|\dot{z}_1 + \frac{z_1}{\tau_1}\right| \le \xi_1, \quad \dot{z}_2 + \frac{z_2}{\tau_2} \le \left|\dot{z}_2 + \frac{z_2}{\tau_2}\right| \le \xi_2, \quad \dot{z}_3 + \frac{z_3}{\tau_3} \le \left|\dot{z}_3 + \frac{z_3}{\tau_3}\right| \le \xi_3, \tag{39}$$

where $\xi_1(e_1, s_1, z_1, x_d, \dot{x}_d, \ddot{x}_d)$, $\xi_2(e_1, s_1, s_2, z_1, z_2, x_d, \dot{x}_d, \ddot{x}_d)$, and $\xi_2(e_1, s_1, s_2, s_3, z_1, z_2, z_3, x_d, \dot{x}_d, \ddot{x}_d)$ are three continuous functions. Due to the fact that the set Ω_0 is compact in R^3 and the set $\Omega_1 = \left\{[e_1, s_1, s_2, s_3, z_1, z_2, z_3]^T : e_1^2 + s_1^2 + s_2^2 + s_3^2 + z_1^2 + z_2^2 + z_3^2 \le 2B_1\right\}$ (where $B_1 > 0$) is compact in R^7, $\Omega_0 \times \Omega_1$ is thus compact in R^{10}. Therefore, ξ_1, ξ_2, and ξ_3 have maximums on $\Omega_0 \times \Omega_1$. Let M_1, M_2, and M_3 be the maximums of ξ_1, ξ_2, and ξ_3 on $\Omega_0 \times \Omega_1$, respectively, one can obtain that:

$$z_1\dot{z}_1 + \frac{z_1^2}{\tau_1} \le M_1|z_1|, \quad z_2\dot{z}_2 + \frac{z_2^2}{\tau_2} \le M_2|z_2|, \quad z_3\dot{z}_3 + \frac{z_3^2}{\tau_3} \le M_3|z_3|. \tag{40}$$

With the use of Young's inequality, one can obtain that:

$$z_1\dot{z}_1 \le -\frac{z_1^2}{\tau_1} + \frac{z_1^2}{2} + \frac{M_1^2}{2}, \quad z_2\dot{z}_2 \le -\frac{z_2^2}{\tau_2} + \frac{z_2^2}{2} + \frac{M_2^2}{2}, \quad z_3\dot{z}_3 \le -\frac{z_3^2}{\tau_3} + \frac{z_3^2}{2} + \frac{M_3^2}{2}. \tag{41}$$

Thus, the following inequalities can be obtained.

$$\dot{V}_{cz} \le -\frac{1}{\tau_1}z_1^2 - \frac{1}{\tau_2}z_2^2 - \frac{1}{\tau_3}z_3^2 + \frac{1}{2}z_1^2 + \frac{1}{2}M_1^2 + \frac{1}{2}z_2^2 + \frac{1}{2}M_2^2 + \frac{1}{2}z_3^2 + \frac{1}{2}M_3^2. \tag{42}$$

Thus, the following inequalities can be obtained.

$$\begin{aligned} \dot{V}_1 \le\ & -(k_1 - 1)e_1^2 - (k_2 - \tfrac{1}{2} - \overline{A}_a)s_1^2 - (k_3 - \tfrac{\overline{A}_a}{2} - \tfrac{RT_s a}{V_a})s_2^2 - (k_4 - \tfrac{RT_s a}{2V_a})s_3^2 - \\ & (\tfrac{1}{\tau_1} - 1)z_1^2 - (\tfrac{1}{\tau_2} - \tfrac{1}{2} - \tfrac{\overline{A}_a}{2})z_2^2 - (\tfrac{1}{\tau_3} - \tfrac{1}{2} - \tfrac{RT_s a}{2V_a})z_3^2 + \tfrac{1}{2}M_1^2 + \tfrac{1}{2}M_2^2 + \tfrac{1}{2}M_3^2 + \eta_1 \end{aligned} \tag{43}$$

By choosing $k_1 > 1$, $k_2 > \frac{1}{2} + \overline{A}_a$, $k_3 > \frac{\overline{A}_a}{2} + \frac{RT_s a}{V_a}$, $k_4 > \frac{RT_s a}{2V_a}$, $\tau_1 < 1$, $\tau_2 < \frac{2}{\overline{A}_a + 1}$, and $\tau_3 < \frac{2V_a}{RT_s a + V_a}$, one has:

$$\gamma = \min\left\{k_1 - 1, k_2 - \frac{1}{2} - \overline{A}_a, k_3 - \frac{\overline{A}_a}{2} - \frac{RT_s a}{V_a}, k_4 - \frac{RT_s a}{2V_a}, \frac{1}{\tau_1} - 1, \frac{1}{\tau_2} - \frac{1}{2} - \frac{\overline{A}_a}{2}, \frac{1}{\tau_3} - \frac{1}{2} - \frac{RT_s a}{2V_a}\right\} > 0 \tag{44}$$

Then, it can be readily obtained that the following inequality holds.

$$\dot{V} \le -2\gamma V + \eta, \tag{45}$$

where $\eta = \frac{1}{2}M_1^2 + \frac{1}{2}M_2^2 + \frac{1}{2}M_3^2 + \eta_1$. □

Clearly, if $\gamma > \eta / 2B_1$, then $\dot{V} \le 0$ on set Ω_1, thus V will remain $V(t) \le B_1$ for all t, provided that the initial conditions satisfy $V(0) \le B_1$. Therefore, the errors $e_1, s_1, s_2, s_3, z_1, z_2, z_3$ are bounded. Hence, one can conclude that the closed loop system is uniformly and ultimately bounded.

4. Experimental Results

In this section, the proposed controller was implemented for the servo control of the pneumatic servo system as shown in Figure 2. The cylinder forward chamber was controlled by the valve through a 10 m long transmission line with 4 mm inside diameter, while the pressure in the return chamber was maintained at about 3 bar by utilizing a tank. A gel phantom was used to perform the following needle insertion experiments. The system physical parameters and the parameters of the controller are given in Table 1.

Table 1. Parameters of the system and the proposed controller.

Symbol	Value	Unit
m	0.32	kg
A_a	7.854×10^{-5}	m^2
A_b	6.597×10^{-4}	m^2
A_r	1.257×10^{-5}	m^2
R	287	N m/(kg K)
T_s	300	K
p_s	6×10^5	Pa
V_{a0}	6×10^{-7}	m^3
L_c	0.125	m
V_l	1.257×10^{-4}	m^3
C_d	$1.099 - 0.1075 \times \frac{p_u}{p_d}$	
p_r	0.29	
A_l	1.257×10^{-5}	m^2
D_l	0.004	m
L_l	10	m
μ	1.79×10^{-5}	$N s/m^2$
p_0	1×10^5	Pa
$\hat{b}(0), b_{min}, b_{max}$	9, 0, 15	N s/m
$\hat{F}_f(0), \hat{F}_{fmin}, \hat{F}_{fmax}$	6, 0, 20	N
$\hat{d}_f(0), d_{min}, d_{max}$	0, −10, 10	N
k_1, τ_1	40, 0.5	
k_2, h_1, η_1, τ_2	50, 40, 0.4, 0.75	
k_3, τ_3	50, 1.2	
k_4	90	
$\gamma_1, \gamma_2, \gamma_3$	100, 10, 10	

The same control algorithm as the proposed controller, but in which the long transmission line was characterized as a part of the cylinder's dead volume and the chamber pressure was directly measured, was first tested for tracking a sinusoidal trajectory and a smooth square trajectory. As shown in Figure 4, the performance was poor for practical application, which indicates the need for an advanced method to address the issue of long transmission line. The performance of the proposed controller was tested on three types of reference trajectories: A 0.5 Hz sinusoidal signal, a smooth square signal, and a 4 s periodic signal. Figure 5 shows the response of the system, and the tracking errors are presented in Figure 6. The maximum absolute tracking errors ($\max_t\{|e_1|\}$) were about 2.51 mm, 2.68 mm, and 1.81 mm, while the final steady-state tracking errors ($\max_{t\geq 5}\{|e_1|\}$) were about 0.96 mm, 1.05 mm, and 1.39 mm. As seen, the proposed controller could significantly improve the system performance, which indicates the effectiveness of the proposed long transmission line compensation method. However, it should be noted that these needle insertion experiments were performed in a gel phantom, whose resisting force behavior was simpler than real soft tissue. The interaction between needle and soft tissue is very complex and may decrease the needle insertion precision in practical. Since the current research focused on addressing the issue of long transmission line and realizing high accuracy control of a pneumatic actuator with a pressure observer, modeling of needle-tissue interaction and further improving needle insertion precision would be the subject of the next phase of this research.

The process of parameter and disturbance estimations is shown in Figure 7. It can be seen that the estimates converged quickly, and the tracking error improvement could be achieved within several seconds. Comparisons between the observed chamber pressure and the measured one are shown in Figure 8. As can be seen, the estimated chamber pressure was close to its actual value, which indicates the effectiveness of the proposed pressure observer. However, the estimation error during the charging process was slightly bigger than the one during the discharging process. This might be due to the fact that charging process was close to adiabatic and the discharging process was close to isothermal.

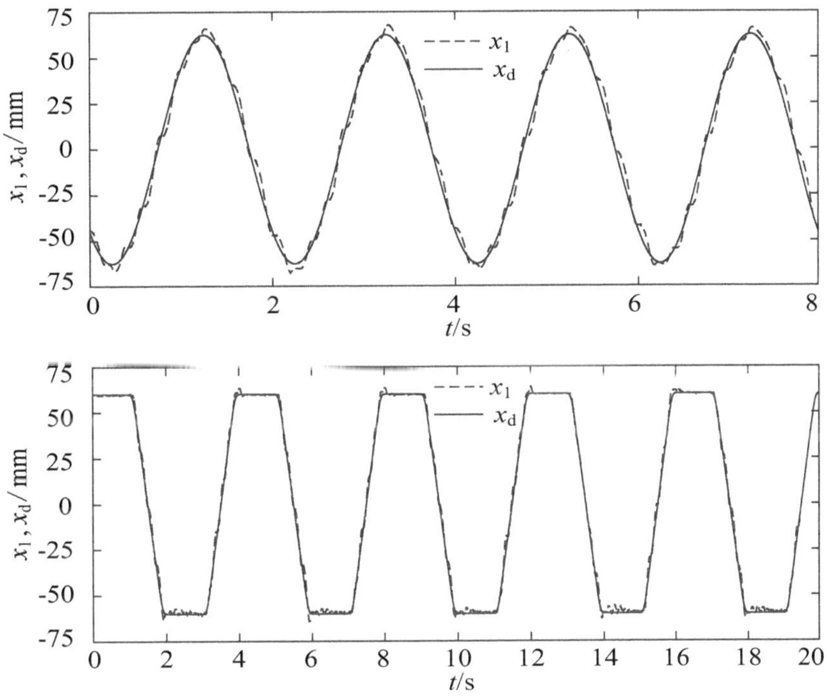

Figure 4. Tracking response of the same control algorithm as the proposed controller but without using long transmission line compensation.

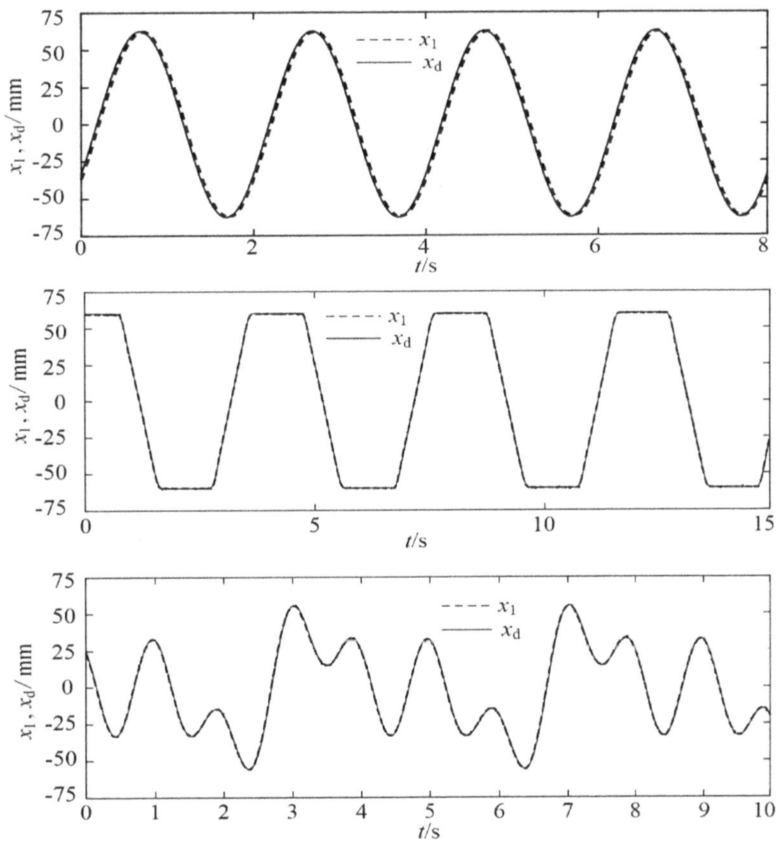

Figure 5. Tracking response of the proposed controller for three different types of trajectories.

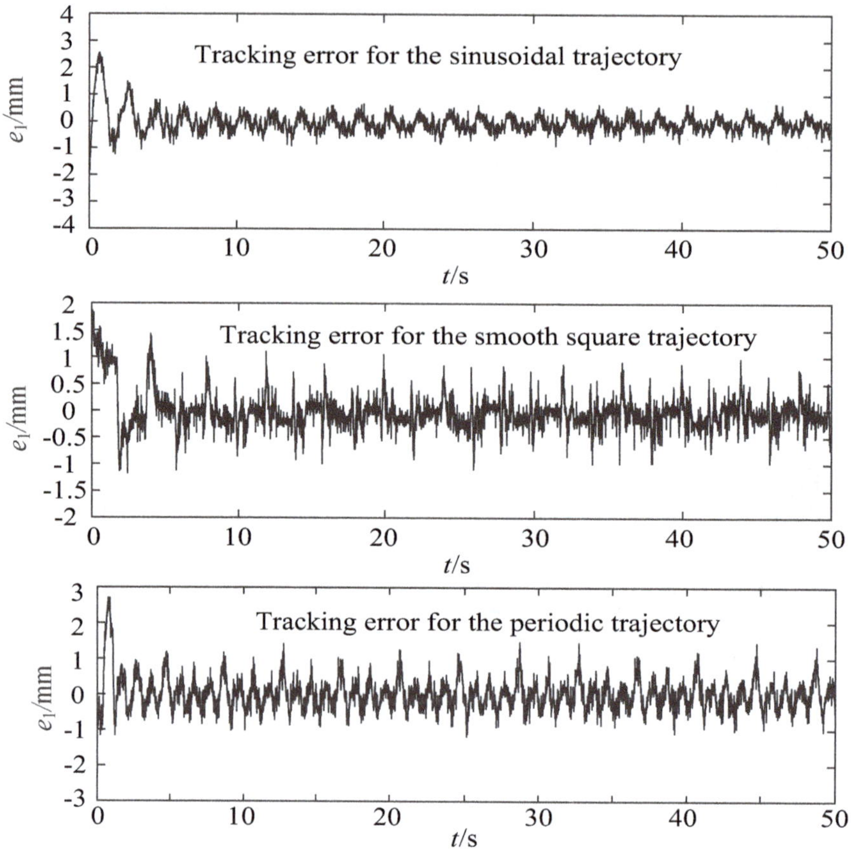

Figure 6. Tracking errors of the proposed controller for three different types of trajectories.

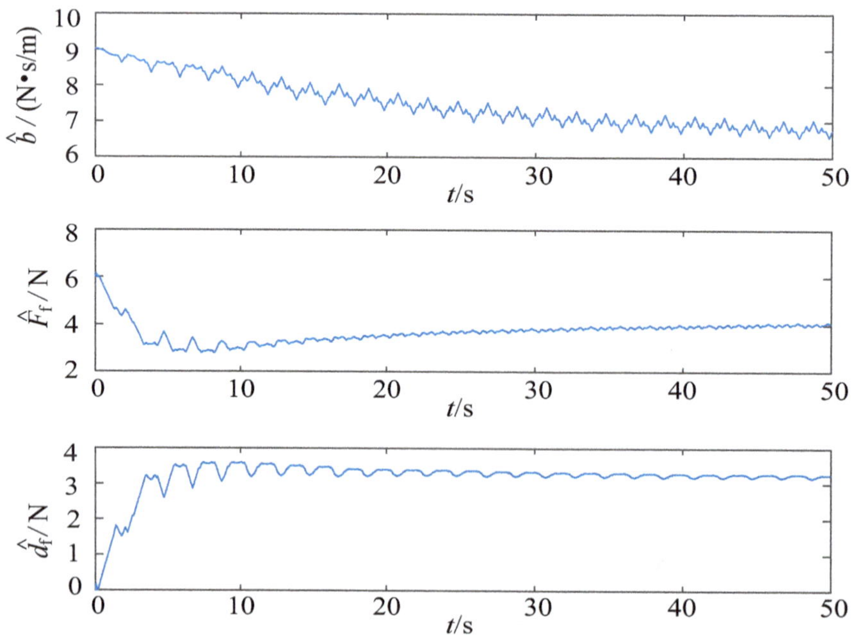

Figure 7. Parameter and disturbance estimations of the proposed controller when the reference is a 0.5 Hz sinusoidal trajectory.

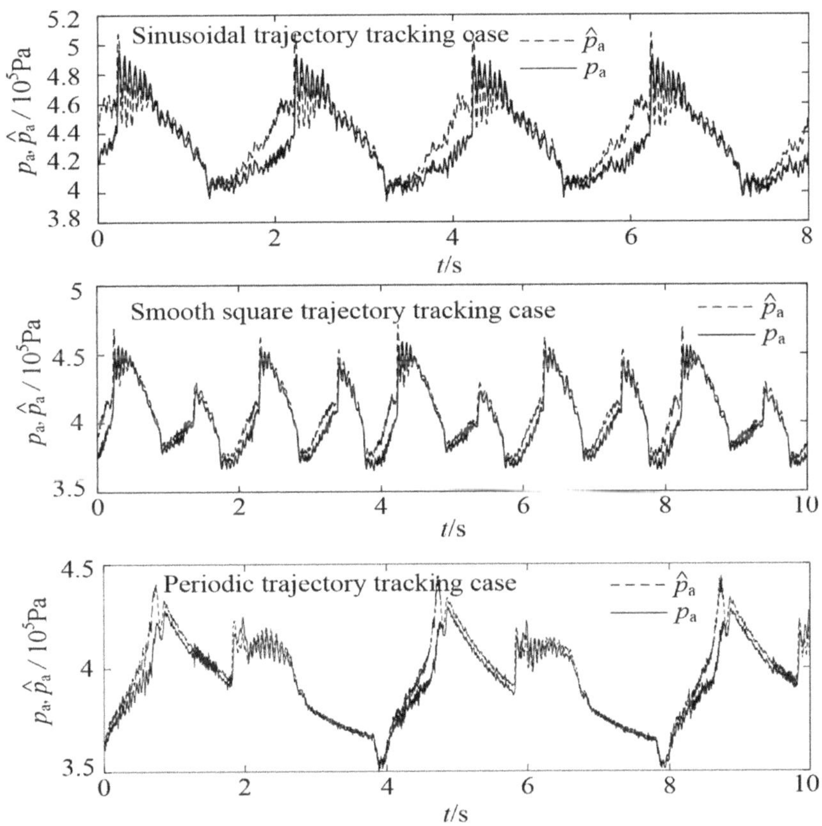

Figure 8. Actual and observed chamber pressure for the system tracking three different types of references.

Experiments were also conducted to verify the performance robustness of the proposed controller. To simulate a sudden disturbance acting on the system, a big step signal was added to the output of the position sensor at $t = 22$ s, and removed 10 s later. Figure 9 shows the control accuracy of the proposed controller in this scenario for tracking a sinusoidal trajectory with a frequency of 0.5 Hz and amplitude of 62.5 mm. It can be seen that the system performance did not deteriorate except the transient spikes when the sudden disturbance was added or removed.

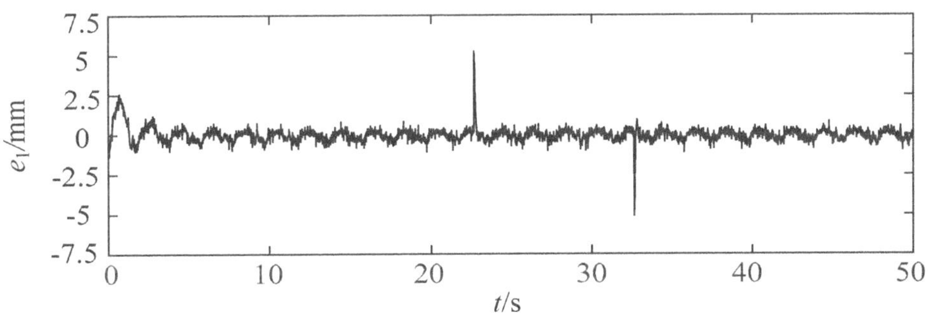

Figure 9. Tracking error of the proposed controller for 0.5 Hz sinusoidal trajectory with disturbance.

5. Conclusions

In this paper, the precise motion control of a MRI compatible 1-DOF pneumatic servo system was considered. The long transmission line was characterized as an intermediate chamber connected between the valve and the cylinder in series, and a nonlinear first order system was used to approximate its dynamics. Simultaneously, a globally stable pressure observer was developed to estimate the chamber pressure. Based on the model of the long transmission line and the pressure observer, a pressure observer based adaptive dynamic surface controller was developed and the stability of the closed-loop system was proved via the Lyapunov method. In contrast to most of the existing nonlinear controllers synthesized with the backstepping method, by employing the dynamic surface control technique, the proposed controller could cope with the problem of "explosion of complexity", since the repeated differentiation of virtual controls was no longer required. The experimental results confirmed that the proposed controller was effective and had good performance robustness to sudden disturbances, thus enabling future application in pneumatically actuated MRI-compatible robots. However, precise motion control of pneumatic actuator did not necessarily lead to precise position control needle tip. Modeling of the interaction between needle and soft tissue, and incorporating a more accurate needle insertion force model in the controller design is an essential requirement for practical robot-assisted needle insertion. Thus, these issues will be explored further in the next phase of this research.

Author Contributions: D.M. and B.L. proposed the pressure observe based dynamic surface controller for precise position tracking control of the MRI-compatible pneumatic servo system. A.L. designed the experiments. J.Y. and Q.L. performed the experiments and analyzed the data. D.M. and A.L. wrote the paper.

Acknowledgments: This work was supported by the National Natural Science Foundation of China (Grant No. 51505474), the Fundamental Research Funds for the Central Universities (Grant No. 2015XKMS020), the China Postdoctoral Science Foundation (Grant No. 2016T90520), and a Project Funded by the Priority Academic Program Development of Jiangsu Higher Education Institutions.

References

1. Fischer, G.; Iordachita, I.; Csoma, C.; Tokuda, J.; DiMaio, S.; Tempany, C.; Hata, N.; Fichtinger, G. MRI-compatible pneumatic robot for transperineal prostate needle placement. *IEEE/ASME Trans. Mechatron.* **2008**, *13*, 295–305. [CrossRef] [PubMed]
2. Stoianovici, D.; Jun, C.; Lim, S.; Li, P.; Petrisor, D.; Fricke, S.; Sharma, K.; Cleary, K. Multi-image compatible, MR safe, remote center of motion needle-guide robot. *IEEE Trans. Biomed. Eng.* **2018**, *65*, 165–177. [CrossRef] [PubMed]
3. Stoianovici, D.; Kim, C.; Srimathveeravalli, G.; Sebrecht, P.; Petrisor, D.; Coleman, J.; Solomon, S.; Hricak, H. MRI-Safe Robot for Endorectal Prostate Biopsy. *Trans. Mechatron.* **2014**, *19*, 1289–1299. [CrossRef]
4. Stoianovici, D.; Patriciu, A.; Petrisor, D.; Mazilu, D.; Kavoussi, L. A new type of motor: Pneumatic step motor. *IEEE/ASME Trans. Mechatron.* **2007**, *12*, 98–106. [CrossRef] [PubMed]
5. Zemiti, N.; Bricault, I.; Fouard, C.; Sanchez, B.; Cinquin, P. LPR: A CT and MR-compatible puncture robot to enhance accuracy and safety of image-guided interventions. *IEEE/ASME Trans. Mechatron.* **2008**, *13*, 306–315. [CrossRef]
6. Schouten, M.; Bomers, J.; Yakar, D.; Huisman, H.; Rothgang, E.; Bosboom, D.; Scheenen, T.; Misra, S.; Futterer, J. Evaluation of a robotic technique for transrectal MRI-guided prostate biopsies. *Eur. Radiol.* **2012**, *22*, 476–483. [CrossRef] [PubMed]
7. Franco, E.; Brujic, D.; Rea, M.; Gedroyc, W.; Ristic, M. Needle-guiding robot for laser ablation of liver tumors under MRI guidance. *IEEE/ASME Trans. Mechatron.* **2016**, *21*, 931–944. [CrossRef]
8. Yang, B.; Tan, U.; McMillan, A.; Gullapalli, R.; Desai, J. Design and control of a 1-DOF MRI-compatible pneumatically actuated robot with long transmission lines. *IEEE/ASME Trans. Mechatron.* **2011**, *16*, 1040–1048. [CrossRef] [PubMed]
9. Yang, B.; Roys, S.; Tan, U.; Philip, M.; Richard, H.; Gullapalli, R.; Desai, J. Design, development, and evaluation of a master–slave surgical system for breast biopsy under continuous MRI. *Int. J. Robot. Res.* **2014**, *33*, 616–630. [CrossRef]
10. Van den Bosch, M.; Moman, M.; van Vulpen, M.; Battermann, J.; Duiveman, E.; van Schelven, L.; de Leeuw, H.; Lagendijk, J.; Moerland, M. MRI-guided robotic system for transperineal prostate interventions: Proof of principle. *Phys. Med. Biol.* **2010**, *55*, 133–140. [CrossRef]

11. Chen, Y.; Squires, A.; Seifabadi, R.; Xu, S.; Agarwal, H.; Bernardo, M.; Pinto, P.; Choyke, P.; Wood, B.; Tse, Z. Robotic system for MRI-guided focal laser ablation in the prostate. *IEEE/ASME Trans. Mechatron.* **2017**, *22*, 107–114. [CrossRef] [PubMed]
12. Chen, Y.; Xu, S.; Squires, A.; Seifabadi, R.; Turkbey, I.; Pinto, P.; Choyke, P.; Wood, B.; Tse, Z. MRI-guided robotically assisted focal laser ablation of the prostate using canine cadavers. *IEEE/ASME Trans. Mechatron.* **2018**, *65*, 1434–1442. [CrossRef] [PubMed]
13. Melzer, A.; Gutmann, B.; Remmele, T.; Wolf, R.; Lukoscheck, A.; Bock, M.; Bardenheuer, H.; Fischer, H. INNOMOTION for percutaneous image-guided interventions. *IEEE Eng. Med. Biol. Mag.* **2008**, *27*, 66–73. [CrossRef] [PubMed]
14. Jiang, S.; Feng, W.; Lou, J.; Yang, Z.; Liu, J.; Yang, J. Modeling and control of a five-degrees-of-freedom pneumatically actuated magnetic resonance-compatible robot. *Int. J. Med. Robot. Comput. Assist. Surg.* **2014**, *10*, 170–179. [CrossRef] [PubMed]
15. Comber, D.; Barth, E.; Webster, R. Design and control of a magnetic resonance compatible precision pneumatic active cannula robot. *J. Med. Dev.* **2014**, *8*, 1011003-1–1011003-7. [CrossRef]
16. Richer, E.; Hurmuzlu, Y. A high performance pneumatic force actuator system: Part 1—nonlinear mathematical model. *J. Dyn. Syst. Meas. Control* **2000**, *122*, 416–425. [CrossRef]
17. Richer, E.; Hurmuzlu, Y. A high performance pneumatic force actuator system: Part II—nonlinear controller design. *J. Dyn. Syst. Meas. Control* **2000**, *122*, 426–434. [CrossRef]
18. Turkseven, M.; Ueda, J. An asymptotically stable pressure observer based on load and displacement sensing for pneumatic actuators with long transmission lines. *IEEE/ASME Trans. Mechatron.* **2017**, *22*, 681–692. [CrossRef]
19. Li, J.; Kawashima, K.; Fujita, T.; Kagawa, T. Control design of a pneumatic cylinder with distributed model of pipelines. *Precis. Eng.* **2013**, *37*, 880–887. [CrossRef]
20. Krichel, S.; Sawodny, O. Non-linear friction modeling and simulation of long pneumatic transmission lines. *Math. Comput. Model. Dyn. Syst.* **2014**, *20*, 23–44. [CrossRef]
21. Turkseven, M.; Ueda, J. Model-based force control of pneumatic actuators with long transmission lines. *IEEE/ASME Trans. Mechatron.* **2018**, *23*, 1292–1302. [CrossRef]
22. Pandian, S.; Takemura, F.; Hayakawa, Y.; Kawamura, S. Pressure observer-controller design for pneumatic cylinder actuators. *IEEE/ASME Trans. Mechatron.* **2002**, *7*, 490–499. [CrossRef]
23. Wu, J.; Goldfarb, M.; Barth, E. On the observability of pressure in a pneumatic servo actuator. *J. Dyn. Syst. Meas. Control* **2004**, *126*, 921–924. [CrossRef]
24. Bigras, P. Sliding-mode observer as a time-variant estimator for control of pneumatic systems. *J. Dyn. Syst. Meas. Control* **2005**, *127*, 499–502. [CrossRef]
25. Gulati, N.; Barth, E. A globally stable, load-independent pressure observer for the servo control of pneumatic actuators. *IEEE/ASME Trans. Mechatron.* **2009**, *14*, 295–306. [CrossRef]
26. Langjord, H.; Kassa, G.; Johansen, T. Adaptive nonlinear observer for electropneumatic clutch actuator with position sensor. *IEEE Trans. Control Syst. Technol.* **2012**, *20*, 1033–1039. [CrossRef]
27. Driver, T.; Shen, X. Pressure estimation-based robust force control of pneumatic actuators. *Int. J. Fluid Power* **2013**, *14*, 37–45. [CrossRef]
28. Swaroop, D.; Hedrick, J.K.; Yip, P.P.; Gerdes, J.C. Dynamic surface control for a class of nonlinear systems. *IEEE Trans. Autom. Control* **2000**, *45*, 1893–1899. [CrossRef]
29. Kheowree, T.; Kuntanapreeda, S. Adaptive dynamic surface control of an electrohydraulic actuator with friction compensation. *Asian J. Control* **2015**, *17*, 855–867. [CrossRef]
30. Peng, Z.; Wang, D.; Chen, Z.; Hu, X.; Lan, W. Adaptive dynamic surface control for formations of autonomous surface vehicles with uncertain dynamics. *IEEE Trans. Control Syst. Technol.* **2013**, *21*, 513–520. [CrossRef]
31. Huang, J.; Ri, S.; Liu, L.; Wang, Y.; Kim, Y.; Pak, G. Nonlinear disturbance observer-based dynamic surface control of mobile wheeled inverted pendulum. *IEEE Trans. Control Syst. Technol.* **2015**, *23*, 2400–2407. [CrossRef]
32. Wu, J.; Huang, J.; Wang, Y.; Xing, K. Nonlinear disturbance observer-based dynamic surface control for trajectory tracking of pneumatic muscle system. *IEEE Trans. Control Syst. Technol.* **2014**, *22*, 440–455. [CrossRef]
33. Wang, M.; Ren, X.; Chen, Q.; Wang, S.; Gao, X. Modified dynamic surface approach with bias torque for multi-motor servomechanism. *Control Eng. Pract.* **2016**, *50*, 57–68. [CrossRef]

34. Li, A.; Meng, D.; Lu, B.; Li, Q. Nonlinear cascade control of single-rod pneumatic actuator based on an extended disturbance observer. *J. Cent. South Univ.* **2019**, *26*, 1637–1648. [CrossRef]
35. Meng, D.; Tao, G.; Chen, J.; Ban, W. Modeling of a pneumatic system for high-accuracy position control. In Proceedings of the International Conference on Fluid Power and Mechatronics, Beijing, China, 17–20 August 2011; pp. 505–510.
36. Goodwin, G.; Mayne, D. A parameter estimation perspective of continuous time model reference adaptive control. *Automatica* **1989**, *23*, 57–70. [CrossRef]

13

Toward Operations in a Surgical Scenario: Characterization of a Microgripper via Light Microscopy Approach

Federica Vurchio [1], Pietro Ursi [2], Francesco Orsini [1], Andrea Scorza [1], Rocco Crescenzi [3], Salvatore A. Sciuto [1] and Nicola P. Belfiore [1,*]

[1] Department of Engineering, University of Roma Tre, via della Vasca Navale 79, 00146 Rome, Italy; federica.vurchio@uniroma3.it (F.V.); francesco.orsini@uniroma3.it (F.O.); andrea.scorza@uniroma3.it (A.S.); salvatore.sciuto@uniroma3.it (S.A.S.)

[2] Department of General Surgery and Surgical Specialties "Paride Stefanini", Sapienza University of Rome, Viale del Policlinico 155, 00161 Rome, Italy; pietro.ursi@uniroma1.it

[3] Department of Information Engineering, Electronic and Telecommunications, Sapienza University of Rome, Via Eudossiana 18, 00184 Roma, Italy; rocco.crescenzi@uniroma1.it

* Correspondence: nicolapio.belfiore@uniroma3.it.

Abstract: Micro Electro Mechanical Systems (MEMS)-Technology based micro mechanisms usually operate within a protected or encapsulated space and, before that, they are fabricated and analyzed within one Scanning Electron Microscope (SEM) vacuum specimen chamber. However, a surgical scenario is much more aggressive and requires several higher abilities in the microsystem, such as the capability of operating within a liquid or wet environment, accuracy, reliability and sophisticated packaging. Unfortunately, testing and characterizing MEMS experimentally without fundamental support of a SEM is rather challenging. This paper shows that in spite of large difficulties due to well-known physical limits, the optical microscope is still able to play an important role in MEMS characterization at room conditions. This outcome is supported by the statistical analysis of two series of measurements, obtained by a light trinocular microscope and a profilometer, respectively.

Keywords: microactuators; microgrippers; MEMS; displacement measurement; comb-drives; microscopy; profilometer; characterization; minimally invasive surgery

---

1. Introduction

The recent developments of the microsystems have been so promising that nowadays they offer a great potential to many applications which require a high grade of miniaturization. Nevertheless, using microsurgery to heal diseases with a minimal invasive approach is still an ambitious challenge because of severe requirements (accuracy, precision, reliability, reduced consumption, limited costs, small size, high performance repeatability, short response time, efficiency in wet or liquid environments). One way of coping with this challenge consists in modifying the common Micro Electro Mechanical Systems (MEMS) to increase their degrees of freedom (usually unitary) and dexterity, for example, providing them with several revolute pairs. These microsystems need to be tested in a significant environment, starting from room environment (in air), but this is not so obvious as it could appear at first sight. In fact, these systems need to be analyzed by means of SEM, which implies putting the mechanisms within a vacuum chamber, rather than a particular environment. Therefore, significant operational tests must be performed by other means of observations, such as microscopy or interferometric profilometry. However, the latter instruments have less resolution than a SEM and their use can be critical to inspect the smallest parts of a microsystem.

This paper shows that microscopy observation can still be very effective in MEMS operational tests under environmental conditions. An effort has been made to assess microscopy observation of MEMS by comparing this means with a higher class, but also a more expensive and difficult-to-use instrument, namely, a profilometer. The statistical treatment of the results of two experimental campaigns (optical microscope and profilometer) shows that the characterization and image acquisition capability of the optical microscope is comparable to that of the profilometer, while the optical microscope maintains a larger degree of freedom in setting the operational parameters.

Given the interdisciplinary nature of the present investigation, it is helpful to give a glimpse to the different types of involved competences. It is particularly important to review some previous contributions concerning the operational conditions that would be required to a micro-electro-mechanical system in surgery.

A first survey of MEMS for surgical applications [1] showed how MEMS technology may improve the functionality of existing surgical devices and also add new capabilities that give rise to new treatments. For example, MEMS can improve surgical outcomes, with lower risk, by providing the surgeon with real-time feedback on the operation. From the mechanical and operational point of view, microgrippers for different applications have been extensively proposed in literature [2,3].

There are many other different applications where MEMS can play a significant role. For a representative example, MEMS-Technology based micro-accelerometers [4] are able to measure the heart wall motion of patients who have undergone coronary artery bypass graft surgery (CABG). Furthermore, there are many other applications where MEMS could be conveniently used to improve success in surgery, such as in laparoscopic sleeve gastrectomy (LSG) with cruroplasty [5], in surgical treatment of gastrointestinal stromal tumors of the duodenum [6] in colovesical fistula surgery with minimally invasive approach [7], in Endoluminal loco-regional resection by Transanal Endoscopic Microsurgery (TEM) [8–10], and in Low Rectal Anterior Resection (LAR) [11].

These kinds of applications require very specific actions during the different stages of design, fabrication and packaging, because their correct working is depending on many physical parameters, such as temperature, humidity of the environment, presence of water or other liquids, chemical reactions and pressure. For example, the influence of temperature and humidity on the adsorbed water layer on micro scale monocrystalline silicon (Si) films has been investigated in air, using an Si-MEMS kHz-frequency resonator [12]. Water proof or water insensitive three-axis MEMS based accelerometers have been presented [13] for encouraging their operation in laboratory scale experiments. The theory of water electrolysis in a closed electrochemical cell has been described [14] to develop a new actuation principle for MEMS. A special apparatus has been employed to study the adhesive friction due to water in the nanometer range, where the water layer thickness greatly affects friction and adhesion [15]. Heat transfer characteristics of isolated bubble of water were investigated by local wall temperature measurement using a novel MEMS based sensor [16]. MEMS-OR-PAM (optical-resolution photoacoustic microscopy) has also been proved [17] to be a powerful tool for studying highly dynamic and time-sensitive biological phenomena.

Although MEMS still have not developed their potential for surgery applications, there are many more examples of their use in biomedical instruments [18–20]. The mechanical characteristics of cells provide information on their functionality and their state of health, while their geometry can be linked to genetic alterations and apoptosis; the importance of these analyses could help in the collection of phenotypic information or for the diagnosis of pathological disorders [21]. For example, a study[22] was conducted about the viscoelasticity of L929 cells, to investigate their cellular structure, notoriously linked to important physiological functions. In addition, applications of microspectroscopic techniques [23] have been conducted to characterize the viscoelastic properties of living cells. The study of the mechanical properties of cells, also concerns the muscle cells: for example the mechanical response, in terms of strength and displacement, of some smooth muscle cells subjected to elongation has been studied [24] with the aim of better understanding the links between their functionalities and their structure. A study [25] on skeletal muscle cells described how the relationship between the stiffness and the force exerted by some actin filaments can indicate the physiological state of the actin cytoskeleton. Moreover, the mechanical properties of tissue-engineered vascular constructs have been studied by monitoring pressure and diameter variations of vascular constructs submitted to hydrostatic loading [26]. A silicon microgripper has also been proposed [27] to characterize the mechanical stiffness of biological tissues, with the wider prospective of developing a professional inspecting instrument for laboratory measurements or surgical operations.

More recently, new emerging MEMS-Technology based instruments for biomedical and surgical applications have been developed. In fact, based on a new concept hinge [28,29], a class of different microgrippers, equipped with rotary comb-drives, has been developed [30–33], also in significant environments [34], and fabricated [35,36]. Thanks to their size, these instruments are expected to be employed in surgery and diagnostics. This class of microsystem is the focus of the present investigation.

2. Experimental Characterization of MEMS-Technology Based Instruments in Operational Environments

In spite of MEMS' great potential for biomedical applications, only a few studies [37] focus on their characterization in an operational environment.

In fact, SEM observation is often a necessity to characterize MEMS, but this means it could be detrimental for the assessment of tests under real operational conditions, basically because tests are performed in vacuum conditions.

Considering the extensively spread biomedical applications, it is also worth mentioning the Optical Coherence Tomography (OCT), which is an optical imaging technique used primarily to investigate the internal microstructure of biological tissues, in ophthalmology and in dentistry [38]. The main advantage of OCT compared to other traditional systems is that this method offers the possibility of a non-invasive in vivo visualization of the tissue with high-resolution three-dimensional images [39]. Despite the axial resolution of some OCT systems (such as Ultrahigh-resolution OCT) [40] that can reach a few micrometers [41], the lateral resolution is affected by the diffraction limits due to the spot size in the focal plane of the probe beam. In fact, the lateral resolution often presents values between 10 and 20 μm [42,43]. Indeed, the above mentioned values of lateral resolution, together with higher costs, make OCTs less attractive than the light microscopy for the characterization of microgrippers in operational conditions.

Considering the above mentioned characteristics for SEM and OCT, traditional light microscopy is quite competitive since it allows test stands to be less expensive in a widespread range of test conditions.

In this investigation a performance characterization of some comb-driven microgrippers in operative condition has been carried out.

The characterization of MEMS-Technology based microgrippers has been recently approached by using a profilometer [44], while the present work will show that a more simple commercial light microscope is still capable to satisfy the same activity with no detriment of measurement significance. Since optical microscopy is widely used in laboratories, it is believed that this paper might have some impact on the future characterizations of microsystems in air, wet or liquid environments. The importance of micromanipulation of mobile micro-particle suspended in liquid well has been recently underlined and a visual-servo automatic micromanipulating system has been presented [45].

Since the intrinsic resolution of optical microscopy is generally rather worse than SEM or profilometer imaging, its real aptitude and efficacy in examining micro-objects remains something that must be validated. Therefore, the present paper will endorse microscopy observation to characterize a microsystem in environmental conditions, by comparing the results obtained by means of both optical microscope and profilometer image analysis techniques. This is justified since the optical devices are the most suitable for carrying out measurements on microsystems without contact and in operative conditions.

In this work, the above mentioned characterization involved the measurements of the angular displacements of a rotary comb-drive embedded into an independently developed microgripper, when a voltage is applied to the device. This is obtained by an in-house Image Analysis Software (IAS) implemented by the authors. The analysis of the measurement results has been achieved by means of uncertainty models for the evaluation of the corresponding error sources. For this purpose, the two image acquisition systems and the corresponding measurement chains will be described, together with the analysis of the relative sources of uncertainty. Finally, the measurements carried out with the Optical Profilometer System (OPS) and Light Trinocular Microscope (LTM) systems will be analyzed to check whether the two groups of results could be considered comparable and consistent within the interval of experimental uncertainties.

3. Materials and Methods

The evolution of MEMS gave rise to different kinds of microsystems that have been based on MEMS Technology. However, despite the relevant elements mentioned above, one cannot help but notice that, in the international technical-scientific panorama, guidelines, protocols and regulations regarding the characterization of these devices are still lacking, both under the metrological and the mechanical point of view. The present investigation is part of a larger project dedicated to the development of new concept microgrippers for surgical applications and it attempts to partially fill this gap and to validate the optical image analysis as a proper means of characterization of the developed microsystems under operative conditions.

The peculiar object of this investigation is a rotary comb-drive depicted in Figure 1. This component consists in an electrostatic actuator that provides motion to the microgripper illustrated in Figure 1a. The rotary comb-drive is composed of a pair of sets of fingers, as shown in the more detailed Figure 1b. The mobile series of fingers rotates as a function of the applied voltage and the determination of the voltage-rotation curve is greatly important for the operational aspects. Two measurement chains have been set up to measure such voltage-rotation function. The first is composed by a Fogale Zoomsurf 3D Optical Profiling System (OPS, Table 1), while the second is composed of a NB50TS Eurotek Light Trinocular Microscope (LTM, Table 2).

For the sake of the present investigation it is convenient to underline that the two sets of images from the two devices have been both processed using the same in-house built software in order to properly discriminate which one, between OPS and LTM, is the most suitable system to characterize the microgripper devices.

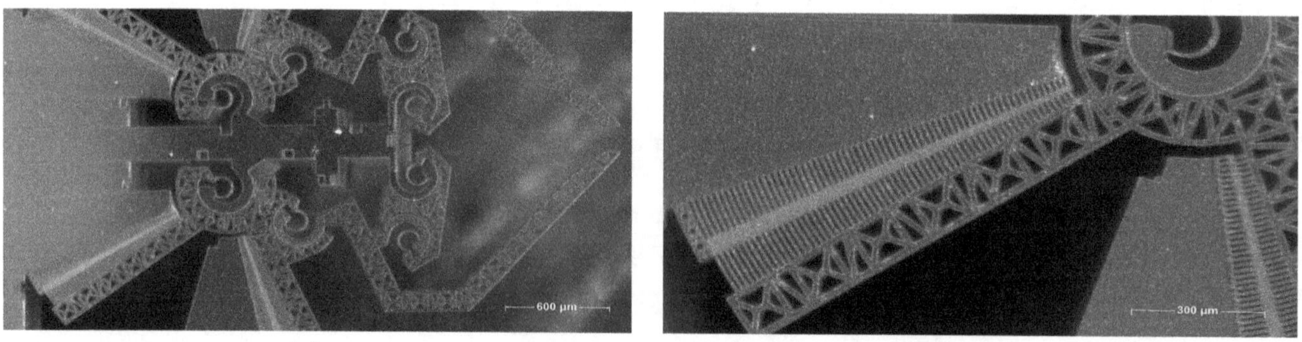

(a) (b)

Figure 1. Image of a microgripper prototype obtained from optical microscope (**a**) and a detail of the rotary comb-drive (**b**).

Table 1. Optical Profilometer System (OPS) experimental setup: specifications of the comb-drive actuated silicon microgripper (Device Under Test, DUT) and of the testing stand.

Device	Characteristics
DUT Material	Silicon type P, dopant Boron, orientation <100>, electrical resistivity 0.005–0.030 Ohm·cm
DUT Geometry	module dimensions 2000 μm ×1500 μm, device thickness 40 μm, insulated layer thickness 3 μm, handle thickness 400 μm
Power Supply	Keithley 236, Range settable to 1.1/11/110/1100 V with respectively 0.1/1/10/100 mV resolution, accuracy 0.06 V (Range ±110.00 V)
Micropositioner	n.1 MP25L, n.1 MP25R, range X/Y/Z 10/10/10 mm with 5 μm resolution
Probes (supply)	PA-C-1M with tungsten needles
DUT Stage	The wafer containing the DUT is placed on the profilometer working surface and fixed by an adhesive tape
3D Optical Profilometer	Fogale Zoomsurf 3D optical profiling system, field of view from 7.2 mm × 5.4 mm to 80 nm × 60 nm, maximum lateral resolution 0.6 μm
Digital Image	768 × 580 pixels, 8 bit, 0.6 px/μm
Image Processing Software	In-house software developed in MATLAB (2017a, MathWorks)
Notebook pc	Intel core i7-2670, 6 Gb RAM, Nvidia GeForce GT 520 MX

Table 2. Light Trinocular Microscope (LTM) experimental setup (DUT, micropositioner, probes and PC as in Table 1).

Device	Characteristics
Power Supply	HP E3631A, DC Output: 0 to +25 V, 0 to −25 V, Resolution 1.5 mV, Accuracy 0.04 V at F.S.
DUT Stage	Instrumented support with micrometric screws for angular and linear movement of the sample, in the 3 orthogonal directions in space (x, y, z)
Light microscope	Eurotek NB50TS NB SOTS, Zoom range 0.8× ...5× (8× ...50×), LED illumination Transmitted-Reflected, B2-1525 additional objective 2×
Digital Image	1920 × 1080 pixels, 24 bit, 1.359 px/μm
Digital camera	MD6iS, 6MP, pixel dimension, 2.8 μm × 2.8 μm, maximum resolution 3264 × 1840 px
Image Processing Software	In-house software developed in MATLAB environment (2017a, MathWorks)

3.1. OPS and LTM Experimental Setups

The Device Under Test (DUT) consists of a microgripper prototype made up of pseudo-rigid beams and flexure hinges. Any jaw of the microgripper is actuated by a capacitive rotary comb-drive that provides a torque when a voltage is applied to the electrodes.

During the first experimental campaign, performed with the Optical Profiling System, a variable voltage source has been used to supply the DUT and to evaluate the angular displacements of its comb drive. In this investigation, a power supply Keithley 236 SMU with 0.06 V output voltage accuracy (Range ±110.00 V) has been used (Figure 2).

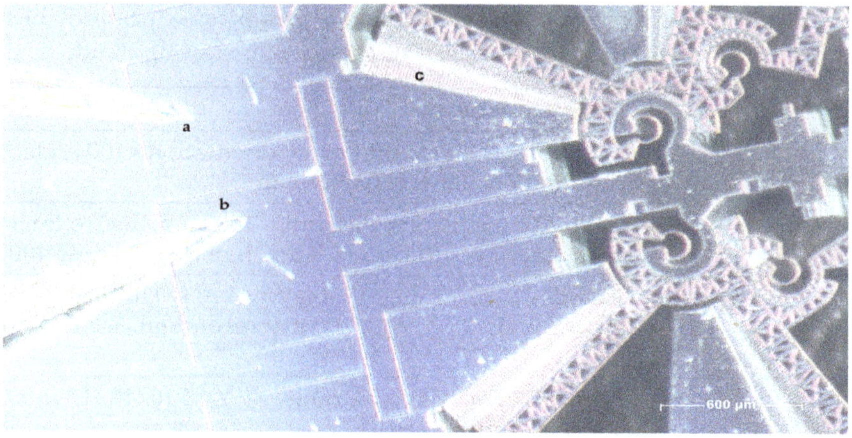

Figure 2. The two micropositioners with probe arms and tungsten needles (*a*) and (*b*), used in both the experimental setups; a voltage is applied to the comb-drive (*c*) of the DUT, in order to supply the device.

Two micropositioners with 5 μm resolution have been used, each one being equipped with tungsten needles, in order to apply the voltage to the DUT electrodes, Figure 3, and a set of digital images have been acquired using a Fogale Zoomsurf 3D OPS. The digital image resolution of 0.6 pixel/μm is provided by the Profilometer embedded software.

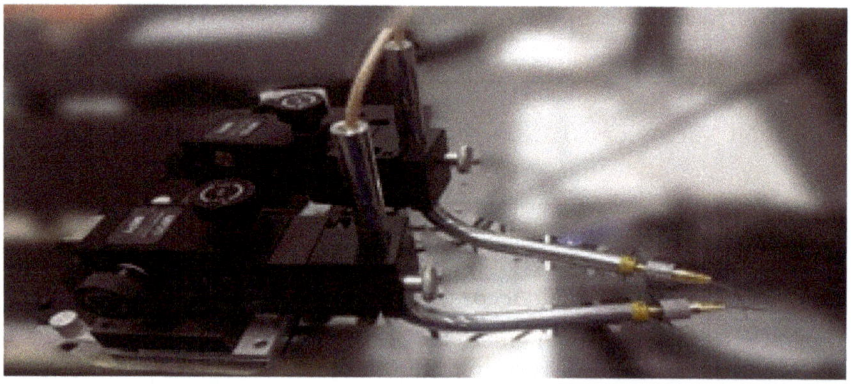

Figure 3. The two micropositioners with probe arms and tungsten needles.

During the image acquisition campaign performed by means of the LTM system the same microgripper sample has been analyzed. The power supply device is a HP E3631A, with 0.04 V output voltage accuracy (Range 0 to +25 V). An electric protection circuit, equipped with a fuse, has also been connected in series, between the power supply and the DUT, to cautiously prevent the passage of a current exceeding 200 mA, which could compromise the device. Two micropositioners have been used (Figure 3) and the microgripper angular displacements have been measured by means of acquired images and collected by a NB50TS Eurotek trinocular microscope system. The optical resolution is limited by the diffraction of the visible light and it is about 0.45–0.6 μm, as in conventional light microscopes [46]; in this study, the worst case of 0.6 μm has been considered. The pixel resolution has been provided by means of calibration procedure; by means of Matlab software, a length of 1000 μm on an image of a micrometer slide was considered and 15 tests were performed. By means of this procedure, the pixel density of 1.359 ± 0.007 pixel/μm was calculated. Furthermore, the sampling constraints (Nyquist limit) and the density of the photo sites on the digital sensor also limit the whole systems resolution. To achieve a *higher level* particle characterization (i.e., differentiation based upon higher order measurements such as circularity), the size of the particle or the object under examination must be greater than 4 μm [46]. In our case, in fact, it is possible to verify that it is impossible to resolve the comb-drive finger gap, that is 3 μm. However, the distance between two fingers, that is 10 μm, is clearly discriminated (see also Ref. [27]); for all these reasons, a overall resolution of about 4 μm for the LTM system is assumed. In Figure 4, the entire LTM setup is shown and some specifications of its main components are reported in Table 2. Once the device has been positioned on the DUT stage, it has been powered by means of two probes with tungsten needles. Through the micropositioners, the tungsten needles are approached to the microgripper electrical connections.

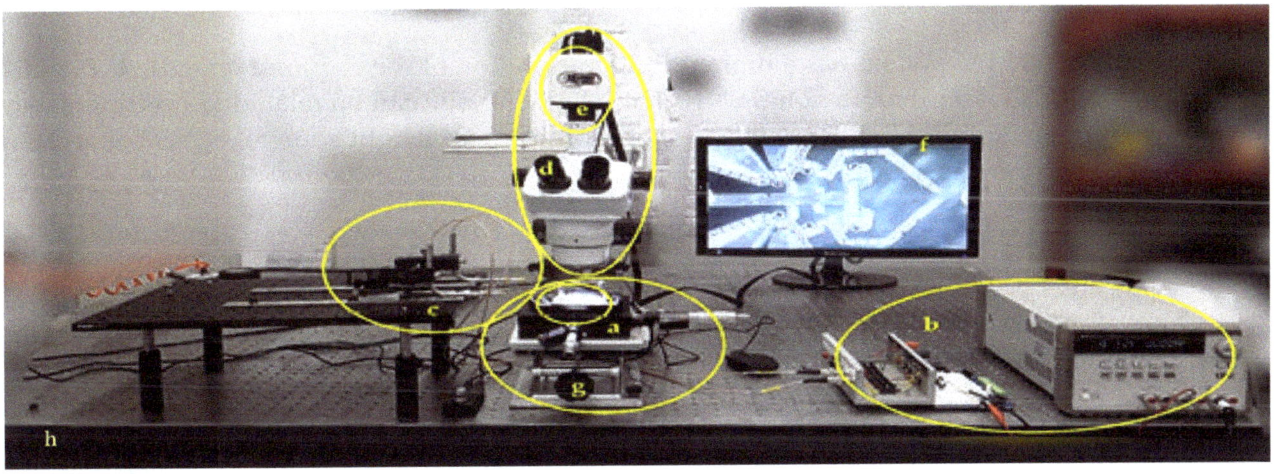

Figure 4. Optical Microscope measurement setup. Microgripper prototype (*a*), Supply voltage with protection circuit (*b*), micropositioners with two embedded probe arms and tungsten needles (*c*), Optical Microscope (*d*), embedded camera for images acquisition (*e*), a monitor for displaying and monitoring the device movement in operating conditions (*f*), instrumented support with micrometric screws (*g*), pneumatic suspension table (*h*).

Considering the OPS measurement chain, a set of images has been acquired, each one corresponding to a specific voltage setting: to calculate the angular displacement of the comb-drive, the first acquired image referred to 0 V, has been compared with the others (i.e., 2 V, 4 V, ..., 28 V); Figure 5a illustrates an example of an image that has been processed by the in-house built software. Considering the LTM measurement chain, the same steps have been carried out. However, in order to calculate the angular displacements, the first acquired image (0 V) has been compared with the other images referred to voltages up to 24 volts (i.e., 2 V, 4 V, ..., 24 V) instead of 28 V (as in the previous case); Figure 5b shows an example of image that has been processed by the in-house software. Considering the OPS, a set of 12 images has been acquired at each voltage, for a total of 180 images; considering the LTM image acquisition system, a set of 16 images has been acquired at each voltage, for a total of 208 images.

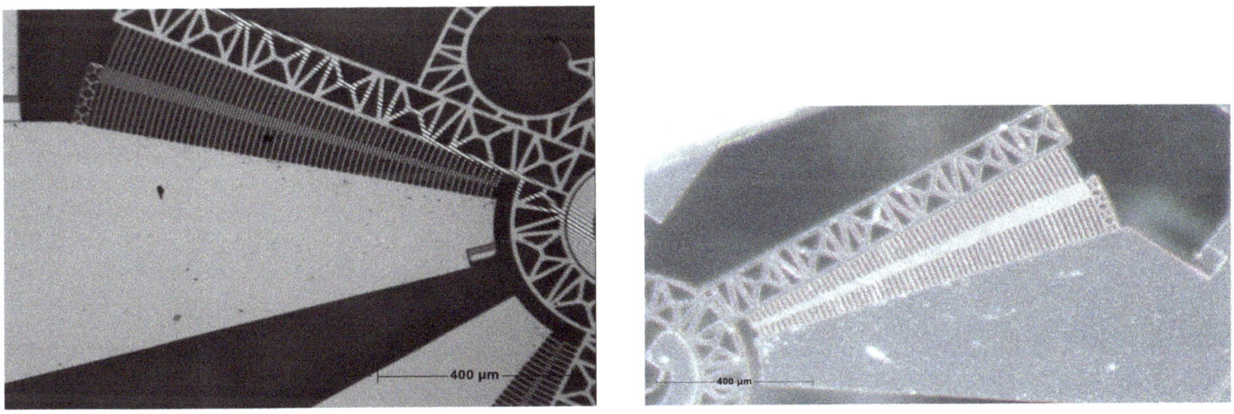

(a) (b)

Figure 5. Two examples of images of the Microgripper comb-drive, acquired by optical profilometer (**a**), and optical microscope (**b**); both images (**a**,**b**) are referred to 0 V.

The OPS experimental investigation was made before the LTM campaign. Therefore, the testing voltages used in the second campaign have been influenced by the need of not imposing values that could damage the comb-drives, avoiding the pull-in effect. Such phenomenon occurred during the OPS campaign when the applied voltage was greater than 25 V. Above this value the fingers were unstable; in fact, they were used to get in contact quite often, inducing a short circuit.

Despite that the LTM system has a higher digital resolution of the acquired images, its Signal-to-Noise Ratio (SNR) is lower than the OPS SNR. This characteristic can be related to multiple factors, such as environmental noise, light source (i.e., non-homogeneous light source), optical aberrations, image A/D conversion and processing.

3.2. Image Analysis Software

A semi-automatic software has been implemented in Matlab according to the following steps.

1. At first, it is important to find the Instant Center of Rotation (ICR) of the DUT comb-drive. Considering the image that corresponds to 0 V (both for OPS and for LTM systems), four point are manually selected (a, a′, b, b′ and c, c′, d, d′) on the edges of the comb-drive and the ICR has been found as the intersection of the two lines (Figure 6).

2. The second step regards the manual selection of a particular Region Of Interest (ROI) on the same image considered previously. The identified ROI is characterized by a particular pixel pattern, which is compared with subsequent images (that correspond to 2 V, 4 V, . . . , 28 V for OPS and 2 V, 4 V, . . . , 24 V for LTM) to identify where this pattern is located. This procedure is carried out through a template-matching algorithm, which identifies for each image the coordinates of the point corresponding to the center of gravity (COG) of the ROI. This point corresponds to one of the three vertices of the triangle necessary to identify the angular aperture of the device comb-drive. The comb-drive has a static part fixed to the structure of the MEMS device and a mobile part. The ROI has been chosen on the mobile part of the microgripper comb-drive (Figure 7).

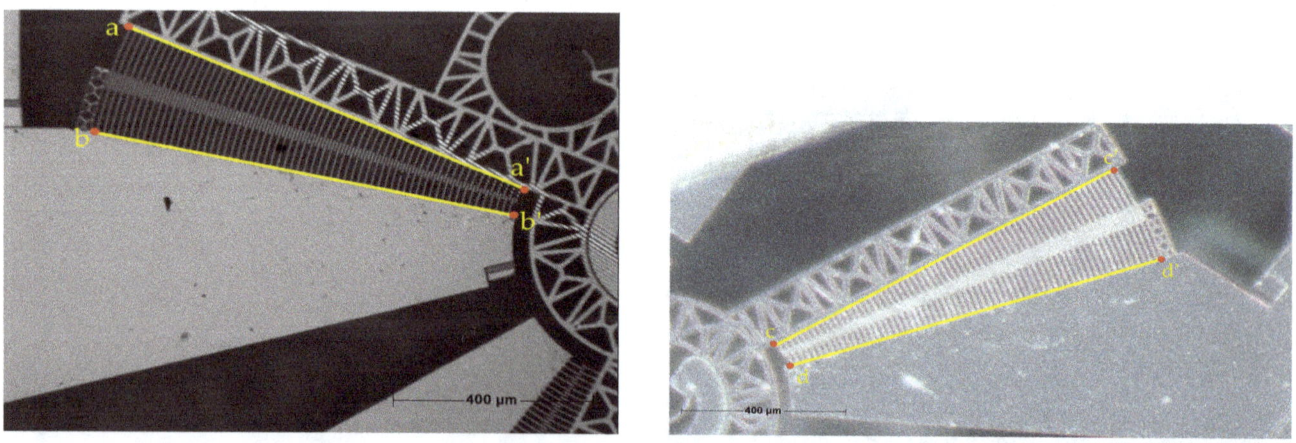

(a) (b)

Figure 6. Two images of the microgripper comb-drive acquired by optical profilometer (**a**) and microscope (**b**), respectively.

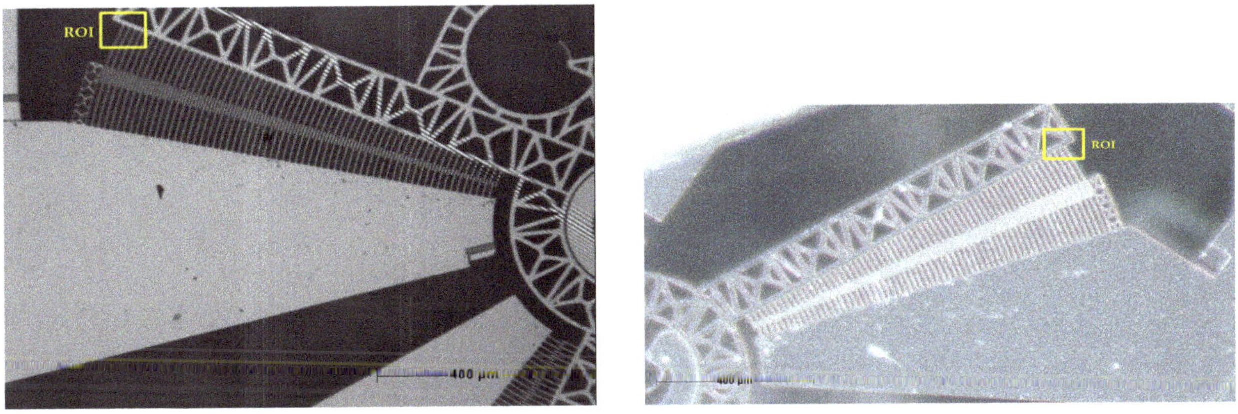

(a) (b)

Figure 7. Manual selection of a particular region of the image (ROI), to find its center of gravity (COG) on OPS image (**a**) and on LTM image (**b**).

The first and second above described steps of the implemented software are the only ones in which the manual selection of an operator is necessary to properly select points on the images and the positions and dimensions of the ROI. The following ones have been automated.

3. As shown in Figure 8, the automatic part of the implemented software considers the coordinates of the following three points on the images:
   - The most distant point from the ICR on the fixed part of the comb-drive (a);
   - The ICR of the comb-drive (b);
   - The center of the ROI (c);

   The first two points remain fixed for all the following images, under the hypothesis of no deformation due to the movement of the comb-drive, while the only point, whose coordinates change for each considered image, is the center of the ROI.

4. These three points determine a triangle, where the vertex ICR corresponds to the angular opening α of the comb-drive. With reference to Figure 9, points a, b and c are considered to be the vertices of an isosceles triangle, where

$$\alpha = 2\arcsin\left(\frac{A}{B}\right) \tag{1}$$

   with $A = \frac{\overline{ca}}{2}$ and $B = \overline{cb}$. Using a template matching algorithm, a match is found between the coordinates of the center of the selected ROI on the first image (i.e., that corresponds to 0 V supply) and on all the subsequent images. Through this operation the in-house software detects the new coordinates of the ROI center of gravity (ROIGC) for each subsequent image and therefore for each applied voltage. The ROIGC changes its coordinates and, consequently, it changes also the shape of the corresponding triangle and the angular aperture of the DUT comb-drive, depending on the different voltage supply.

5. The angular displacement is obtained from the comb-drive angular aperture at each voltage value.

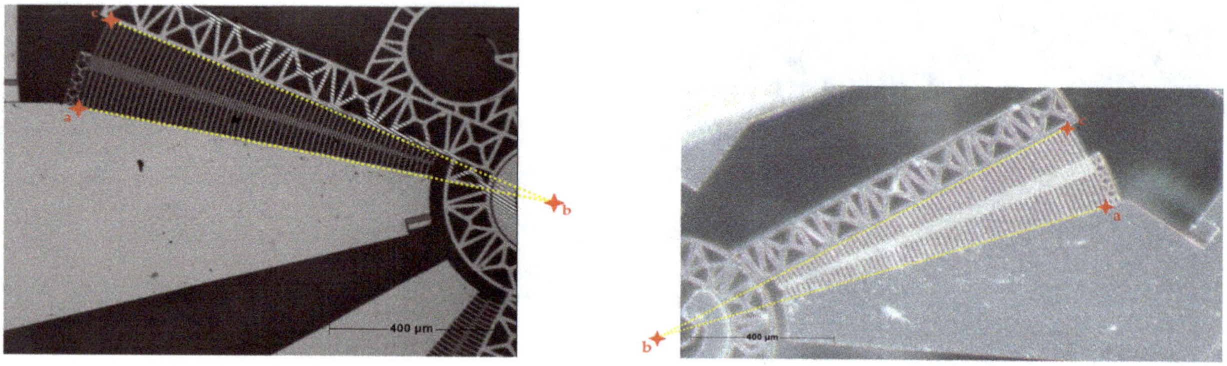

(a) (b)

Figure 8. The determination of three points on the profilometer (**a**) and the microscope (**b**) images: the most distant point from the ICR on the fixed part of the comb-drive, the ICR of the comb-drive and the center of the ROI.

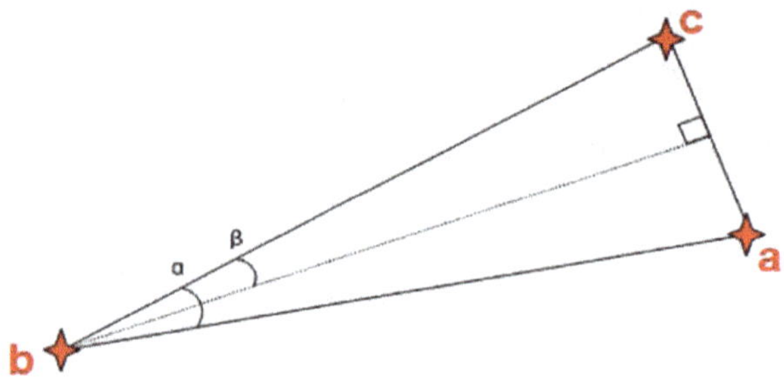

Figure 9. The triangle used by the software to evaluate the comb-drive angular displacement.

The above described software can be used with any type of image. For example, in this study two sets of images have been considered, acquired by the optical profilometer and the light microscope, respectively. The limit associated with this type of analysis is that the procedure provides a first semi-automatic part, which must be carried out by the operator. This approach introduces some sources of uncertainty, due to the variability in selecting the initial points for the determination of the comb-drive ICR, as well as the variability in the selection of the size and position of the Region of Interest, together with the uncertainty of the code itself. These sources of uncertainty will be considered in the next section, where a model will be proposed for the analysis of the uncertainty of both the entire measurement chains.

3.3. A Model for the Uncertainty Analysis of the Measurements

The purpose of this section is to estimate the overall uncertainty associated with the two measurement systems and for this reason a model for measurement uncertainty analysis is proposed; an analysis of the main uncertainty sources of the two measurement setups is carried out and the calculation of the measurement uncertainty relative to the angular displacements of the comb-drive device is performed, both for the profilometer and the light microscope.

For each value of the angular displacements, the mean $\bar{x}$ and standard deviation of the mean $S_{\bar{x}}$ have been obtained, based on a statistical analysis conducted on a number of observations $N = 12$ for the profilometer and $N = 16$ for the light microscope, for each considered voltage. On the hypothesis that the sample comes from a normal population, a Student's t-distribution has been used. For the calculation of the overall uncertainty of the measurement systems considered, it is necessary to combine the type A and type B uncertainties [47], using the following expression:

$$\delta_T = \sqrt{\delta_A^2 + \delta_B^2}\,. \quad (2)$$

First, the main uncertainty sources for both measurement systems have been identified and evaluated, as shown in Table 3, where for each source a probability density function PDF together with the uncertainty type and mean m is determined.

Table 3. OPS and LTM measurement setup uncertainty sources.

Uncertainty Source	Probability Density Function (PDF) [1]	Type [2]	m	δ (OPS)	δ (LTM)	Unit
Power Supply: voltage accuracy	$N(m,\sigma)$	B		0.06	0.04	V
Optical System: maximal lateral resolution due to diffraction	$U(m,\sigma)$	B	0	0.57	0.57	μm
Digital Image: digital conversion	$U(m,\sigma)$	B	0	3.14	1.43	μm
Image Processing Software: uncertainty in point identification	$U(m,\sigma)$	A		±1.9	±1.9	pixel
Uncertainty in ROI position (template-matching [3])				±1.9	±1.9	pixel
Uncertainty in ROI size (template-matching [3])				±1.9	±1.9	pixel
Uncertainty in the template-matching algorithm	Monte Carlo Simulation	B		0.02	0.02	°

Notes: [1] $N(\mu,\sigma)$ is a Gaussian PDF with mean m and standard deviation σ; $U(\mu,\sigma)$ is a uniform PDF with mean m and standard deviation σ; [2] Type A and type B uncertainty as in standard [47]; [3] the uncertainty value δ for OPS and LTM is referred to 95% of confidence level.

3.3.1. Uncertainty Analysis for OPS Measurement Setup

Type A, namely δ_A, uncertainty are evaluated by statistical methods (statistical analysis of a series of observations) and have been calculated from standard deviation of the experimental measurements; Type B, δ_B, uncertainty are evaluated by means other than the statistical analysis of series of observations. The main sources of type B uncertainty considered are:

- Power Supply uncertainty has been evaluated through the data sheet and a Gaussian distribution has been assumed;
- OPS uncertainty has been evaluated considering its maximal lateral resolution, limited by diffraction of the light; a uniform distribution with 0.6 μm semi-amplitude has been assumed;
- Digital image uncertainty has been evaluated considering the digital resolution of the acquired images (0.6 px/μm). A uniform distribution with 2 pixels semi-amplitude has been assumed [44,48,49];

3.3.2. Uncertainty Analysis for LTM Measurement Setup

In this case, δ_A still represents Type A uncertainty, whereas δ_B are the Type B uncertainty. The main sources of type B uncertainty considered are:

- Power Supply uncertainty has been evaluated through the data sheet and a Gaussian distribution has been assumed;
- LTM system uncertainty has been evaluated considering its maximal lateral resolution, limited by diffraction of the light; a uniform distribution with 0.6 μm semi-amplitude has been assumed.
- Digital image uncertainty has been evaluated considering the digital resolution of the acquired images (1.359 px/μm). A uniform distribution with 2 pixels semi-amplitude has been assumed.
- Uncertainty due to the plane planarity, the focusing plane variation, and the vibration of the DUT have been considered negligible, thanks to optical table with pneumatic vibration isolators that increase the stability of the device and reduce vibrations that could cause an incorrect characterization.

To evaluate the total uncertainty of the two measurement systems, according to Equation (2), two contributions have been determined: the first is related to the uncertainty contribution evaluable with a statistic analysis of the measurements dispersion obtained with the measurement system (δ_A), while the other is due to the overall uncertainty from the main error sources related to the experimental setup (δ_B). In order to evaluate the δ_B uncertainty, two main contributions have been determined: the first is associated to the derivative of the function that expresses the angular displacement θ of the comb-drive with respect to the applied voltage $\frac{\partial\theta}{\partial V}$, multiplied by the uncertainty due to the power supply δ_V, while the other is related to the measurement of the comb-drive angle $\delta\alpha_t$ [47]

$$\delta_B = \delta_\alpha = \sqrt{\left(\frac{\partial\theta}{\partial V}\delta_V\right)^2 + (\delta\alpha_t)^2} \tag{3}$$

In particular, a second order polynomial function

$$\vartheta = a \cdot V^2 + b \cdot V + c\,, \tag{4}$$

where a, b, and c are obtained experimentally, approximates the trend of the angular displacements.

The term δ_{α_t} is composed by two terms, the first δ_{α_p} is the angle measurement uncertainty due to the OPS and LTM system, associated to the variability of the parameters related to the manual measurement of the lengths Δx_a, Δx_b,Δy_a, and Δy_b, carried out by the operator; while the other δ_{α_s}, is the angle measurement uncertainty due to the template-matching algorithm of image processing software. This last contribution is evaluated [44] by means of a Monte Carlo Simulation (with 10,000 iterations) implemented in MATLAB©; δ_{α_s} corresponds to $\pm 0.02°$, at 95% confidence level.

$$\delta\alpha_t = \sqrt{\left(\frac{\delta\alpha_p}{\alpha} \cdot \alpha\right)^2 + (\delta\alpha_s)^2} \tag{5}$$

The angle measurement uncertainty δ_{α_p} has been measured by means of the triangular properties as shown in Figure 10. For the measurement of values Δx_a, Δx_b, Δy_a and Δy_b, 10 tests were carried out for each of the segments and their mean value has been considered.

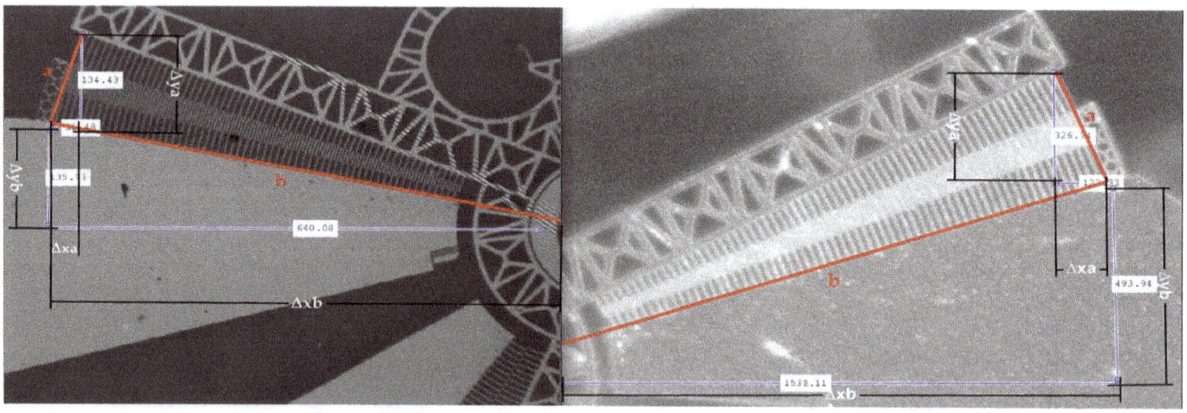

Figure 10. Angle measurement for the uncertainty evaluation related to the profilometer image, on the **left** and microscope image, on the **right**.

The uncertainty related to the light microscope and profilometer error can be obtained as approximated in [44]:

$$\frac{\delta\alpha_p}{\alpha} = \sqrt{\left(\frac{\delta a}{a}\right)^2 + \left(\frac{\delta b}{b}\right)^2}\,, \tag{6}$$

where

$$a = \sqrt{\Delta x_a{}^2 + \Delta y_a{}^2}$$
$$b = \sqrt{\Delta x_b{}^2 + \Delta y_b{}^2} \tag{7}$$

and

$$\delta a = \sqrt{\left(\frac{\partial a}{\partial x}\delta x\right)^2 + \left(\frac{\partial a}{\partial y}\delta y\right)^2} = \sqrt{\left(\frac{\Delta x_a}{\sqrt{\Delta x_a^2 + \Delta y_a^2}}\delta x\right)^2 + \left(\frac{\Delta y_a}{\sqrt{\Delta x_a^2 + \Delta y_a^2}}\delta y\right)^2}$$
$$\delta b = \sqrt{\left(\frac{\partial b}{\partial x}\delta x\right)^2 + \left(\frac{\partial b}{\partial y}\delta y\right)^2} = \sqrt{\left(\frac{\Delta x_b}{\sqrt{\Delta x_b^2 + \Delta y_b^2}}\delta x\right)^2 + \left(\frac{\Delta y_b}{\sqrt{\Delta x_b^2 + \Delta y_b^2}}\delta y\right)^2} \tag{8}$$

The quantities a and b in (7) depend on the image resolution and size. For this study, the lengths of the comb-drive triangle in the profilometer image are considered for the maximum rotation (1.3°), i.e., $\Delta x_a = 25$ pixel, $\Delta y_a = 150$ pixel, $\Delta x_b = 680$ pixel, and $\Delta y_b = 150$ pixel, therefore $a = 152$ pixel, and $b = 696$ pixel. Instead, the lengths of the comb-drive triangle in the microscope image are considered for the maximum rotation (0.93°), i.e., $\Delta x_a = 130$ pixel, $\Delta y_a = 330$ pixel, $\Delta x_b = 1550$ pixel, and $\Delta y_b = 450$ pixel, therefore $a = 355$ pixel, and $b = 1614$ pixel.

4. A Comparison between the Two Measurement Systems

At first, a comparison between the results obtained from the uncertainty analysis for both image acquisition systems has been carried out; from the results obtained through the analysis software it has been possible to collect a series of measurements attributable to the comb-drive angular displacement depending on the voltage supply. In particular, 12 measurements were obtained for each applied voltage value, for the OPS, and 16 measurements for each applied voltage value, for the LTM system. In a second stage, it has been necessary to verify whether the two sets of results are comparable, within the interval of the experimental uncertainties.

To verify the initial hypothesis that, using two different measurement systems, the angular displacement measurement of the comb-drive is the same, the approach described in Ref. [50] has been followed. Considering the average values, the total uncertainties δ_T of OPS and LTM have been obtained by using Equation (2) and then reported in the form of standard deviations in Table 4. The available data are expressed in the form:

$$\hat{X} = \bar{X} \pm \delta_X \tag{9}$$
$$\hat{Y} = \bar{Y} \pm \delta_Y \tag{10}$$

where $\bar{X}$ and $\bar{Y}$ are the mean values of X and Y (OPS and LTM measurements, respectively), while $\hat{X}$ and $\hat{Y}$ represent the measured values according to the standard [47]. To evaluate whether the two different measurements can be considered consistent or not, it is necessary to find the best estimate for the difference $\Delta_{XY} = \hat{X} - \hat{Y}$ and establish the highest and the lowest probable values of Δ_{XY}. The highest probable value for Δ_{XY} is obtained if $\bar{X}$ assumes its higher probable value, $\bar{X} + \delta_X$, and at the same time $\hat{Y}$ assumes its lowest probable value, $\bar{Y} - \delta_Y$. In this way the highest probable value for Δ_{XY} is

$$p_{\max} = (\bar{X} + \delta_X) - (\bar{Y} - \delta_Y) = (\bar{X} - \bar{Y}) + (\delta_X + \delta_Y)\ . \tag{11}$$

Similarly, the lowest probable value for Δ_{XY} is obtained if $\hat{X}$ assumes its lowest probable value, $\bar{X} - \delta_X$, and at the same time $\hat{Y}$ assumes its highest probable value, $\bar{Y} + \delta_Y$,

$$p_{\max} = (\bar{X} - \delta_X) - (\bar{Y} + \delta_Y) = (\bar{X} - \bar{Y}) - (\delta_X + \delta_Y)\ . \tag{12}$$

Combining (11) and (12), the difference between the measured values is

$$\Delta_{XY} = (\bar{X} - \bar{Y}) \pm (\delta_X + \delta_Y) . \tag{13}$$

The evaluation of the difference $|\bar{X} - \bar{Y}|$ and the sum $\delta_X + \delta_Y$ is fundamental for the sake of our investigation. In fact, if the difference $|\bar{X} - \bar{Y}|$ has the same order of magnitude as, or even less than, the sum $|\bar{X} - \bar{Y}|$, then the two different systems, namely OPS and LTM, measure the angular displacement of the comb-drive without significant difference.

5. Results

All the measurement data have been processed and interpolated to provide a curve fitting of the motion of the comb-drive depending on the voltage supply; in Figure 11 the two curves related to the two measurement setups are shown, while the detailed results are reported in Tables 4.

Table 4. Angular rotation, Total Uncertainty, expressed as standard deviation, and Total Relative Uncertainty of comb-drive depending on the applied voltage.

Supply Voltage (V)	Angular Displ. Mean Value (°) (OPS)	Angular Displ. Mean Value (°) (LTM)	Total Uncertainty (°) (OPS)	Total Uncertainty (°) (LTM)	Total Relative Uncertainty (%) (OPS)	Total Relative Uncertainty (%) (LTM)
2	0.005	0.011	0.010	0.019	206.5%	170.7%
4	0.003	0.023	0.013	0.023	460.1%	99.0%
6	0.065	0.060	0.011	0.023	16.7%	39.2%
8	0.110	0.108	0.015	0.028	13.8%	25.6%
10	0.160	0.168	0.010	0.025	6.5%	14.8%
12	0.227	0.237	0.011	0.028	4.8%	11.8%
14	0.319	0.321	0.011	0.025	3.5%	7.9%
16	0.427	0.414	0.017	0.030	4.0%	7.2%
18	0.543	0.533	0.013	0.034	2.3%	6.4%
20	0.696	0.642	0.016	0.024	2.2%	3.7%
22	0.810	0.787	0.017	0.019	2.1%	2.5%
24	0.952	0.926	0.021	0.030	2.2%	3.2%
26	1.122		0.023		2.0%	
28	1.308		0.021		1.6%	

For low values of the voltage, the observations reveal that the microgripper mobile parts face a certain resistance while attempting to move, showing a certain instability. In fact, the torque-voltage function presents an increasing rate of change. This phenomenon is one of the main source of a high dispersion of the results at low values of voltage, while this problem does not occur for higher values (>4 V).

In Table 5 the results of the comparison between the OPS and LTM systems are shown.

As already observed in Ref. [44], for the optical profilometer, even if we consider the image acquisition system of the light microscope, it is possible to observe a concordant behavior with the results reported in Refs. [35,37].

Second order polynomial regression curves have been determined by a least squares fitting method to describe the outcome from the OPS and the LTM systems: the fitting capacity is confirmed by the high value R^2 coefficients [51], equal to 0.999 for both the OPS and LTM systems.

The Equations (3) and (4) have been used to calculate the type B uncertainty δ_B.

Table 5. Applied voltage vs parameters differences.

Applied Voltage (V)	$\bar{X} \pm \delta_{T_X}$ [°]	$\bar{Y} \pm \delta_{T_Y}$ [°]	$\lvert\bar{X}_V - \bar{Y}_V\rvert$ [°]	$\delta_{T_X} + \delta_{T_Y}$ [°]
2	0.005 ± 0.010	0.011 ± 0.019	0.006	0.029
4	0.003 ± 0.013	0.023 ± 0.023	0.02	0.04
6	0.065 ± 0.011	0.060 ± 0.023	0.005	0.03
8	0.110 ± 0.015	0.108 ± 0.028	0.002	0.04
10	0.160 ± 0.010	0.168 ± 0.025	0.008	0.04
12	0.227 ± 0.011	0.237 ± 0.028	0.01	0.04
14	0.319 ± 0.011	0.321 ± 0.025	0.002	0.04
16	0.427 ± 0.017	0.414 ± 0.03	0.013	0.05
18	0.543 ± 0.013	0.533 ± 0.03	0.01	0.05
20	0.696 ± 0.016	0.642 ± 0.024	0.054	0.04
22	0.810 ± 0.017	0.787 ± 0.019	0.023	0.04
24	0.952 ± 0.021	0.926 ± 0.03	0.026	0.05

Table 4 shows that above 16 V the total relative uncertainty of the optical profilometer is less than 4.0%, while for the microscope it is less than 7.2%. Since the same software for digital image processing has been used, these results may be mainly related to the two different setups. The greatest contribution in the calculation of uncertainty is given by the δ_{α_t} uncertainty, composed by the angle measurement uncertainty due to the OPS and LTM, $\left(\frac{\delta_{\alpha p}}{\alpha} \cdot \alpha\right)$, and the angle measurement uncertainty due to the template-matching algorithm of the image processing software δ_{α_s}, that correspond to 0.02° both for OPS and LTM systems. As mentioned above, the OPS and the LTM generally have different typical values of SNR and this fact is also affecting uncertainty in the two measurement systems.

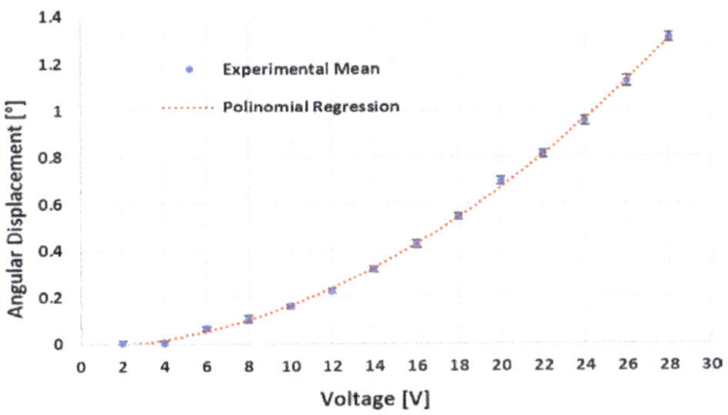

(a)

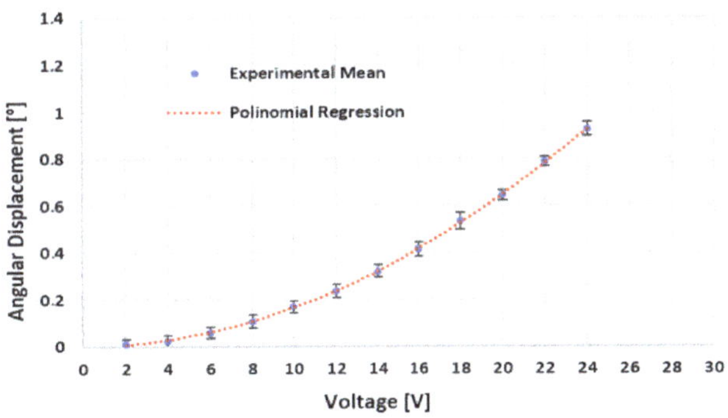

(b)

Figure 11. Relationship between angular displacement vs the applied voltage for the OPS (**a**) and the LTM (**b**) systems.

A second evaluation of the two experimental setups has been conducted; indeed, it has been necessary to evaluate whether the different results relative to the mean values of the angular displacement of the comb drive for the two experimental setups are comparable or not, to properly establish if the two measurement systems produce the same results, based on the verification that the differences between the measured mean values are smaller or comparable with the sum of the original uncertainties. Table 5 shows that, for each applied voltage value, there is no significant difference between the results obtained by the two methods. It is therefore possible to conclude that the measurements carried out with the OPS and LTM systems can be considered consistent, within the interval of the experimental uncertainties. From the point of view of total relative uncertainty, the results obtained with the profilometer appear to be better than those obtained with the microscope. However, considering the high costs of a profilometer system (about two times higher than the light microscope here used) and also the ease of use of a system such as the light microscope, the latter appears to be the best trade-off system able to carry out performance characterization of a device like microgripper for biomedical application. Furthermore, despite both image acquisition systems being able to characterize the microgripper in operating conditions, only the microscope permits a real-time study; this last feature is certainly the most important because it allows LTM to characterize the device in static and dynamic conditions.

6. Discussion

The first step of this investigation has been the mechanical characterization of a microgripper prototype. The comb-drive angular displacement has been expressed as a function of the applied voltage. Two different measurement systems, OPS and LTM, have been used. Both systems showed that the two rotation-voltage curves follow the same quadratic trend. In order to perform the measurements, a systematic approach has been developed based on in-house built software. This gave rise to a system which has quite high repeatability and low-operator-dependence. Moreover, an analysis of the uncertainties has been carried out, with the construction of a model that considers the main sources of uncertainty present in the measuring setups. The evaluation of the accuracy of the considered setups has shown that for voltages greater than 14 V, the total relative uncertainty of OPS is less than 4.0%, while for the LTM is less than 7.2%. A verification to check whether the two sets of results are consistent, within the interval of the experimental uncertainties has been carried out.

The same in-house software has been used for image processing and therefore the differences in the obtained results are due to the uncertainty of the two image acquisition systems. The main considered contributions were:

- Type A uncertainty δ_A evaluated by means of a statistic analysis of the measurements results;
- the angle measurement uncertainty δ_{α_p} due to the OPS and LTM systems;
- the angle measurement uncertainty δ_{α_s} due to the template-matching algorithm of image processing software and
- the power supply uncertainty δ_V.

Despite the obtained results showing that the OPS system has a total relative uncertainty lower than those of the LTM system, the light microscope is still the image acquisition system that will best suit the characterization of MEMS-Technology based microgrippers. In fact, profilometer or electronic microscopy are not practical or even unfeasible for the characterization of these devices in working or in real-time conditions. Therefore, the light microscope is the most promising image acquisition system because it may perform a mechanical characterization, and because of its use in biomedical or surgical real-time scenarios.

7. Conclusions

Nowadays there is a growing need of more accurate and precise devices, especially in microsurgery or diagnostics. The developments of the manufacturing technology offer new tools, such as microgrippers, suitable for a variety of biomedical applications, including minimally invasive surgery. However, SEM observation is impossible in air, wet or liquid environments, while profilometer or OCT measurements are often unpractical or more expensive in operational or real-time scenarios. The aim of this paper is therefore encouraging the use of light microscopes in future investigations, by validating, for the test case, light microscopy as the best trade-off among the characterization accuracy and the need of a large operational range and real time response. The validation method has been applied to a MEMS-technology based microgripper developed earlier by the research group.

Author Contributions: Conceptualization and investigation, all the Authors; methodology, A.S.; software, data curation and validation, F.V. and F.O.; formal analysis, F.V., F.O. and A.S.; writing, N.P.B.; supervision, S.A.S. and P.U.; resources, S.A.S. and R.C.

Acknowledgments: The microgrippers under study have been fabricated by MTLAB-FBK, Micro Technology Laboratory-Fondazione Bruno Kessler.

Abbreviations

The following abbreviations are used in this manuscript:

SEM	Scanning Electron Microscope
MEMS	Micro Electro Mechanical System
IAS	Image Analysis Software
OPS	Optical Profilometer System
LTM	Light Trinocular Microscope

References

1. Rebello, K.J. Applications of MEMS in surgery. *Proc. IEEE* **2004**, *92*, 43–55. [CrossRef]
2. Verotti, M.; Dochshanov, A.; Belfiore, N. A Comprehensive Survey on Microgrippers Design: Mechanical Structure. *J. Mech. Des. Trans. ASME* **2017**, *139*, 060801. [CrossRef]
3. Dochshanov, A.; Verotti, M.; Belfiore, N. A Comprehensive Survey on Microgrippers Design: Operational Strategy. *J. Mech. Des. Trans. ASME* **2017**, *139*, 070801. [CrossRef]
4. Lowrie, C.; Desmulliez, M.P.Y.; Hoff, L.; Elle, O.J.; Fosse, E. Fabrication of a MEMS accelerometer to detect heart bypass surgery complications. *Sens. Rev.* **2009**, *29*, 319–325. [CrossRef]
5. Balla, A.; Quaresima, S.; Ursi, P.; Seitaj, A.; Palmieri, L.; Badiali, D.; Paganini, A.M. Hiatoplasty with crura buttressing versus hiatoplasty alone during laparoscopic sleeve gastrectomy. *Gastroenterol. Res. Pract.* **2017**, *2017*, 6565403. [CrossRef]
6. Popivanov, G.; Tabakov, M.; Mantese, G.; Cirocchi, R.; Piccinini, I.; D'Andrea, V.; Covarelli, P.; Boselli, C.; Barberini, F.; Tabola, R.; Ursi, P.; Cavaliere, D.; Surgical treatment of gastrointestinal stromal tumors of the duodenum: A literature review. *Transl. Gastroenterol. Hepatol.* **2018**, *3*, 71. [CrossRef] [PubMed]
7. Cochetti, G.; Del Zingaro, M.; Boni, A.; Cocca, D.; Panciarola, M.; Tiezzi, A.; Gaudio, G.; Balzarini, F.; Ursi, P.; Mearini, E. Colovesical fistula: Review on conservative management, surgical techniques and minimally invasive approaches. *G. Chir.* **2018**, *39*, 195–207.
8. Quaresima, S.; Balla, A.; Dambrosio, G.; Bruzzone, P.; Ursi, P.; Lezoche, E.; Paganini, A.M. Endoluminal loco-regional resection by TEM after R1 endoscopic removal or recurrence of rectal tumors. *Minim. Invasive Ther. Allied Technol.* **2016**, *25*, 134–140. [CrossRef] [PubMed]
9. Paci, M.; Scoglio, D.; Ursi, P.; Barchetti, L.; Fabiani, B.; Ascoli, G.; Lezoche, G. Transanal Endocopic Microsurgery (TEM) in advanced rectal cancer disease treatment [Il ruolo della TEM nel trattamento dei tumori del retto extraperitoneale]. *Ann. Ital. Chir.* **2010**, *81*, 269–274.
10. Lezoche, E.; Fabiani, B.; D'Ambrosio, G.; Ursi, P.; Balla, A.; Lezoche, G.; Monteleone, F.; Paganini, A.M. Nucleotide-guided mesorectal excision combined with endoluminal locoregional resection by transanal endoscopic microsurgery in the treatment of rectal tumors: Technique and preliminary results. *Surg. Endosc.* **2013**, *27*, 4136–4141. [CrossRef] [PubMed]
11. Ursi, P.; Santoro, A.; Gemini, A.; Arezzo, A.; Pironi, D.; Renzi, C.; Cirocchi, R.; Di Matteo, F.; Maturo, A.; D'Andrea, V.; et al. Comparison of outcomes following intersphincteric resection vs low anterior resection for low rectal cancer: A systematic review. *G. Chir.* **2018**, *39*, 123–142.
12. Theillet, P.O.; Pierron, O.N. Quantifying adsorbed water monolayers on silicon MEMS resonators exposed to humid environments. *Sens. Actuators A Phys.* **2011**, *171*, 375–380. [CrossRef]
13. Bhattacharya, S.; Murali Krishna, A.; Lombardi, D.; Crewe, A.; Alexander, N. Economic MEMS based 3-axis water proof accelerometer for dynamic geo-engineering applications. *Soil Dyn. Earthq. Eng.* **2012**, *36*, 111–118. [CrossRef]
14. Neagu, C.; Jansen, H.; Gardeniers, H.; Elwenspoek, M. Electrolysis of water: An actuation principle for MEMS with a big opportunity. *Mechatronics* **2000**, *10*, 571–581. [CrossRef]
15. Scherge, M.; Li, X.; Schaefer, J.A. The effect of water on friction of MEMS. *Tribol. Lett.* **1999**, *6*, 215–220. [CrossRef]

16. Yabuki, T.; Nakabeppu, O. Heat transfer mechanisms in isolated bubble boiling of water observed with MEMS sensor. *Int. J. Heat Mass Transf.* **2014**, *76*, 286–297. [CrossRef]
17. Yao, J.; Huang, C.H.; Wang, L.; Yang, J.; Gao, L.; Maslov, K.I.; Zou, J.; Wang, L.V. Wide-field fast-scanning photoacoustic microscopy based on a water-immersible MEMS scanning mirror. *J. Biomed. Opt.* **2012**, *17*, 080505. [CrossRef]
18. Bashir, R. BioMEMS: State-of-the-art in detection, opportunities and prospects. *Adv. Drug Deliv. Rev.* **2004**, *56*, 1565–1586. [CrossRef]
19. Bhushan, B. Nanotribology and nanomechanics of MEMS/NEMS and BioMEMS/BioNEMS materials and devices. *Microelectron. Eng.* **2007**, *84*, 387–412. [CrossRef]
20. Grayson, A.; Shawgo, R.; Johnson, A.; Flynn, N.; Li, Y.; Cima, M.; Langer, R. A BioMEMS review: MEMS technology for physiologically integrated devices. *Proc. IEEE* **2004**, *92*, 6–21. [CrossRef]
21. Bragheri, F.; Minzioni, P.; Martinez Vazquez, R.; Bellini, N.; Paiè, P.; Mondello, C.; Ramponi, R.; Cristiani, I.; Osellame, R. Optofluidic integrated cell sorter fabricated by femtosecond lasers. *Lab Chip* **2012**, *12*, 3779–3784. [CrossRef]
22. Wu, H.; Kuhn, T.; Moy, V. Mechanical properties of L929 cells measured by atomic force microscopy: Effects of anticytoskeletal drugs and membrane crosslinking. *Scanning* **1998**, *20*, 389–397. [CrossRef]
23. Mattana, S.; Mattarelli, M.; Urbanelli, L.; Sagini, K.; Emiliani, C.; Serra, M.; Fioretto, D.; Caponi, S. Non-contact mechanical and chemical analysis of single living cells by microspectroscopic techniques. *Light Sci. Appl.* **2018**, *7*, 17139. [CrossRef]
24. Mulvany, M.J.; Halpern, W. Mechanical properties of vascular smooth muscle cells in situ. *Nature* **1976**, *260*, 617–619. [CrossRef]
25. Wakatsuki, T.; Schwab, B.; Thompson, N.; Elson, E. Effects of cytochalasin D and latrunculin B on mechanical properties of cells. *J. Cell Sci.* **2001**, *114*, 1025–1036.
26. Levesque, P.; Gauvin, R.; Larouche, D.; Auger, F.; Germain, L. A Computer-Controlled Apparatus for the Characterization of Mechanical and Viscoelastic Properties of Tissue-Engineered Vascular Constructs. *Cardiovasc. Eng. Technol.* **2011**, *2*, 24–34. [CrossRef]
27. Bagolini, A.; Bellutti, P.; Di Giamberardino, P.; Rudas, I.J.; D'Andrea, V.; Verotti, M.; Dochshanov, A.; Belfiore, N.P. Stiffness Characterization of Biological Tissues by Means of MEMS-Technology Based Micro Grippers Under Position Control. In *Advances in Service and Industrial Robotics*; Ferraresi, C., Quaglia, G., Eds.; Springer International Publishing: Cham, Switzerland, 2018; pp. 939–947.
28. Belfiore, N.; Broggiato, G.; Verotti, M.; Balucani, M.; Crescenzi, R.; Bagolini, A.; Bellutti, P.; Boscardin, M. Simulation and construction of a mems CSFH based microgripper. *Int. J. Mech. Control* **2015**, *16*, 21–30.
29. Verotti, M.; Crescenzi, R.; Balucani, M.; Belfiore, N.P. MEMS-based conjugate surfaces flexure hinge. *J. Mech. Des. Trans. ASME* **2015**, *137*, 012301. [CrossRef]
30. Botta, F.; Verotti, M.; Bagolini, A.; Bellutti, P.; Belfiore, N.P. Mechanical response of four-bar linkage microgrippers with bidirectional electrostatic actuation. *Actuators* **2018**, *7*, 78. [CrossRef]
31. Cecchi, R.; Verotti, M.; Capata, R.; Dochshanov, A.; Broggiato, G.; Crescenzi, R.; Balucani, M.; Natali, S.; Razzano, G.; Lucchese, F.; et al. Development of micro-grippers for tissue and cell manipulation with direct morphological comparison. *Micromachines* **2015**, *6*, 1710–1728. [CrossRef]
32. Di Giamberardino, P.; Bagolini, A.; Bellutti, P.; Rudas, I.; Verotti, M.; Botta, F.; Belfiore, N.P. New MEMS tweezers for the viscoelastic characterization of soft materials at the microscale. *Micromachines* **2017**, *9*, 15. [CrossRef] [PubMed]
33. Verotti, M.; Dochshanov, A.; Belfiore, N.P. Compliance Synthesis of CSFH MEMS-Based Microgrippers. *J. Mech. Des. Trans. ASME* **2017**, *139*, 022301. [CrossRef]
34. Potrich, C.; Lunelli, L.; Bagolini, A.; Bellutti, P.; Pederzolli, C.; Verotti, M.; Belfiore, N.P. Innovative silicon microgrippers for biomedical applications: Design, mechanical simulation and evaluation of protein fouling. *Actuators* **2018**, *7*, 12. [CrossRef]
35. Bagolini, A.; Ronchin, S.; Bellutti, P.; Chistè, M.; Verotti, M.; Belfiore, N.P. Fabrication of Novel MEMS Microgrippers by Deep Reactive Ion Etching With Metal Hard Mask. *J. Microelectromech. Syst.* **2017**, *26*, 926–934. [CrossRef]
36. Bertini, S.; Verotti, M.; Bagolini, A.; Bellutti, P.; Ruta, G.; Belfiore, N.P. Scalloping and stress concentration in DRIE-manufactured comb-drives. *Actuators* **2018**, *7*, 57. [CrossRef]

37. Crescenzi, R.; Balucani, M.; Belfiore, N. Operational characterization of CSFH MEMS technology based hinges. *J. Micromech. Microeng.* **2018**, *28*, 5. [CrossRef]
38. Prasad, P. *Introduction to Biophotonics*; John Wiley and Sons, Inc.: Hoboken, NJ, USA, 2003.
39. Strathman, M.; Liu, Y.; Keeler, E.G.; Song, M.; Baran, U.; Xi, J.; Sun, M.T.; Wang, R.; Li, X.; Lin, L.Y. MEMS scanning micromirror for optical coherence tomography. *Biomed. Opt. Express* **2015**, *6*, 211–224. [CrossRef]
40. Werkmeister, R.M.; Sapeta, S.; Schmidl, D.; Garhöfer, G.; Schmidinger, G.; dos Santos, V.A.; Aschinger, G.C.; Baumgartner, I.; Pircher, N.; Schwarzhans, F.; et al. Ultrahigh-resolution OCT imaging of the human cornea. *Biomed. Opt. Express* **2017**, *8*, 1221–1239. [CrossRef]
41. Huang, D.; Swanson, E.A.; Lin, C.P.; Schuman, J.S.; Stinson, W.G.; Chang, W.; Hee, M.R.; Flotte, T.; Gregory, K.; Puliafito, C.A. Optical Coherence Tomography. *Science* **1991**, *254*, 1178–1181. [CrossRef]
42. Lee, J.; Shirazi, M.F.; Park, K.; Jeon, M.; Kim, J. Defect inspection of actuator lenses using swept-source optical coherence tomography. *Opt. Rev.* **2018**, *25*, 403–409. [CrossRef]
43. Kim, S.; Lee, C.; Kim, J.Y.; Kim, J.; Lim, G.; Kim, C. Two-axis polydimethylsiloxane-based electromagnetic microelectromechanical system scanning mirror for optical coherence tomography. *J. Biomed. Opt.* **2016**, *21*, 106001. [CrossRef]
44. Orsini, F.; Vurchio, F.; Scorza, A.; Crescenzi, R.; Sciuto, S.A. An image analysis approach to microgrippers displacement measurement and testing. *Actuators* **2018**, *7*, 64. [CrossRef]
45. Chang, R.J.; Chien, Y.C. Polymer microgripper with autofocusing and visual tracking operations to grip particle moving in liquid. *Actuators* **2018**, *7*, 27. [CrossRef]
46. Brown, L. Imaging Particle Analysis: Resolution and Sampling Considerations. 2009. Accessed online: http://www.fluidimaging.com/resource-center-whitepapers (accessed on 12 June 2015).
47. International Organization for Standardization; International Electrotechnical Commission. *ISO/IEC Guide 98-3: Uncertainty of Measurement. Part 3: Guide to the Expressión of Uncertainty in Measurement (GUM:1995). Partie 3: Guide pour L'expression de L'incertitude de Mesure (GUM:1995)*; Number pt. 3; ISO Standard Catalogue: Geneva, Switzerland, 2008.
48. Pawley, J. *Handbook of Biological Confocal Microscopy*; Springer US: New York, NY, USA, 2010.
49. Waters, J. Accuracy and precision in quantitative fluorescence microscopy. *J. Cell Biol.* **2009**, *185*, 1135–1148. [CrossRef] [PubMed]
50. Taylor, J.R. *An Introduction to Error Analysis. Uncertainty Stuty in Physical Measurements. (in Italian) Introduzione all'analisi degli Errori. Lo Studio delle Incertezze Nelle Misure Fisiche*; Collana di Fisica. Testi e Manuali; Zanichelli: Bologna, Italy, 1986.
51. Navidi, W. *Statistics for Engineers and Scientists*; McGraw-Hill: New York, NY, USA, 2014.

The Effect of Patellar Tendon Release on the Characteristics of Patellofemoral Joint Squat Movement

Jianping Wang, Yongqiang Yang, Dong Guo, Shihua Wang, Long Fu and Yu Li *

School of Mechanical and Power Engineering, Henan Polytechnic University, Jiaozuo 454000, China; wjp@hpu.edu.cn (J.W.); y17864208259@163.com (Y.Y.); 15538949519@163.com (D.G.); 211805020010@home.hpu.edu.cn (S.W.); fl1@gaokowl.com (L.F.)

* Correspondence: liyu@hpu.edu.cn

Abstract: Objectives: This paper studies the patellar tendon release's effect on the movement characteristics of the artificial patellofemoral joint squat to provide reference data for knee joint surgery. Methods: Firstly, the dynamic finite element model of the human knee joint under squatting was established. Secondly, in the above no-release models, the release of 30% of the attachment area at the upper end, the lower end, or both ends of the patellar tendon were conducted, respectively. Then the simulations of all above four models were conducted. Finally, the results of the simulation were compared and analyzed. Results: The simulation results show that, after releasing the patellar tendon (compared with the no-release simulation's results), the relative flexion, medial-lateral rotation, medial-lateral tilt, and superior-inferior shift of the patella relative to the femur increased; the medial-lateral shift and anterior-posterior shift of the patella relative to the femur decreased. Conclusion: In this paper, the maximum flexion angle of the patella increased after the patellar tendon being released (compared with the no-release model), which indicated that the mobility of knee joint was improved after the patellar tendon release. The simulation data in this paper can provide technical reference for total knee arthroplasty.

Keywords: total knee arthroplasty; patellar tendon; patellofemoral joint; squat movement; dynamic finite element analysis

1. Introduction

With the application of prostheses in total knee arthroplasty (TKA), post-operative complications concomitantly usually occur [1]. One of these complications, often being ignored, is patella baja [2–4]. At the same time, relevant studies [5–9] show that, after TKA, the patellar tendon suffers certain reductions. Other studies [6,10] indicate that the patellar tendon can be shortened, the position of the patella lowered, reducing the knee joint movement and variation. A slightly low patella does not, however, affect the function of the knee joint. Check points during surgery must include patella contracture syndrome [11] and true patella baja [10], which can be treated by release of scar operation, patellar tendon lengthening, and patellar ligament insertion. Patients with pseudo-patella baja and slight joint line up, and those that do not affect knee function, are treated with follow-up observation. However, excessive upward movement of the joint line can result in serious symptoms [12], such as the need for surgery to replace a thin pad [13] and/or patellar ligament release. This paper is for studying the patellar tendon release's effect on the movement characteristics of the artificial patellofemoral joint squat to provide reference data for knee joint surgery.

2. Materials and Methods

2.1. The Establishment of a Finite Element Model

In this paper, a healthy male volunteer with a height of 173 cm and a weight of 60 kg was scanned by medical instrument computed tomography (CT) in the range of 10 cm above and below the knee joint center. The correlative parameter was set to 120 kVp and 150 mA, with a scanning interval of 1 mm. The volunteer was scanned with magnetic resonance imaging (MRI). MR (GE Sigma HD1.5T, Boston, MA, USA) was used for proton density weighting (PDWI) and chemical shift fat suppression weighted scanning, and the image coordinates of each layer of different weighted phases were consistent. Flux density is 1.5 T, and slide thickness is 1 mm [14]. Based on the CT and MRI images of the healthy volunteer, a three-dimensional geometric anatomical model including all bone tissues and main soft tissues was established (as shown in Figure 1). A three-dimensional solid model of press fit condylar (PFC) femoral prosthesis (PFC sigma, DePuy orthopaedics, Warsaw, IN, USA.) commonly used in TKA was established. Then the total knee replacement operation was simulated, and the prosthesis was assembled on the three-dimensional geometric anatomical model of the knee joint (as shown in Figure 2a). The model of the knee joint was divided into finite element meshes after TKA. In the finite element model of the knee joint, most of the unit types were hexahedrons (c3d8r, an eight-node linear brick element with reduced integration), and very few were pentahedrons (C3D6, a six-node linear triangular prism element) and tetrahedrons (C3D4, a four-node linear tetrahedron element), with a total unit number of 31,767, and 37,031 nodes (as shown in Figure 2b). The volunteer was provided details of the study and signed an informed consent form.

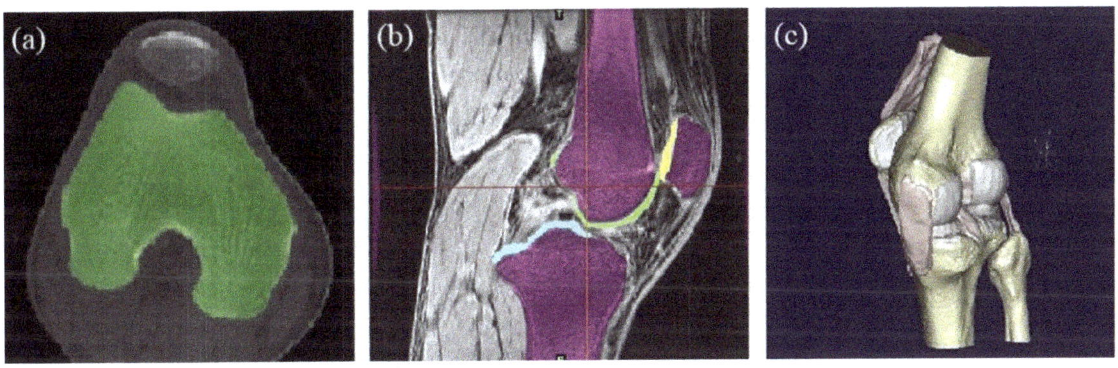

Figure 1. (**a**) Contour tracing of bone from CT; (**b**) MRI image; (**c**) the geometric anatomy model of human knee.

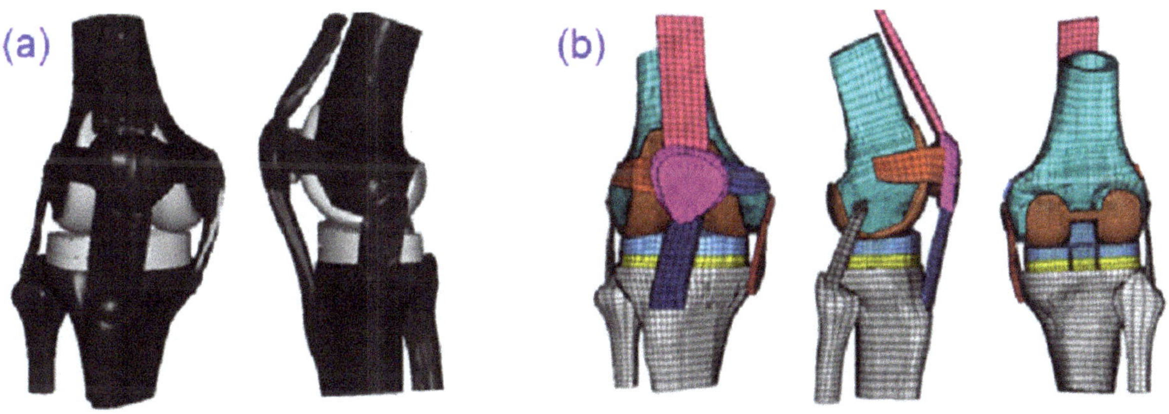

Figure 2. (**a**) 3D geometric anatomical model of knee joint after TKA; (**b**) finite element model of knee joint after TKA.

Hypermesh software, version 11.0 (Altair Engineering Corp, MI, USA) was used to simulate the release at ends of the patellar tendon. The width of the patellar tendon at the upper end was

6.84 mm before release (Figure 3a) and 4.788 mm after release (Figure 3b). The height of the patellar tendon at the lower end was 8.09 mm before release (Figure 3c) and 5.633 mm after release (Figure 3d). Figure 3 shows the finite element models before and after release the 30% of the patellar tendon at both ends (clinically, one-third of the central patellar tendon is often transplanted to repair damaged ligaments [15–18]. Therefore, 30% of the patellar tendon was used as an example). Figure 3a represents the model before release of the patellar tendon at the upper end. Figure 3b represents the model released the patellar tendon at the upper end. Figure 3c represents the model before releasing the patellar tendon at the lower end. Figure 3d represents the model releasing the patellar tendon at the lower end. The establishment of the model was based on the model built by Wang Jian-ping, and the validity of the model was verified by in vitro cadaveric experiments [19].

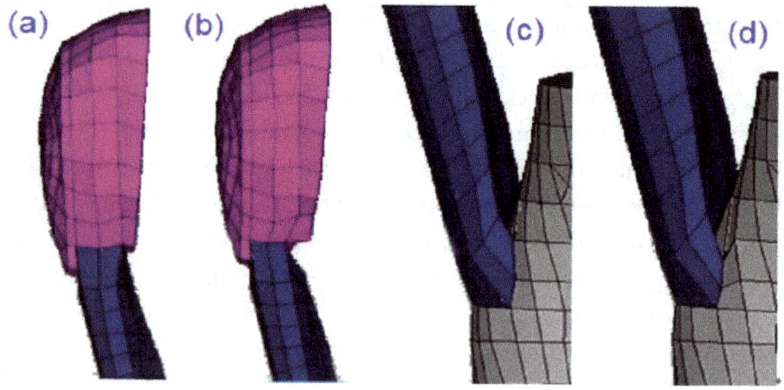

Figure 3. The finite element model of patellar tendon: (**a**) the upper before release; (**b**) the upper released; (**c**) the lower before release; (**d**) the lower released.

2.2. *The Establishment of a Coordinate System for the Knee Joint's Motion*

The corresponding reference coordinate systems of femur, tibia and patella are established by the following methods: (1) The femur posterior condylar cortical bone was contour-fitted to two laps, with one line through the center of two circles as the X axis of the femur. Parallel with lines of force and through the centerline of the femoral medial condyle represent the Z axis of the femur. Regarding the line, this passes through the center of the femoral medial condyle and perpendicular to the X-axis and Z-axis, as the Y-axis. (2) The intersection point of the Z-axis and the plane of the tibial joint line serves as the origin of the tibial coordinate system, and the femoral coordinate system moves to this point to obtain the tibial coordinate system. (3) The center of the patellar anterior surface moves inward 10 mm, then the center serves as the origin of the patellar coordinate system. The coordinate system of the femur was relocated to the origin, and the patellar coordinate system can be obtained [20]. The bone coordinate systems are shown in Figure 4.

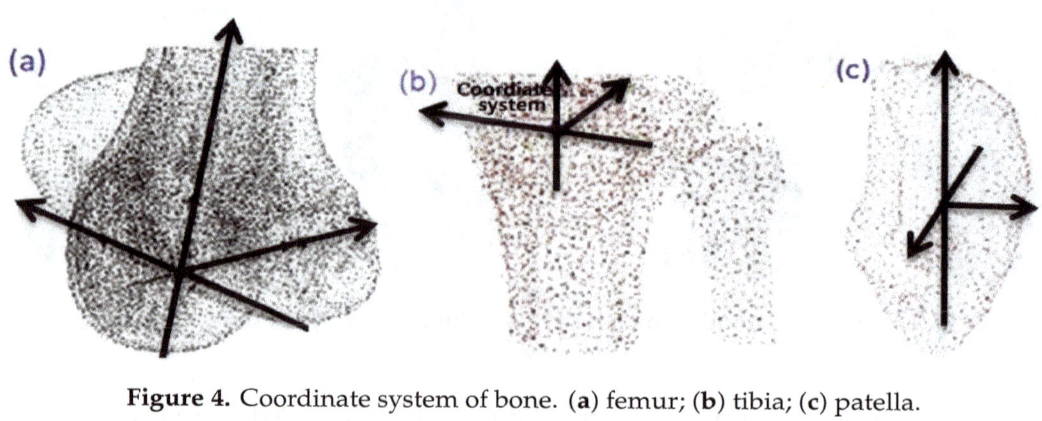

Figure 4. Coordinate system of bone. (**a**) femur; (**b**) tibia; (**c**) patella.

2.3. *Loading Conditions and the Setting of Material Properties*

For this study, 400 N [19,21] of force was applied to the quadriceps, and the direction of the force was parallel with the femoral shaft, pointing to the starting point of the quadriceps. At the same time, half of the body's weight (0.5BW) was applied along the force line of the knee joint, that is, a force of 300 N perpendicular to the ground was applied to the center of the femoral head. The boundary conditions were defined: the reference point of the ankle corresponding to the rotation center was fully fixed with six degrees of freedom. The material properties of bone tissue and femoral prosthesis were defined as isotropic and linear elastic, respectively. The material properties of polymer polyethylene pad were defined as non-linear elastic-plastic deformability [22,23]. The material properties of soft tissue were defined as nonlinear elastic [24]. The friction coefficient of polymer polyethylene and cobalt chromium molybdenum material was defined as 0.04 [22]. The penalty function with weighted factor was adopted [25,26]. For the femur, polymer polyethylene pad, tibial plateau, patellar prosthesis, and other soft tissues, seven surface contact pairs were defined in the finite element model after TKA. Moreover, nine surface contact pairs were defined in the finite element model of normal human.

3. Results

The four different knee joint finite element models were imported into the finite element analysis ABAQUS software, version 6.10 (Dassault SIMULIA Corp., Paris, France). Within 0–135 degrees, the data of motion characteristics at different flexion degrees were calculated and analyzed, as shown in Figure 5.

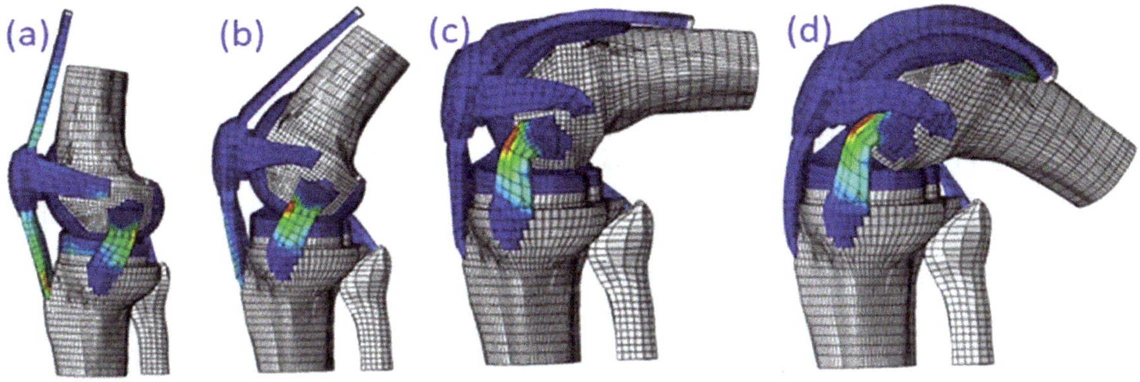

Figure 5. A sample of simulation results after TKA. Flexion degrees: (**a**) 0°; (**b**) 30°; (**c**) 90°; (**d**) 135°.

3.1. *Medial-Lateral Shift and Flexion of Patella Along the Inner and Outer Axes*

Figure 6a shows the medial-lateral shift data of the patellofemoral joint within 0–135 degrees of knee flexion. As the figure shows, from 0 to 30 degrees of flexion, the patella relative to the femur shifted outward. After releasing the patellar tendon, the patella shifted outward greatly. The lateral shift of the patellar tendon released at the lower end was larger than that of release at the upper end. The lateral shift was the largest when both ends were released simultaneously. From 40 degrees to 135 degrees of flexion, the patella relative to the femur shifted inward. After releasing the patellar tendon, the patella medial shift was smaller than that of no-release. The medial shift of the patellar tendon released at different ends was basically balanced. After the upper end of the patellar tendon was released, the maximum of the patella medial shift was 2.62 mm at 110 degrees of flexion, which was 11% lower than that of 2.94 mm at 100 degrees of flexion for the no-release model. After the lower end of the patellar tendon was released, the maximum medial shift of the patella was 2.63 mm at 110 degrees of flexion, and decreased 11% by compared with the no-release model. After both ends of the patellar tendon were released, the maximum medial shift of the patella was 2.61 mm at 110 degrees of flexion, and decreased 11% by compared with the no-release model.

Figure 6b shows the changes of patella flexion before and after the release. At the same flexion degree of the knee, the release of the patellar tendon at the upper end and lower end was compared with the no-release model, the flexion of the patella relative to femur was slightly larger. The patella flexion after both ends release (compared with the no-release model), in the same flexion degree of the knee, showed a smaller degree of patella flexion (within 130–135 degrees of flexion, being slightly larger than the no-release model). At 135 degrees of knee flexion, for the three releasing models: the upper end release, lower end release, and both ends release models, the patellar flexion reached maximums of 92, 92.73, and 93.17 degrees, respectively. Compared with the no-release model of 89 degrees, this shows an increase of 3%, 4%, and 5%, respectively.

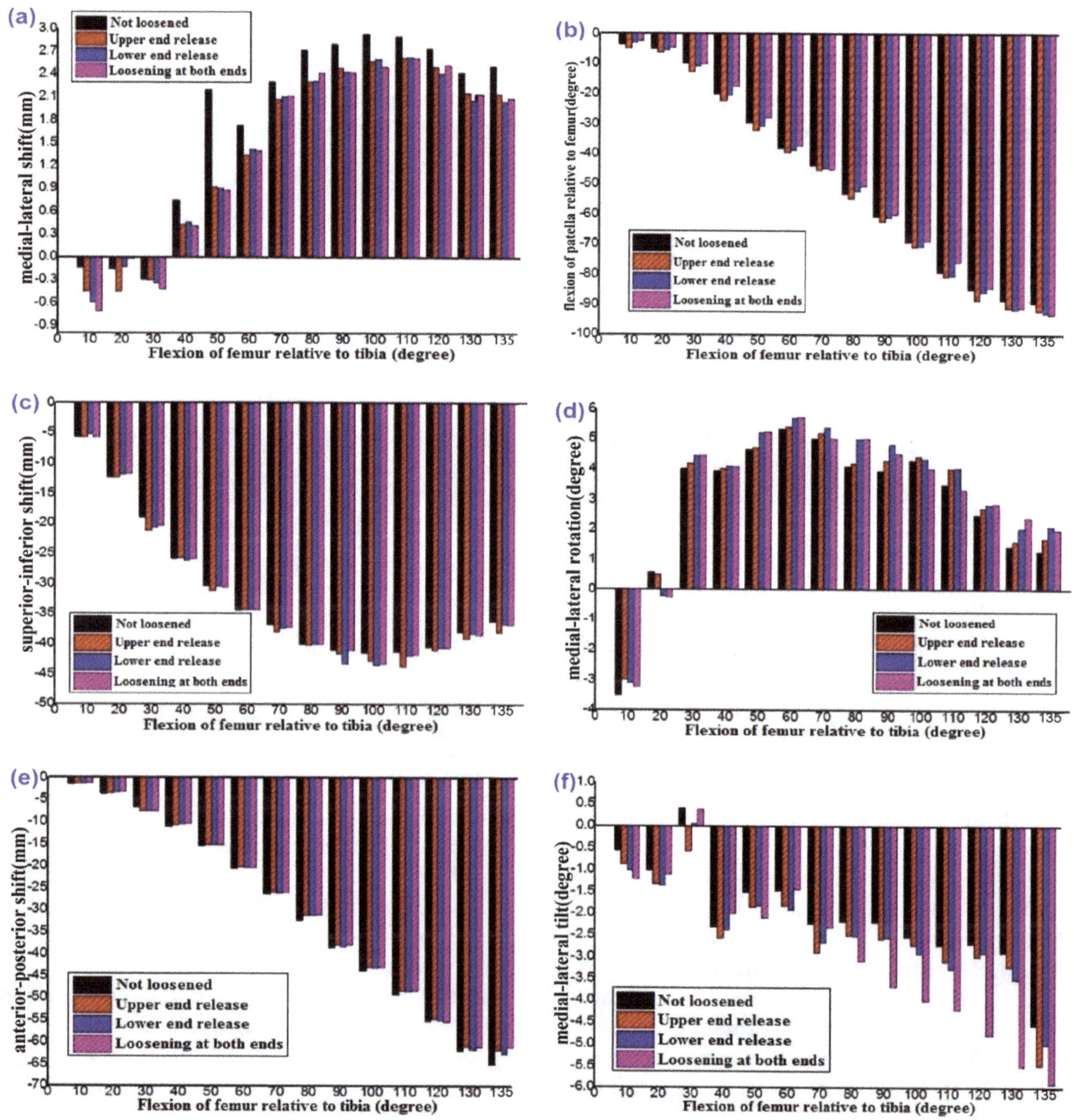

Figure 6. Patellofemoral movement data at different flexion degrees before and after the patellar tendon was released. (**a**) Medial-lateral shift; (**b**) flexion of patella relative to femur; (**c**) superior-inferior shift; (**d**) medial-lateral rotation; (**e**) anterior-posterior shift; (**f**) medial-lateral tilt.

3.2. *Superior-Inferior Shift and Medial-Lateral Rotation of the Patella Along Its Upper and Lower Axes*

As Figure 6c shows, during the knee joint's squatting movement, the patella relative to the femur shifted downward. The patella inferior shift of no-release model was slightly smaller than that of the upper end release. For the lower end release simulation, the patella inferior shift was slightly smaller within early 0–20 degrees of flexion and slightly larger after the 20-degree flexion than that of the no-release model. Within all flexion degrees, the patella inferior shift of the both ends release was slightly larger than that of no-release model, other than 20-degree flexion. After releasing the upper end of the patellar tendon, the maximum inferior shift of the patella was 43.80 mm at 110-degree flexion, which increased 6% compared with 41.42 mm at 100-degree flexion of the no-release model. For the lower end release model, the maximum inferior shift of the patella was 43.49 mm at 100-degree flexion, which increased 5% compared with the no-release model. After releasing the patellar tendon at both ends, the maximum inferior shift of the patellar was 43.43 mm at 100-degree flexion, which increased 5% compared with the no-release model.

Figure 6d shows the data of medial-lateral rotation. The data of the patella relative to the femur showed lateral rotation first and then medial rotation. Compared to the no-release model and the upper end model, the knee flexion degree of the initial patella medial rotation was greater for the lower end model and both-ends model. Meanwhile, it is shown that the patella medial-rotation for all three release models as larger than that of the no-release model. At 60 degrees of knee flexion, the patella medial-rotation reached the maximum of 5.41 degrees, 5.70 degrees, and 5.72 degrees, respectively, for the upper-end, lower-end and both-ends models, which increased 1%, 7%, and 7%, respectively, compared with the 5.34 degree value of the no-release model.

3.3. *Anterior-Posterior Shift and Medial-Lateral Tilt of Patella Along the Anteroposterior Axis*

Figure 6e shows the patella translated backward relative to the femur. During the knee joint's squatting movement, the patella relative to the femur translated backward. Within all flexion degrees, the patella backward translations of all three release models were smaller than that of no-release model, other than the 30-degree flexion, and the patella posterior shift was the least when both ends were released. At 135 degrees of knee flexion, the patella posterior shift reached the maximum values of 61.82 mm, 62.57 mm, and 61.07 mm, respectively, for the upper-end, lower-end, and both-ends models, which decreased 5%, 4%, and 6% compared with the value 64.97 mm of the no-release model.

Figure 6f shows the data of medial-lateral tilt. Before and after patellar tendon release, within all flexion degrees, the patella showed an inward movement pattern relative to the femur other than 30-degree flexion. At the same degree of knee flexion, after the release of the patella tendon, the medial tilt angle of the patella relative to the femur was larger than that of no release. After 80 degrees of knee flexion, when both ends of the patellar tendon were released at the same time, the patella medial tilt angle was the largest. At 135 degrees of knee flexion, the patella medial tilt angle reached the maximum values of 5.51 degrees, 5.01 degrees, and 5.92 degrees, respectively, for the upper-end, lower-end, and both-ends models, which increased 21%, 10%, and 30%, respectively, compared with the 4.55 degree value of the no-release model.

4. Discussion

This paper investigates the patellar tendon release's effect on the movement characteristics of the artificial patellofemoral joint squat. The simulation results show that, after the patellar tendon being released, respectively, at the upper end, the lower end, and both ends, being compared with the no-release simulation results, the relative flexion, medial-lateral rotation, medial-lateral tilt, and superior-inferior shift of the patella relative to the femur increased, and the medial-lateral shift and anterior-posterior shift of the patella relative to the femur decreased. Different release models have different effects on the squatting motion characteristics of the patellofemoral joint. In this study, the data of patellofemoral joint squatting after TKA of the no-release model was analyzed and compared with those of all three release models and other related research results of the natural knee joint.

4.1. *Medial-Lateral Shift and Flexion of the Patella*

For the medial-lateral shift of the patella relative to the femur the maximum patella medial-shift of all three release models were balanced, and the maximum medial-shift was decreased compared with that of the no-release model (the maximum reduction was about 11% for the both-ends model). The patella shifted outward first and then inward relative to the femur, which is similar to the related studies [27,28].

For the flexion movement of the patella, relative to the femur, previous studies [27,28] showed that the flexion of patella changes linearly with the flexion of the patellofemoral joint. It is consistent with the results of this study. In this study, the maximum flexion angle of the patella increased after the patellar tendon being released (compared with the no-release model, the maximum of the both-ends model increased by 5%), which indicated that the mobility of the knee joint was improved after the patellar tendon release.

4.2. *Superior-Inferior Shift and Medial-Lateral Rotation of Patella*

For the superior-inferior shift of the patella, relative to the femur, after the patellar tendon was released in different ends, the patella shifted downward relative to the femur. In the high flexion, the patella was moved up slightly, and the maximum inferior shift (about 43.5 mm at 110 degrees) was increased 5% compared with that of no-release model. The maximum increase occurred in the upper-end release model and the minimum one occurred at both-ends release model. Related studies [27,29] also showed that the patella, with the knee flexion, shifted downward relative to the femur, and the maximum flexion angle of the knee was 110 degrees in their studies (the maximum inferior shift was about 50 mm), which was basically similar to this paper (in this paper, the maximum flexion angle of the knee was 135 degrees, and the maximum inferior shift was 43.8 mm).

For the medial-lateral rotation of the patella, relative to the femur, after the patellar tendon was released at different ends, the motion pattern of the patella relative to the femur was lateral rotation first and then medial rotation, which is consistent with that of the no-release model. For all the above three release models, the maximum medial rotation of the patella increased; among them, the increase of the upper end release was the minimum (1%), and the increase of the both-ends release were the maximum (7%). Heegaard et al. [30] showed that within 0–110 degrees of knee flexion, the patellar rotation pattern changed from medial to lateral rotation, and then lateral rotation within 110–135 degrees of knee flexion. This phenomenon indicates that the patellar motion changes during the high flexion, which might be related to the way of femoral fixation and passive loading.

4.3. *Anterior-Posterior Shift and Medial-Lateral Tilt of the Patella*

For the anterior-posterior shift of the patella, relative to the femur, the results of Azmy et al.'s [31] in vitro experiments showed that with the flexion of the knee joint, the patella shifted backward; after 30 degree knee flexion, posterior movement rate of the patella increased, and the maximum posterior movement of the patella reached 32 mm. The results of Baldwin et al. [29], based on the experimental dynamic finite element model, also show that the patella continues to shift backward with the knee flexion, and the maximum posterior movement of the patella is about 30 mm. The motion analysis results of patella anterior-posterior shift in this paper are consistent with those of the above studies; with knee flexion, patella continued to shift backward. Meanwhile, the analysis results of this paper gave the data of the posterior shift of the patella during high knee flexion. At 135 degree knee flexion, the posterior shift of the patella after the upper end, the lower end, and both ends of the patellar tendon were released to reach the maximum values of 61.82 mm, 62.57 mm, and 61.07 mm, respectively, which was 5%, 4%, and 6% lower than the no-release values of 64.97 mm.

For the medial-lateral tilt of the patella relative to the femur with the flexion of the knee joint, the patella relative to the femur exhibits an inward motion pattern before and after release. At the same degree of flexion, the medial tilt angle of the patella relative to the femur was larger than that of the no-release model, the increase of the both ends release was the maximum (30%), and the increase of the lower end release was the minimum (10%). The relevant findings [27,29,31,32] also showed that the patella, with the flexion of knee, tilted inward relative to the femur, which is consistent with the results of this study. At the same time, there are different research results for the medial-lateral tilt motion of the patella [33]. The results of Amis et al. [33] showed that the patella continued to tilt outward with knee flexion, which may be related to the loading method that the quadriceps were divided into six bundles. There are differences in related studies, which may be related to the fact that the patella was less constrained by the femoral articular surface in the direction of patella medial-lateral tilt.

Several limitations of the present study should be noted. In this study, only 30% of the patella was released, and others were not analyzed. The finite element model of the human knee joint after TKA was established in this paper, based on the consideration of all bone tissue and the main soft tissue of the knee; although the transverse patellar ligaments, which play an important role in the movement of the patella, are added, the effect of the joint capsule, hamstring, or gastrocnemius on knee joint activity was not considered. In the subsequent analysis of the knee joint, these tissues could be taken into account to make the model more in line with human physiology.

The anterior cruciate ligament (ACL) has the functions of restricting the forward movement of the tibia and controlling the internal and external valgus of the knee [34–36]. The ACL is extremely vulnerable during exercise and it is difficult to repair itself. If not treated in time, the patient's daily activities will be seriously affected [37]. The posterior cruciate ligament (PCL), aside from providing restraint to posterior tibial translation, is reported to have a considerable role in providing rotational stability to the knee [38]. Injuries to the PCL are far less common than injuries to other knee structures, such as the ACL or the menisci [39]. In addition, it has been found that the clinical outcomes of PCL reconstruction are less satisfactory and less predictable relative to those of ACL reconstruction [39]. The medial patellofemoral ligament (MPFL) is one of the most important restraints to lateral displacement of the patella from 0° to 30° of flexion, providing up to 60% of lateral patellofemoral stability [40]. In the last decade, the understanding of the pathoanatomic mechanisms involved in lateral patellar dislocation (LPD) has evolved tremendously and reconstruction of the medial patellofemoral ligament (MPFL), as the most important passive restraint against LPD, has evolved to become an established operative procedure [41]. This paper mainly investigates the patellar tendon release's effect on the movement characteristics of the artificial patellofemoral joint squat. However, different knee ligaments play different roles. Based on the models used in this study, we will further study the ligaments' reconstruction and other related issues.

5. Conclusions

This paper investigates the patellar tendon release's effect on the movement characteristics of the artificial patellofemoral joint squat. The post-TKA patellofemoral joint's motion characteristics in different patellar tendon release pattern were obtained. Compared with the no-release model, the flexion, medial-lateral rotation, medial-lateral tilt, and superior-inferior shift of the patella relative to the femur increased; and the medial-lateral shift and anterior-posterior shift of the patella relative to the femur decreased. In this paper, the maximum flexion angle of the patella increased after the patellar tendon being released (compared with the no-release model), which indicated that the mobility of knee joint was improved after the patellar tendon release. Different release models have different effects on the squatting motion characteristics of patellofemoral joint. In this paper, the simulation results can be used to moderately release the ends of the patellar tendon in the TKA surgery, in order to improve the motility of the patella relative to the femur. The results of this paper can provide a reference for the study of the pathology and rehabilitation of the knee joint, as well as related operations.

Author Contributions: Conceptualization: J.W.; data curation: L.F. and Y.L.; investigation: J.W. and L.F.; methodology: J.W. and Y.L.; resources: J.W.; software: J.W., Y.Y., and D.G.; supervision: J.W. and Y.L.; validation: Y.Y., D.G., and S.W.; writing—original draft: J.W.; writing—review and editing: Y.Y., D.G., S.W. and Y.L.

References

1. Adravanti, P.; Tecame, A.; De Girolamo, L.; Ampollini, A.; Papalia, R. Patella Resurfacing in Total Knee Arthroplasty: A Series of 1280 Patients at Midterm Follow-Up. *J. Arthroplast.* **2018**, *33*, 696–699. [CrossRef] [PubMed]
2. Chonko, D.J.; Lombardi, A.V.; Berend, K.R. Patella baja and total knee arthroplasty (TKA): Etiology, diagnosis, and management. *Surg. Technol. Int.* **2004**, *12*, 231–238. [PubMed]
3. Ali, S.A.; Helmer, R.; Terk, M.R. Patella Alta: Lack of Correlation Between Patellotrochlear Cartilage Congruence and Commonly Used Patellar Height Ratios. *J. Am. Roentgenol.* **2009**, *193*, 1361–1366. [CrossRef] [PubMed]
4. Nakagawa, S.; Arai, Y.; Inoue, H.; Atsumi, S.; Ichimaru, S.; Ikoma, K.; Fujiwara, H.; Kubo, T. Two Patients with Osteochondral Injury of the Weight-Bearing Portion of the Lateral Femoral Condyle Associated with Lateral Dislocation of the Patella. *Case Rep. Orthop.* **2014**, *2014*, 876410. [CrossRef] [PubMed]
5. Chougule, S.S.; Stefanakis, G.; Stefan, S.C.; Rudra, S.; Tselentakis, G. Effects of fat pad excision on length of the patellar tendon after total knee replacement. *J. Orthop.* **2015**, *12*, 197–204. [CrossRef]
6. Weale, A.E.; Murray, D.W.; Newman, J.H.; Ackroyd, C.E. The length of the patellar tendon after unicompartmental and total knee replacement. *Bone Jt. J.* **1999**, *81*, 790–795. [CrossRef]
7. Davies, G.S.; Van Duren, B.; Shorthose, M.; Roberts, P.G.; Morley, J.R.; Monk, A.P. Changes in patella tendon length over 5 years after different types of knee arthroplasty. *Knee Surg. Sports Traumatol. Arthrosc.* **2016**, *24*, 3029–3035. [CrossRef]
8. FlORen, M.; Davis, J.; Peterson MG, E.; Laskin, R.S. A mini-midvastus capsular approach with patellar displacement decreases the prevalence of patella baja. *J. Arthroplast.* **2007**, *22*, 51–57. [CrossRef]
9. Meneghini, R.M.; Ritter, M.A.; Pierson, J.L.; Meding, J.B.; Berend, M.E.; Faris, P.M. The effect of the Insall-Salvati ratio on outcome after total knee arthroplasty. *J. Arthroplast.* **2006**, *21*, 116–120. [CrossRef]
10. Kazemi, S.M.; Daftari, B.L.; Eajazi, A.; Miniator Sajadi, M.R.; Okhovatpoor, M.A.; Farhang, Z.R. Pseudo-patella baja after total knee arthroplasty. *Med. Sci. Monit. Int. Med. J. Exp. Clin. Res.* **2011**, *17*, CR292. [CrossRef]
11. Krishnan, S.G.; Steadman, J.R.; Millett, P.J.; Hydeman, K.; Close, M. *Lysis of Pretibial Patellar Tendon Adhesions (Anterior Interval Release) to Treat Anterior Knee Pain After ACL Reconstruction*; Springer: London, UK, 2006.
12. Seo, J.G.; Moon, Y.W.; Kim, S.M.; Park, S.H.; Lee, B.H.; Chang, M.J.; Jo, B.C. Prevention of pseudo-patella baja during total knee arthroplasty. *Knee Surg. Sports Traumatol. Arthrosc.* **2015**, *23*, 3601–3606. [CrossRef] [PubMed]
13. Bugelli, G.; Ascione, F.; Cazzella, N.; Franceschetti, E.; Franceschi, F.; Dell'Osso, G.; Giannotti, S. Pseudo-patella baja: A minor yet frequent complication of total knee arthroplasty. *Knee Surg. Sports Traumatol. Arthrosc.* **2017**, *26*, 1831–1837. [CrossRef] [PubMed]
14. Wang, J.-P.; Qian, L.-W.; Wang, C.-T. Simulation of Geometric Anatomy Model of Human Knee Joint. *J. Syst. Simul.* **2009**, *21*, 2806–2809.
15. Matava, M.J.; Hutton, W.C. A biomechanical comparison between the central one-third patellar tendon and the residual tendon. *Br. J. Sports Med.* **1995**, *29*, 178–184. [CrossRef]
16. Mansson, O.; Sernert, N.; Rostgard-Christensen, L.; Kartus, J. Long-term clinical and radiographic results after delayed anterior cruciate ligament reconstruction in adolescents. *Am. J. Sports Med.* **2015**, *43*, 138–145. [CrossRef]
17. George, D.S.L.M.; Pampolha, A.G.M.; Orlando Junior, N. Functional results from reconstruction of the anterior cruciate ligament using the central third of the patellar ligament and flexor tendons. *Rev. Bras. Ortop. (Engl. Ed.)* **2015**, *50*, 705–711.
18. Haviv, B.; Yassin, M.; Rath, E.; Bronak, S. Prevalence and clinical implications of nerve injury during bone patellar tendon bone harvesting for anterior cruciate ligament reconstruction. *J. Orthop. Surg.* **2017**, *25*, 230949901668498. [CrossRef]

19. Wang, J.; Tao, K.; Li, H.; Wang, C. Modelling and analysis on biomechanical dynamic characteristics of knee flexion movement under squatting. *Sci. World J.* **2014**, *2014*, 321080.
20. Grood, E.S.; Suntay, W.J. A joint coordinate system for the clinical description of three-dimensional motions: Application to the knee. *J. Biomech. Eng.* **1983**, *105*, 136–144. [CrossRef]
21. Li, G.; Most, E.; Otterberg, E.; Sabbag, K.; Zayontz, S.; Johnson, T.; Rubash, H. Biomechanics of Posterior-Substituting Total Knee Arthroplasty: An In Vitro Study. *Clin. Orthop. Relat. Res.* **2002**, *404*, 214–225. [CrossRef]
22. Godest, A.C.; Beaugonin, M.; Haug, E.; Taylor, M. Simulation of a knee joint replacement during a gait cycle using explicit finite element analysis. *J. Biomech.* **2002**, *35*, 267–275. [CrossRef]
23. Taylor, M.; Barrett, D.S. Explicit finite element simulation of eccentric loading in total knee replacement. *Clin. Orthop. Relat. Rec* **2003**, *414*, 162–171. [CrossRef] [PubMed]
24. Pena, E.; Calvo, B.; Martinez, M.A.; Doblare, M. A three-dimensional finite element analysis of the combined behavior of ligaments and menisci in the healthy human knee joint. *J. Biomech.* **2006**, *39*, 1686–1701. [CrossRef] [PubMed]
25. Halloran, J.P.; Petrella, A.J.; Rullkoetter, P.J. Explicit finite element modeling of total knee replacement mechanics. *J. Biomech.* **2005**, *38*, 323–331. [CrossRef]
26. Bustince, H.; Fernandez, J.; Burillo, P. *Penalty Function in Optimization Problems: A Review of Recent Developments*; Springer: Cham, Switzerland, 2018.
27. Tang, T.S.; MacIntyre, N.J.; Gill, H.S.; Fellows, R.A.; Hill, N.A.; Wilson, D.R. Accurate assessment of patellar tracking using fiducial and intensity-based fluoroscopic techniques. *Med. Image Anal.* **2004**, *8*, 343–351. [CrossRef] [PubMed]
28. Fellows, R.A.; Hill, N.A.; Gill, H.S.; MacIntyre, N.J.; Harrison, M.M.; Ellis, R.E.; Wilson, D.R. Magnetic resonance imaging for in vivo assessment of three-dimensional patellar tracking. *J. Biomech.* **2005**, *38*, 1643–1652. [CrossRef]
29. Baldwin, M.A.; Clary, C.; Maletsky, L.P.; Rullkoetter, P.J. Verification of predicted specimen-specific natural and implanted patellofemoral kinematics during simulated deep knee bend. *J. Biomech.* **2009**, *42*, 2341–2348. [CrossRef]
30. Heegaard, J.; Leyvraz, P.F.; Curnier, A.; Rakotomanana, L.; Huiskes, R. The biomechanics of the human patella during passive knee flexion. *J. Biomech.* **1995**, *28*, 1265–1279. [CrossRef]
31. Azmy, C.; Guerard, S.; Bonnet, X.; Gabrielli, F.; Skalli, W. EOS (R) orthopaedic imaging system to study patellofemoral kinematics: Assessment of uncertainty. *Orthop. Traumatol. Surg. Res.* **2010**, *96*, 28–36. [CrossRef]
32. McWalter, E.J.; Hunter, D.J.; Wilson, D.R. The effect of load magnitude on three-dimensional patellar kinematics in vivo. *J. Biomech.* **2010**, *43*, 1890–1897. [CrossRef]
33. Amis, A.A.; Senavongse, W.; Bull, A.M.J. Patellofemoral kinematics during knee flexion-extension: An in vitro study. *J. Orthop. Res.* **2006**, *24*, 2201–2211. [CrossRef] [PubMed]
34. Testa, R. Knee rotational laxity and proprioceptive function 2A years after partial ACL reconstruction. *Knee Surg. Sports Traumatol. Arthrosc.* **2012**, *20*, 762–766.
35. Gokeler, A.; Benjaminse, A.; Hewett, T.E.; Lephart, S.M.; Engebretsen, L.; Ageberg, E.; Dijkstra, P.U. Proprioceptive deficits after ACL injury: Are they clinically relevant? *Br. J. Sports Med.* **2012**, *46*, 180–192. [CrossRef] [PubMed]
36. Smith, C.K.; Howell, S.M.; Hull, M.L. Anterior laxity, slippage, and recovery of function in the first year after tibialis allograft anterior cruciate ligament reconstruction. *Am. J. Sports Med.* **2011**, *39*, 78. [CrossRef]
37. Tianqu, H. Finite Element Analysis of the Influence of Femoral Tunnel Locating Points on the Isometricity of Grafts in Anterior Cruciate Ligament Reconstruction. Master's Thesis, Central South University, Changsha, China, 24 May 2014.
38. Laprade, C.M.; Civitarese, D.M.; Rasmussen, M.T.; Laprade, R.F. Emerging Updates on the Posterior Cruciate Ligament: A Review of the Current Literature. *Am. J. Sports Med.* **2015**, 0363546515572770. [CrossRef]
39. Narvy, S.J.; Pearl, M.; Vrla, M.; Yi, A.; Hatch, G.F.R. Anatomy of the Femoral Footprint of the Posterior Cruciate Ligament: A Systematic Review. *Arthrosc. J. Arthrosc. Relat. Surg.* **2015**, *31*, 345–354. [CrossRef]

40. Tucker, A.; Mcmahon, S.; Mcardle, B.; Rutherford, B.; Acton, D. Synthetic versus autologous reconstruction (Syn-VAR) of the medial patellofemoral ligament: A study protocol for a randomised controlled trial. *Trials* **2018**, *19*, 268. [CrossRef]
41. Balcarek, P.; Rehn, S.; Howells, N.R.; Eldridge, J.D.; Kita, K.; Dejour, D.; Friede, T. Results of medial patellofemoral ligament reconstruction compared with trochleoplasty plus individual extensor apparatus balancing in patellar instability caused by severe trochlear dysplasia: A systematic review and meta-analysis. *Knee Surg. Sports Traumatol. Arthrosc.* **2016**, *25*, 3869–3877. [CrossRef]

15

A Feasibility Study of a Novel Piezo MEMS Tweezer for Soft Materials Characterization

Fabio Botta *, Andrea Rossi and Nicola Pio Belfiore

Dipartimento di Ingegneria, Università degli Studi Roma Tre, Via della Vasca Navale, 79, 00146 Roma, Italy; andrea.rossi@uniroma3.it (A.R.); nicolapio.belfiore@uniroma3.it (N.P.B.)

* Correspondence: fabio.botta@uniroma3.it.

Abstract: The opportunity to know the status of a soft tissue (ST) in situ can be very useful for microsurgery or early diagnosis. Since normal and diseased tissues have different mechanical characteristics, many systems have been developed to carry out such measurements locally. Among them, MEMS tweezers are very relevant for their efficiency and relative simplicity compared to the other systems. In this paper a novel piezoelectric MEMS tweezer for soft materials analysis and characterization is presented. A theoretical approach has developed in order to carry out the values of the stiffness, the equivalent Young's modulus, and the viscous damping coefficients of the analyzed samples. The method has been validated by using both Finite Element Analysis and data from the literature.

Keywords: MEMS; tweezer; piezoelectric; soft tissue; microsurgery

---

1. Introduction

Early diagnosis is crucial to prevent disease progressions [1]. The correlation between the mechanical characteristics of a soft tissue and its status has been highlighted by several studies in many cell types like cancer cells, epithelial cells and laminopathies associated with diseases of the nuclear membrane [2]. In cancer cells, for example, the malignant transformation influences the mechanical properties by disruption and/or reorganization of cytoskeleton [3]. The stiffness, the elastic modulus, and the dynamic viscosity are among the most commonly used mechanical quantities to evaluate the state of a soft tissue. However the possibility to identify a diseased soft tissue in situ, at the microscale, can increase significantly the possibility of the cure.

Different techniques are used to perform such measurements as micropipette aspiration [4], magnetic bead twisting [5], atomic force microscopy [6], optical tweezers [7] or mechanical tweezers [8]. In recent years, researchers focused on the developing of micro-electro-mechanical systems (MEMS) tweezers because of their efficiency and relative simplicity with respect to other systems [9]. New gripping tweezers have been built taking cue from the kinematics of articulated mechanisms [10] as the property of parallelograms [11–15]. More complex motion, with an increasing of the number of degrees of freedom, can be obtained adopting the concept of lumped compliance. In fact, concentrated flexibility has been used in flexure hinges in several investigations [16–20]. In order to improve the displacement accuracy and to lower the stress levels in the flexible elements a new conjugate surfaces flexure hinge (CSFH) flexure has been proposed [21–25] and optimized [26,27]. The system has shown promising results in terms of of versatility and applicability to different types of tissue [28]. Thanks to their high level of miniaturization, MEMS-Technology based tweezers can be employed also in minimal invasive [29–31] or gastrointestinal surgery [32], and more generally speaking, in endoluminal surgery, for example, in TEM [33–35].

The actuation of the tweezer can be obtained by different systems, such as linear electrostatic actuators [36,37], rotatory electrostatic actuators [38,39] or electrothermal actuation [40–46]. However the advent of smart materials in the last decades has greatly increased the possibilities of development of new smart structures [47–49] with the ability, not possible for the traditional systems, to adapt to external conditions variations. Because of their speed of response, low power consumption and high operating bandwidth the piezoelectric materials are, among the smart materials, the most promising ones for active vibration control [50–53] and MEMS applications [54]. However the research in the latter field mainly focuses on the energy harvesting [55–58] or MEMS tweezers for manipulating micro-objects and microassembly [59–61].

This paper presents the design of a novel piezoMEMS tweezer for the analysis and characterization of soft materials. Each jaw can be built as a sandwich composite beam and activated by an electric field.

The tweezer is supposed to be force controlled because the piezoelectric materials produce a stress proportional to the applied electrical field. Furthermore, a sensor is supposed to be integrated into the structure for displacement control. This gives rise to improve the analysis of the cell properties. In fact, the displacement-controlled actuator is able to identify the beginning of a rupture during straining or softening, while a force-controlled system maintains a constant force regardless of the required displacement [62]. The action of the piezoelectric material has been modeled by the Pin Force Model [63].

By applying symmetric electric fields to the composite jaws, they will bend in opposite directions allowing the gripping of the soft tissue.

A new mathematical model to measure the stiffness, the equivalent Young's modulus, and the viscous damping coefficient of the soft tissue has been developed. The model has been tested on three different soft test specimens and the results were in good agreement with those obtained by COMSOL finite elements code.

2. The Adopted Piezo-Mems Microgripper

The purpose of this paper is to develop a theoretical model of a piezo-MEMS microgripper, which can be used to characterize a grasped sample tissue. Therefore, the actual fabrication process of this instrument will not be herein considered. However, for the sake of completeness, a selection of possible materials and technological processes is briefly recalled.

In the last decades, several actuation methods have been proposed to induce motion in MEMS devices such as electrostatic, thermal and piezoelectric. The electrostatic devices are widely adopted but the piezoelectric MEMS's offer some attractive advantages: lower power consumption, broader bandwidth and approximately ten times lower voltages to obtain the same given displacement [64]. Furthermore the piezoelectric materials can be manufactured using the same MEMS conventional technologies and for this reason these materials have been preferred to develop piezo-MEMS devices in the last decades. Typical applications include vibration energy harvesters [65,66], resonators [67], capacitors [68], micro sensors/actuators [69,70], micromachined ultrasonic transducer [71], gyroscopic sensors [72], microlens [73,74], 1D and 2D micro-scanners [75,76].

The piezoelectric materials can be gathered into two groups: ferroelectric (lead zirconate titanate, PZT compounds) and non-ferroelectric (ZnO and AlN). The piezoelectric characteristics (piezoelectric coefficient, Q factor, dielectric constant, etc.) rely on the crystalline structure. In fact ZnO and AlN thin-films show wurtzite structure that entails lower piezoelectricity if compared to PZT materials (perovskite structure). Nevertheless ZnO and AlN exhibit large mechanical stiffness, high Q factor and do not require a polarization process so they can be attractive for sensors applications. PZT thin-films provide high piezoelectric properties, lower cost and stability against temperature but require a poling process before using the piezo-MEMS device [77]. The electric field poling direction depends on the functional configuration of the piezo-MEMS.

Usually the piezoelectric MEMS actuators/sensors are based on cantilever structures and the number of active layers identifies their working configuration:

- unimorph (one piezoelectric layer coupled with an inactive structural layer) or
- bimorph (a structural layer sandwiched by two active layers).

When a PZT bimorph bending beam and the transverse piezoelectric effect (d_{31}) are considered, the PZT layers must be poled in opposite directions in order to maximize the bending action. Then the electrodes of the PZT layers in contact with the structural layer share the same electric potential, whereas the outer electrodes share the same opposite sign potential (see Section 3). The design and fabrication process of piezo-MEMS devices have been extensively explored for the above mentioned unimorph and bimorph cantilever configurations using the aforementioned materials:

- AlN [67,68,71];
- ZnO [70]; and
- PZT [66,69,75,78].

Various technologies can be applied to deposit piezoelectric thin-films such as

- pulsed laser deposition (PLD);
- chemical vapour deposition (CVD);
- screen printing;
- sol-gel and
- radio frequency sputtering.

Usually the sol-gel and sputtering methods are the preferred ones both for research and commercial production because they allow the piezoelectric thin-film to be homogeneously deposited on large Si wafers [79]. The beam structural layer can be metal-based or silicon-based and the etching processes could be accomplished relying on conventional techniques (RIE, D-RIE, ECR).

A schematic view of the target piezo-MEMS tweezer is qualitatively depicted in Figure 1. The system can be obtained by using a multilayer wafer that can be built by using the above mentioned techniques. At the end of the process, the whole microsystem is composed of two bimorph beams (**a**)-(**b**)-(**c**) (see Figure 1). The two bimorph beams are supported by the handle layer (**d**). The specific steps of the process (deposition, etching, exposure, etc.) will depend on the peculiar materials and technology selected for the construction. In the case under study, the system is conceived in such a way that the mask geometry could be quite elementary for any etching step.

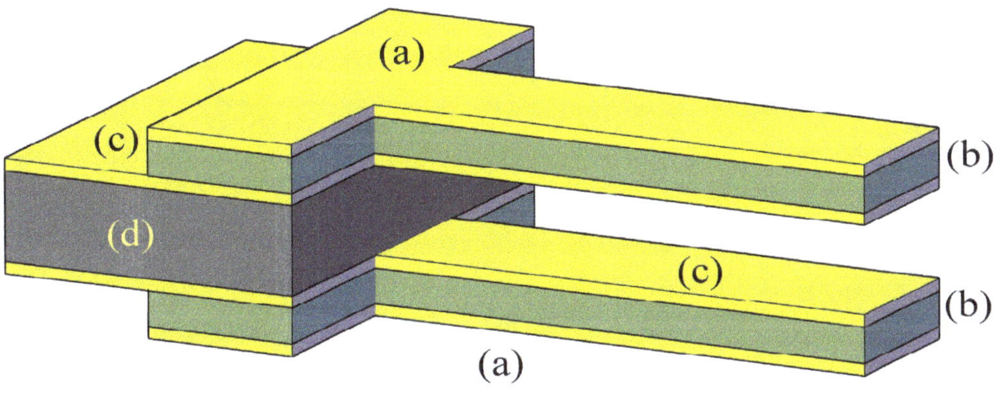

Figure 1. A schematic view of the microsystem: outer layers with a same voltage V_0 (**a**); structural material for the beams (**b**); internal layers with voltage V_i (**c**) and structural layer for the handle (**d**).

Another possible layout is represented in Figure 2, where two new layers (**e**) have been added with respect to the previous example of fabrication. Layers (**a**), (**b**), (**c**), and (**d**) have the same function as described for the previous layout. The second design is better for the operational aspects because a clamping tooth has been added for each jaw. However, these two teeth are more difficult to obtain during the process because they require at least two more deposition layers (**e**) and also a more complex series of intermediate etching-deposition steps that depend on the selected materials.

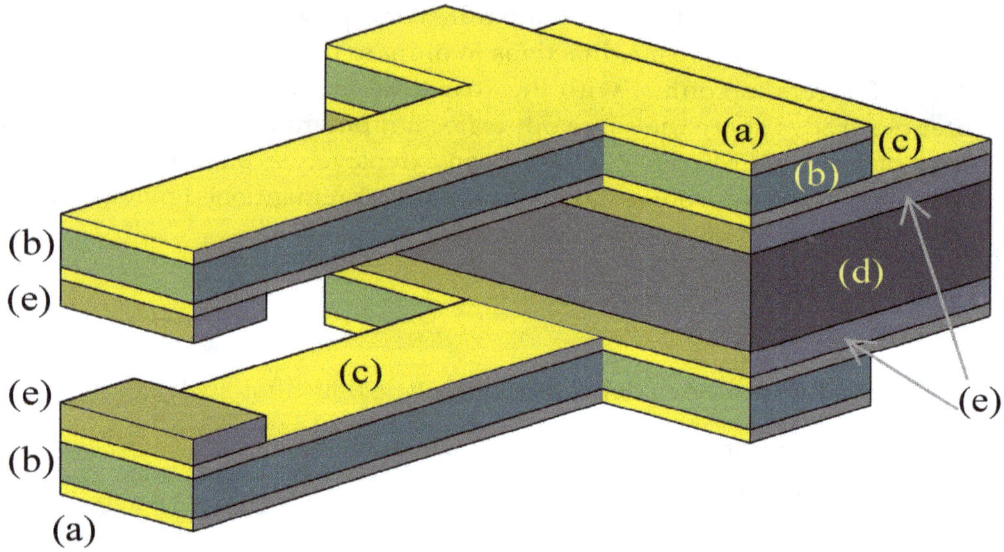

Figure 2. An alternative layout for the microgripper: outer layers with a same voltage V_0 (**a**); structural material for the beams (**b**); internal layers with voltage V_i (**c**) and structural layer for the handle (**d**).

3. Modeling Piezoelectric Actions on the Microbeams

Concerning the piezoelectric actions, many studies [63,80–82] have confirmed that, under certain assumptions (piezoelectric plates are perfectly bonded to the structure, the ratio between their thickness and the thickness of the beam is very low and their inertia and mass negligible with respect to those of the beam) the stresses applied to the beam can be considered as they were concentrated at the piezoelectric plate ends. Moreover, if the electric field to the upper plate is opposite in sign to the one applied to the lower plate, such action is equivalent to a flexural moment (see Figure 3) applied to the end of the beam of magnitude equal to:

$$M_a(t) = \frac{\psi}{6+\psi} E_a c T_a T_b \Lambda(t) \tag{1}$$

with

$$\begin{cases} \Lambda(t) = \frac{d_{31}}{T_a} V(t) \\ \psi = \frac{E_b T_b}{E_a T_a} \end{cases} \tag{2}$$

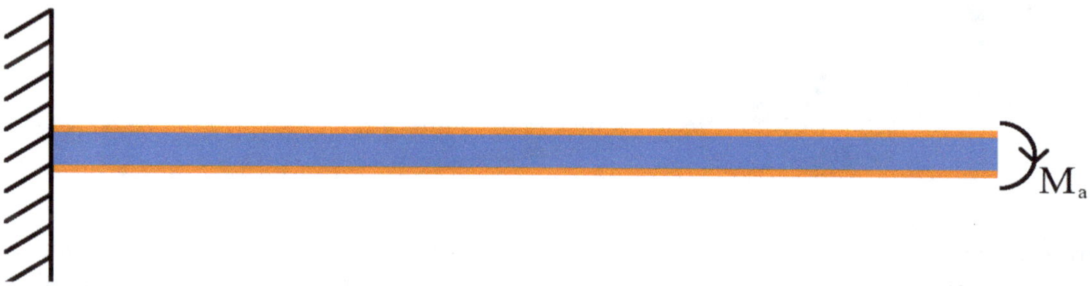

Figure 3. Piezoelectric action (PIN force model).

By activating the piezoelectric plates pairs on the two jaws-beams of the tweezer in opposite manner the two moments M_a will have opposite sign and the beams will bend in opposite direction allowing the gripper to grasp the soft tissue, as depicted in Figure 4.

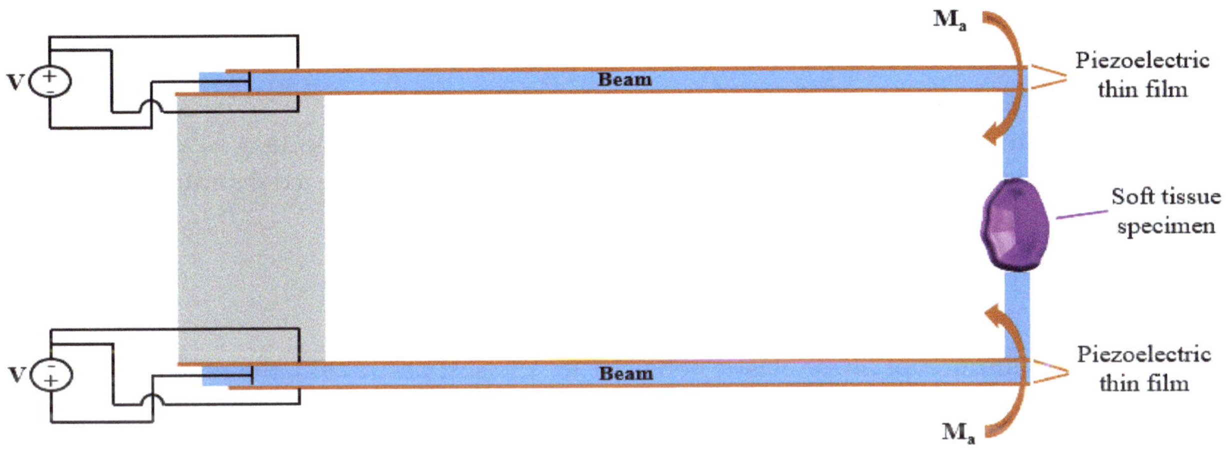

Figure 4. PiezoMEMS grip of the soft tissue.

3.1. Static Model

The value of the stiffness K_{ST} and of the equivalent Young's modulus E_{ST} can be established by a static test with a constant voltage V_0 applied to the piezoelectric plates: $V(t) = V_0$. In this case, the bending of the beams will cause the compression of the soft tissue and consequently a reaction force F_{ST} will be applied from the soft tissue to the beams, through the clamp teeth (see Figure 5).

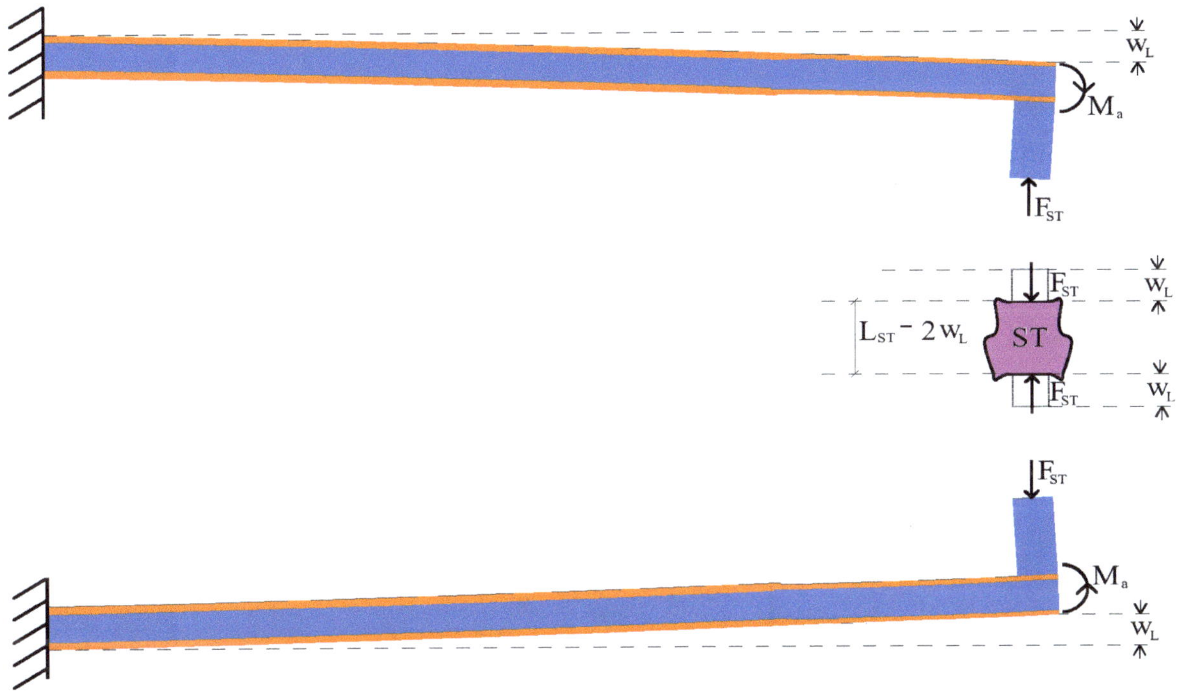

Figure 5. Scheme for the calculation of the tip displacement.

Considering that the Euler Bernoulli model is appropriate for the present case because of the high length-to-thickness aspect ratio of the beams, the tip deflection:

$$w_L = \frac{M_a L^2}{2E_b I_b} - \frac{F_{ST} L^3}{3E_b I_b}, \tag{3}$$

is due to a combination of the loads F_{ST} and M_a. Therefore, the first load

$$F_{ST} = \frac{3E_b I_b}{L^3}\left(\frac{M_a L^2}{2E_b I_b} - w_L\right) \tag{4}$$

can be obtained by measuring w_L.

Due to the high value of the axial stiffness of the clamp teeth, the deflection w_L can be considered equal to the axial displacement of the soft tissue (see Figure 5) so that the axial strain

$$\epsilon_{ST} = \frac{2w_L}{L_{ST}} \tag{5}$$

is calculated.

Under the assumption of linear elastic behavior for the soft tissue (ST), the relationship between the normal stress σ_{ST} applied to the cross section of the soft tissue and ϵ_{ST} can be written as:

$$\sigma_{ST} = \frac{F_{ST}}{S_{ST}} = E_{ST}\frac{2w_L}{L_{ST}} \tag{6}$$

from which the equivalent Young's modulus

$$E_{ST} = \frac{F_{ST} L_{ST}}{2S_{ST} w_L} \tag{7}$$

is evaluated. Moreover, the stiffness

$$K_{ST} = \frac{2E_{ST} S_{ST}}{L_{ST}} \tag{8}$$

is calculated given the dimensions of the ST sample.

3.2. Dynamics Model

To determine the value of the viscous damping C_{ST}, a dynamic test has been conceived by applying a variable harmonic excitation voltage $V(t) = V_0 sin(\omega t)$.

By referring to δL_{int}, δL_{in}, δL_a and δL_{ST} as the virtual works of internal, inertial, actuator and ST forces, respectively, and to δL_{in_m} as the virtual work of the inertial forces of the clamp teeth, the virtual work principle can be written as:

$$\delta L_{int} = \delta L_{in} + \delta L_a + \delta L_{in_m} + \delta L_{ST} \tag{9}$$

where (the quantities over signed by a tilde are virtual quantities):

$$\begin{cases} \delta L_{int} = E_b I_b \int_0^L \frac{\partial^2 w}{\partial x^2}\frac{\partial^2 \widetilde{w}}{\partial x^2} dx \\ \delta L_{in} = -\rho S \int_0^L \frac{\partial^2 w}{\partial t^2}\ \widetilde{w}\ dx \\ \delta L_a = M_a \frac{\partial \widetilde{w}}{\partial x}\Big|_{x=L} \\ \delta L_{in_m} = -m \frac{\partial^2 w_L}{\partial t^2}\ \widetilde{w}_L \\ \delta L_{ST} = F_{ST}\ \widetilde{w}_L \end{cases} \tag{10}$$

with (see Figure 6):

$$F_{ST} = K_{ST} w_L + C_{ST}\ \dot{w}_L \tag{11}$$

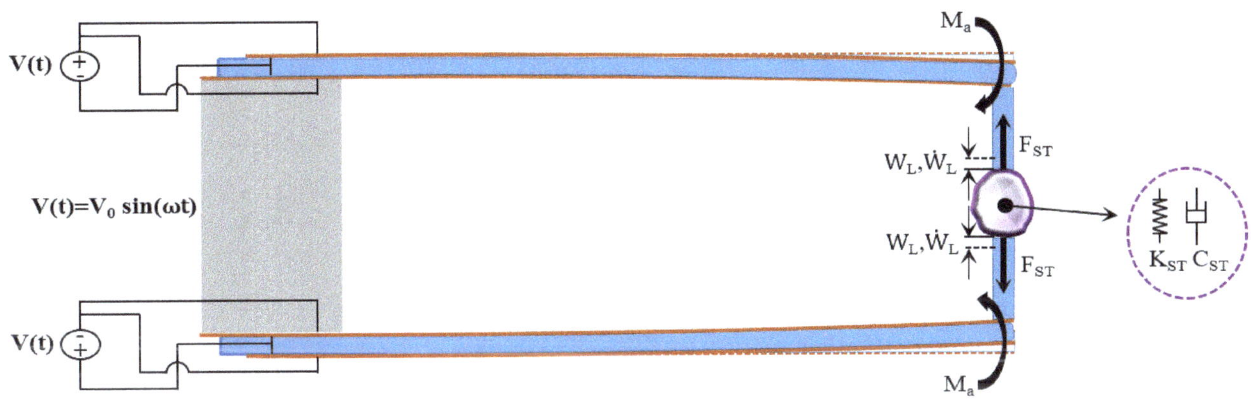

Figure 6. Scheme for the calculation of the stiffness and viscous damping of the soft tissue.

The viscous damping coefficient C_{ST} can be identified by measuring the amplitude $|w_L|$ in correspondence of the i-th vibration mode of the structure that has been excited by means of the piezoelectric elements, where the flexural modes of the beams are obtained as

$$\varphi(x) = B_1 \sin(\lambda x) + B_2 \cos(\lambda x) + B_3 \sinh(\lambda x) + B_4 \cosh(\lambda x) \tag{12}$$

with

$$\begin{cases} \varphi(0) = 0 \\ \left.\frac{\partial\varphi(x)}{\partial x}\right|_{x=0} = 0 \\ \left.\frac{\partial^2\varphi(x)}{\partial x^2}\right|_{x=L} = 0 \\ EI\left.\frac{\partial^3\varphi(x)}{\partial x^3}\right|_{x=L} = K_{ST}\varphi(L) - \omega^2 m\varphi(L) \end{cases} \tag{13}$$

By substituting Equation (12) in (13), a system of four equations in four unknowns (B_1, B_2, B_3, B_4) is obtained. The eigenfrequencies are obtained setting to zero the determinant of the matrix coefficient (with $\omega^2 = \lambda^4 \frac{EI}{\rho S}$) and then the eigenmodes can be calculated.

The i-th flexural mode can be excited by applying a potential function

$$V(t) = V_0 \sin(\omega_i t) \tag{14}$$

where $\varphi_i(x)$ and ω_i are the i-th flexural mode and its related frequency, respectively. In these conditions the displacement $w(x,t)$ and the virtual displacement $\tilde{w}(x,t)$ can be written as:

$$\begin{cases} w(x,t) = A_i(t)\varphi_i(x) \\ \tilde{w}\ (x,t) = \varphi_i(x) \end{cases} \tag{15}$$

By substituting Equations (15) and (10) in (9), the following equation is obtained:

$$\begin{aligned} E_b I_b A_i(t) \int_0^L \frac{\partial^2\varphi_i(x)}{\partial x^2}^2 dx = -\rho S\ \ddot{A}_i\ (t) \int_0^L \varphi_i(x)^2 dx - m\ \ddot{A_i}(t)\ \varphi_i(L)^2 + \\ + M_a \left.\frac{\partial\varphi_i(x)}{\partial x}\right|_{x=L} - K_{ST} A_i(t)\varphi_i(L)^2 - C_{ST}\ \dot{A_i}(t)\ \varphi_i(L)^2 \end{aligned} \tag{16}$$

assuming (see Equation (1)):

$$\begin{cases} M = \rho S \int_0^L \varphi_i(x)^2 dx + m\varphi_i(L)^2 \\ C = C_{ST}\varphi_i(L)^2 \\ K = E_b I_b \int_0^L \frac{\partial^2 \varphi_i(x)}{\partial x^2}^2 dx + K_{ST}\varphi_i(L)^2 \\ Q = \frac{\psi}{6+\psi} E_a c T_b d_{31} \left. \frac{\partial \varphi_i(x)}{\partial x} \right|_{x=L} V_0 \end{cases} \tag{17}$$

and therefore Equation (16) becomes:

$$M\ddot{A}_i(t) + C\,\dot{A}_i\,(t) + KA_i(t) = Q\sin(\omega_i t) \tag{18}$$

By neglecting the transient part (see Equation (15.1)), the amplitude of the free end displacement is:

$$\left|w_L\right| = A_{i_f}\varphi_i(L) \tag{19}$$

where

$$A_{i_f} = \frac{Q}{C\omega_i}. \tag{20}$$

Finally, the damping coefficient of the soft tissue

$$C_{ST} = \frac{Q}{\left|w_L\right|\omega_i\varphi_i(L)} \tag{21}$$

can be found from Equation (17.2).

4. Results and Discussion

To validate the proposed model, numerical simulations have been done. The dimensions and the material characteristics are summarized in Table 1:

Table 1. Beams, piezoelectric plates and end masses specifications; lengths are expressed in μm.

	Material	Length	Thickness	Width	Young's mod. [GPa]	Density $[\mathrm{kg/m^3}]$
Beams	Silicon	750	2	80	170	2329
Piezoel. pl.	AlN	750	$2 * 10^{-2}$	80	350	3300
Clamp teeth	Silicon	36	7.5	80	170	2329

In this work, the FEM results have been chosen as the reference values. Three typical soft tissues (liver, muscle and uterus) of known characteristics [83], have been considered. The value of the beam tip displacement, obtained by the FEM simulations, has been included in the mathematical model to calculate the equivalent Young's modulus and the viscous damping coefficient. The ST sample stiffness can be calculated by means of Equation (8). The values of the Young's modulus and the viscous coefficients reported in the literature have been compared with the ones calculated by the new method. Because of the symmetry of the structure with respect to its mid-plane (see Figure 7) only the upper part has been considered in the simulations.

In Table 2 the results of the static simulations, obtained by the above described procedure, have been reported. It is possible to observe that the model results are in good agreement with the real values with a percentage error less than 6% in all the cases.

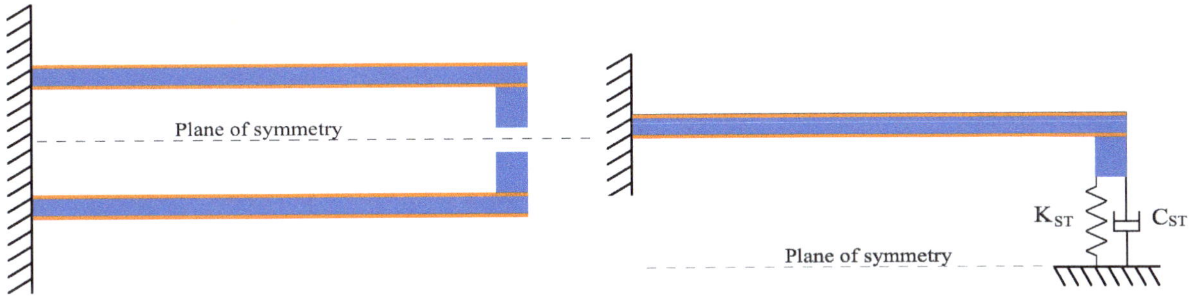

Figure 7. Scheme used for the simulations.

Table 2. Comparison between the actual Young's modules and those obtained by the model; E_{mm} is the Young's modulus obtained by the mathematical model.

	E [kPa]	E_{mm} [kPa]	*Err* %
Liver	10	9.47	5.3%
Muscle	20	19.43	2.8%
Uterus	30	29.64	1.2 %

To obtain the viscous damping coefficient, dynamics simulations are necessary. As described above, the chosen strategy consists in exciting, by the piezoelectric plates, the *i*-th mode of the structure, in order to obtain the amplitude of the free end displacement $|w_L|$ and then in including this in the model.

A comparison between the eigenfrequencies obtained by the COMSOL FEM code and the proposed model is reported in Table 3.

Table 3. Comparison between the eigenfrequencies obtained by the COMSOL FEM code and the proposed model.

	Liver		
	FEM	***Model***	***Err%***
$f_1[Hz]$	15,523.50	15,856.40	2.14%
$f_2[Hz]$	30,701.40	29,487.60	3.95%
$f_3[Hz]$	82,116.70	75,668.50	7.85%
$f_4[Hz]$	162,877.10	151,620.00	6.91%
	Muscle		
	FEM	***Model***	***Err%***
$f_1[Hz]$	18,768.20	18,686.20	0.44%
$f_2[Hz]$	35,437.60	34,681.70	2.13%
$f_3[Hz]$	82,674.80	76,297.90	7.71%
$f_4[Hz]$	162,995.20	151,781	6.88%
	Uterus		
	FEM	***Model***	***Err%***
$f_1[Hz]$	20,066.80	19,721.70	1.72%
$f_2[Hz]$	40,190.2	39,660.70	1.32%
$f_3[Hz]$	83,255.70	77,038.00	7.47%
$f_4[Hz]$	163,118.00	151,949.00	6.85%

In the FEM simulations the first mode has been chosen to excite the structure with the values of the electrical potential reported in Table 4.

Table 4. Electrical potential used for the simulations.

	$V_0[V]$
Liver	8
Muscle	5
Uterus	5

By neglecting the initial transient part, the axial displacements for the various soft tissues have been reported in Figure 8.

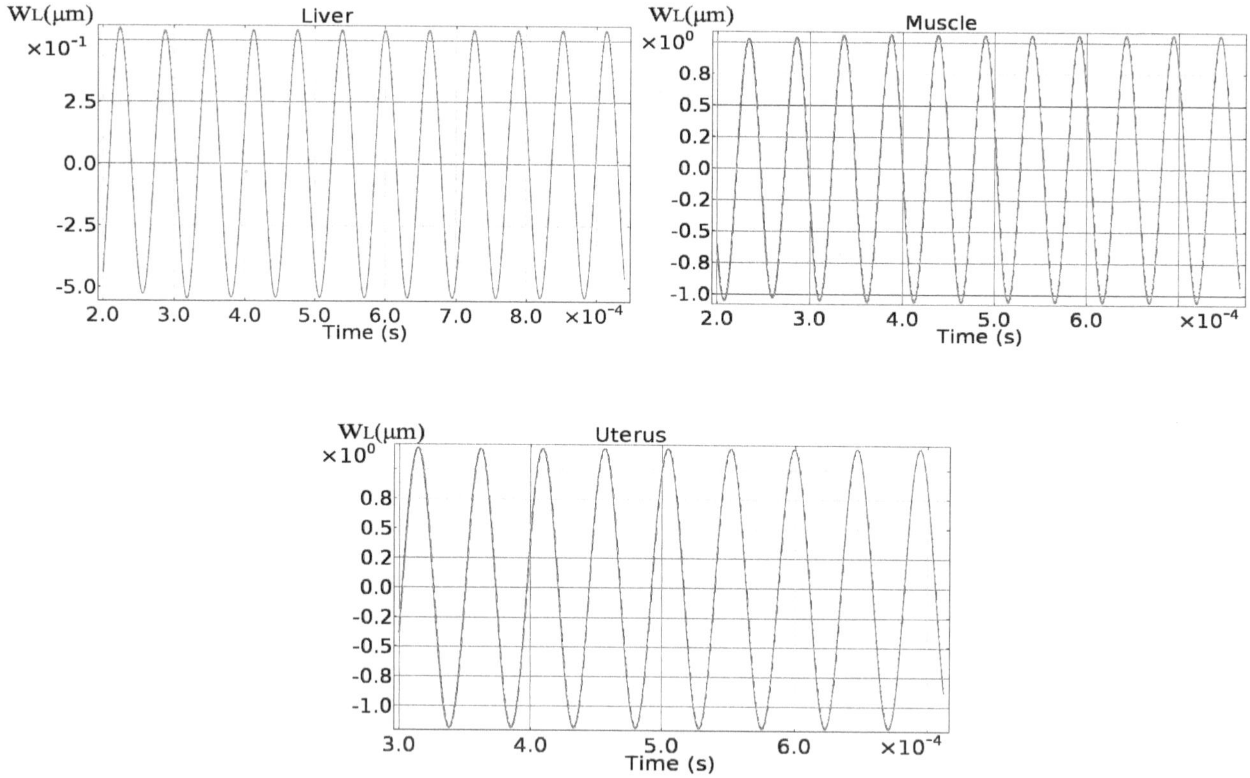

Figure 8. Axial displacement for the various soft tissues.

Finally, the comparison between the actual viscous damping coefficients and those obtained by the model results have been highlighted in Table 5.

Table 5. Comparison between the effective viscous damping and those obtained by the model.

	$C[Ns/m]$	$C_{mm}[Ns/m]$	$Err\%$
Liver	$3.07 * 10^{-5}$	$2.94 * 10^{-5}$	4.2%
Muscle	$5.09 * 10^{-5}$	$4.98 * 10^{-5}$	2.2%
Uterus	$7.14 * 10^{-5}$	$7.26 * 10^{-5}$	1.7%

A good agreement between the relative coefficients is also observed with a percentage error always less than 5%.

5. Conclusions

In this paper a novel piezo MEMS tweezer for soft materials characterization has been proposed. The tweezer mechanical structure is compatible with the known fabrication processes. A new mathematical model to calculate the stiffness, the equivalent Young's modulus and the viscous damping coefficient of the soft tissues is suggested. The method has been tested by comparing its results with Finite Element

Analysis based on experimental data from the literature. The two sets of data are in good agreement with a difference less than 6% in all the considered cases.

Author Contributions: F.B. has designed and developed the mathematical model. A.R. and F.B. carried out the numerical simulations. N.P.B. has reviewed the theoretical approach and the compatibility of the structure with some technological fabrication process.

Abbreviations

The following abbreviations are used in this manuscript:

C	damping coefficient
C_{ST}	damping coefficient of the soft tissue
d_{31}	piezoelectric coefficient
E_a	Young's modulus of the piezoelectric material
E_b	Young's modulus of the beam
E_{ST}	equivalent Young's modulus of the soft tissue
F_{ST}	force applied from the soft tissue to the tweezers
I_b	inertia moment of the beam
K	stiffness coefficient
K_{ST}	stiffness coefficient of the soft tissue
L	beam length
m	mass applied at the end of the tweezer
M_a	piezoelectric bending moment
M	mass coefficient
S_{ST}	cross-sectional area of the soft tissue
ST	soft tissue
T_a	piezoelectric thickness
T_b	beam thickness
V	electric potential applied to the piezoelectric plates
w	transverse displacement
w_L	transverse displacement of the free end
$\tilde{w}$	virtual transverse displacement
$\phi_i(x)$	i-th flexural mode of the beam
ρ	mass density of the beam
ω_i	natural frequency of the i-th flexural mode

References

1. Tang, M.; Xia, L.; Wei, D.; Yan, S.; Du, C.; Cui, H.L. Distinguishing Different Cancerous Human Cells by Raman Spectroscopy Based on Discriminant Analysis Methods. *Appl. Sci.* **2017**, *7*, 900. [CrossRef]
2. Rianna, C.; Radmacher, M. Comparison of viscoelastic properties of cancer and normal thyroid cells on different stiffness substrates. *Eur. Biophys. J.* **2017**, *46*, 309–324. [CrossRef] [PubMed]
3. Lekka, M.; Gil, D.; Pogoda, K.; Dulińska-Litewka, J.; Jach, R.; Gostek, J.; Klymenko, O.; Prauzner-Bechcicki, S.; Stachura, Z.; Wiltowska-Zuber, J.; et al. Cancer cell detection in tissue sections using AFM. *Arch. Biochem. Biophys.* **2012**, *518*, 151–156. [CrossRef] [PubMed]
4. Discher, D.E.; Boal, D.H.; Boey, S.K. Simulations of the erythrocyte cytoskeleton at large deformation. II. Micropipette aspiration. *Biophys. J.* **1998**, *75*, 1584–1597. [CrossRef]
5. Bausch, A.R.; Ziemann, F.; Boulbitch, A.A.; Jacobson, K.; Sackmann, E. Local measurements of viscoelastic parameters of adherent cell surfaces by magnetic bead microrheometry. *Biophys. J.* **1998**, *75*, 2038–2049. [CrossRef]
6. Weisenhorn, A.L.; Khorsandi, M.; Kasas, S.; Gotzos, V.; Butt, H.J. Deformation and height anomaly of soft surfaces studied with an AFM. *Nanotechnology* **1993**, *4*, 106. [CrossRef]
7. Guck, J.; Ananthakrishnan, R.; Cunningham, C.C.; Käs, J. Stretching biological cells with light. *J. Phys. Condens. Matter* **2002**, *14*, 4843. [CrossRef]

8. Adldoost, H.; Jouibary, B.R.; Zabihollah, A. Design of SMA micro-gripper for minimally invasive surgery. In Proceedings of the 2012 19th Iranian Conference of Biomedical Engineering, Tehran, Iran, 20–21 December 2012.
9. Botta, F.; Verotti, M.; Bagolini, A.; Bellutti, P.; Belfiore, N.P. Mechanical response of four-bar linkage microgrippers with bidirectional electrostatic actuation. *Actuators* **2018**, *7*, 78. [CrossRef]
10. Tsai, Y.C.; Lei, S.H.; Sudin, H. Design and analysis of planar compliant microgripper based on kinematic approach. *J. Micromech. Microeng.* **2004**, *15*, 143. . [CrossRef]
11. Wierzbicki, R.; Adda, C.; Hotzendorfer, H. Electrostatic silicon microgripper with low voltage of actuation. In Proceedings of the 2007 International Symposium on Micro-NanoMechatronics and Human Science, Nagoya, Japan, 11–14 November 2007.
12. Hamedi, M.; Salimi, P.; Vismeh, M. Simulation and experimental investigation of a novel electrostatic microgripper system. *Microelectron. Eng.* **2012**, *98*, 467–471. [CrossRef]
13. Piriyanont, B.; Moheimani, S.R.; Bazaei, A. Design and control of a MEMS micro-gripper with integrated electro-thermal force sensor. In Proceedings of the 2013 Australian Control Conference, Fremantle, WA, Australia, 4–5 November 2013.
14. Wierzbicki, R.; Houston, K.; Heerlein, H.; Barth, W.; Debski, T.; Eisinberg, A.; Dario, P. Design and fabrication of an electrostatically driven microgripper for blood vessel manipulation. *Microelectron. Eng.* **2006**, *83*, 1651–1654. [CrossRef]
15. Zhang, Y.; Chen, B.K.; Liu, X.; Sun, Y. Autonomous robotic pick-and-place of microobjects. *IEEE Trans. Robot.* **2010**, *26*, 200–207. [CrossRef]
16. Scalari, G.; Eisinberg, A.; Mazzoni, M.; Menciassi, A.; Dario, P. A sensorized μelectro discharge machined superelastic alloy microgripper for micromanipulation. In Proceedings of the IEEE/RSJ International Conference on Intelligent Robots and Systems, Lausanne, Switzerland, 30 September–4 October 2002; pp. 1591–1595.
17. Greminger, M.A.; Sezen, A.S.; Nelson, B.J. A four degree of freedom MEMS microgripper with novel bi-directional thermal actuators. In Proceedings of the 2005 IEEE/RSJ International Conference on Intelligent Robots and Systems, Edmonton, AB, Canada, 2–6 August 2005.
18. Chang, R.J.; Chen, C.C. Using microgripper for adhesive bonding in automatic microassembly system. In Proceedings of the International Conference on Mechatronics and Automation, Harbin, China, 5–8 August 2007.
19. Chronis, N.; Lee, L.P. Polymer MEMS-based microgripper for single cell manipulation. In Proceedings of the 17th IEEE International Conference on Micro Electro Mechanical Systems. Maastricht MEMS 2004 Technical Digest, Maastricht, The Netherlands, 25–29 January 2004.
20. Sun, X.; Chen, W.; Fatikow, S.; Tian, Y.; Zhou, R.; Zhang, J.; Mikczinski, M. A novel piezo-driven microgripper with a large jaw displacement. *Microsyst. Technol.* **2015**, *21*, 931–942. [CrossRef]
21. Belfiore, N.P.; Broggiato, G.B.; Verotti, M.; Balucani, M.; Crescenzi, R.; Bagolini, A.; Bellutti, P.; Boscardin, M. Simulation and construction of a mems CSFH based microgripper. *Int. J. Mech. Control* **2015**, *16*, 21–30.
22. Verotti, M.; Crescenzi, R.; Balucani, M.; Belfiore, N.P. MEMS-based conjugate surfaces flexure hinge. *J. Mech. Des.* **2015**, *137*, 012301. [CrossRef]
23. Cecchi, R.; Verotti, M.; Capata, R.; Dochshanov, A.; Broggiato, G.; Crescenzi, R.; Balucani, M.; Natali, S.; Razzano, G.; Lucchese, F.; et al. Development of micro-grippers for tissue and cell manipulation with direct morphological comparison. *Micromachines* **2015**, *6*, 1710–1728. [CrossRef]
24. Verotti, M.; Dochshanov, A.; Belfiore, N.P. Compliance Synthesis of CSFH MEMS-Based Microgrippers. *J. Mech. Des.* **2017**, *139*. [CrossRef]
25. Crescenzi, R.; Balucani, M.; Belfiore, N.P. Operational characterization of CSFH MEMS technology based hinges. *J. Micromech. Microeng.* **2018**, *28*, 055012. [CrossRef]
26. Verotti, M. Analysis of the center of rotation in primitive flexures: Uniform cantilever beams with constant curvature. *Mech. Mach. Theory* **2016**, *97*, 29–50. [CrossRef]
27. Verotti, M. Effect of initial curvature in uniform flexures on position accuracy. *Mech. Mach. Theory* **2018**, *119*, 106–118. [CrossRef]
28. Di Giamberardino, P.; Bagolini, A.; Bellutti, P.; Rudas, I.; Verotti, M.; Botta, F.; Belfiore, N.P. New MEMS tweezers for the viscoelastic characterization of soft materials at the microscale. *Micromachines* **2018**, *9*, 15. [CrossRef] [PubMed]

29. Ursi, P.; Santoro, A.; Gemini, A.; Arezzo, A.; Pironi, D.; Renzi, C.; Cirocchi, R.; Di Matteo, F.; Maturo, A.; D'Andrea, V.; et al. Comparison of outcomes following intersphincteric resection vs low anterior resection for low rectal cancer: A systematic review. *G. Di Chir.* **2018**, *39*, 123–142.
30. Balla, A.; Quaresima, S.; Ursi, P.; Seitaj, A.; Palmieri, L.; Badiali, D.; Paganini, A.M. Hiatoplasty with crura buttressing versus hiatoplasty alone during laparoscopic sleeve gastrectomy. *Gastroenterol. Res. Pract.* **2017**, *2017*. [CrossRef] [PubMed]
31. Cochetti, G.; Del Zingaro, M.; Boni, A.; Cocca, D.; Panciarola, M.; Tiezzi, A.; Gaudio, G.; Balzarini, F.; Ursi, P.; Mearini, E. Colovesical fistula: Review on conservative management, surgical techniques and minimally invasive approaches. *G. Di Chir.* **2018**, *39*, 195–207.
32. Popivanov, G.; Tabakov, M.; Mantese, G.; Cirocchi, R.; Piccinini, I.; D'Andrea, V.; Covarelli, P.; Boselli, C.; Barberini, F.; Tabola, R.; et al. Surgical treatment of gastrointestinal stromal tumors of the duodenum: A literature review. *Transl. Gastroenterol. Hepatol.* **2018**, *3*. [CrossRef] [PubMed]
33. Paci, M.; Scoglio, D.; Ursi, P.; Barchetti, L.; Fabiani, B.; Ascoli, G.; Lezoche, G. Transanal Endocopic Microsurgery (TEM) in advanced rectal cancer disease treatment [Il ruolo della TEM nel trattamento dei tumori del retto extraperitoneale]. *Ann. Ital. Di Chir.* **2010**, *81*, 269–274.
34. Quaresima, S.; Balla, A.; Dambrosio, G.; Bruzzone, P.; Ursi, P.; Lezoche, E.; Paganini, A.M. Endoluminal loco-regional resection by TEM after R1 endoscopic removal or recurrence of rectal tumors. *Minim. Invasive Ther. Allied Technol.* **2016**, *25*, 134–140. [CrossRef]
35. Lezoche, E.; Fabiani, B.; D'Ambrosio, G.; Ursi, P.; Balla, A.; Lezoche, G.; Monteleone, F.; Paganini, A.M. Nucleotide-guided mesorectal excision combined with endoluminal locoregional resection by transanal endoscopic microsurgery in the treatment of rectal tumors: Technique and preliminary results. *Surg. Endosc.* **2013**, *27*, 4136–4141. [CrossRef]
36. Legtenberg, R.; Groeneveld, A.W.; Elwenspoek, M. Comb-drive actuators for large displacements. *J. Micromech. Microeng.* **1996**, *6*, 320. [CrossRef]
37. Chen, T.; Sun, L.; Chen, L.; Rong, W.; Li, X. A hybrid-type electrostatically driven microgripper with an integrated vacuum tool. *Sens. Actuators A Phys.* **2010**, *158*, 320–327. [CrossRef]
38. Yeh, J.A.; Chen, C.N.; Lui, Y.S. Large rotation actuated by in-plane rotary comb-drives with serpentine spring suspension. *J. Micromech. Microeng.* **2004**, *15*, 201. [CrossRef]
39. Yeh, J.A.; Jiang, S.S.; Lee, C. MOEMS variable optical attenuators using rotary comb drive actuators. *IEEE Photonics Technol. Lett.* **2006**, *18*, 1170–1172. [CrossRef]
40. Kim, K.; Liu, X.; Zhang, Y.; Sun, Y. Nanonewton force-controlled manipulation of biological cells using a monolithic MEMS microgripper with two-axis force feedback. *J. Micromech. Microeng.* **2008**, *18*. [CrossRef]
41. Kim, K.; Liu, X.; Zhang, Y.; Cheng, J.; Wu, X.Y.; Sun, Y. Elastic and viscoelastic characterization of microcapsules for drug delivery using a force-feedback MEMS microgripper. *Biomed. Microdevices* **2009**, *11*, 421–427. [CrossRef]
42. Solano, B.; Wood, D. Design and testing of a polymeric microgripper for cell manipulation. *Microelectron. Eng.* **2007**, *84*, 1219–1222. [CrossRef]
43. Zeman, M.J.; Bordatchev, E.V.; Knopf, G.K. Design, kinematic modeling and performance testing of an electro-thermally driven microgripper for micromanipulation applications. *J. Micromech. Microeng.* **2006**, *16*, 1540. [CrossRef]
44. Zhang, R.; Chu, J.; Wang, H.; Chen, Z. A multipurpose electrothermal microgripper for biological micro-manipulation. *Microsyst. Technol.* **2013**, *19*, 89–97. [CrossRef]
45. Cauchi, M.; Grech, I.; Mallia, B.; Mollicone, P.; Sammut, N. The effects of cold arm width and metal deposition on the performance of a U-beam electrothermal MEMS microgripper for biomedical applications. *Micromachines* **2019**, *10*, 167. [CrossRef]
46. Cauchi, M.; Grech, I.; Mallia, B.; Mollicone, P.; Sammut, N. The effects of structure thickness, air gap thickness and silicon type on the performance of a horizontal electrothermal MEMS microgripper. *Actuators* **2018**, *7*, 38. [CrossRef]
47. Ren, H.; Wu, S.T. Adaptive Lenses Based on Soft Electroactive Materials. *Appl. Sci.* **2018**, *8*, 1085. [CrossRef]
48. Yan, B.; Wang, K.; Hu, Z.; Wu, C.; Zhang, X. Shunt damping vibration control technology: A review. *Appl. Sci.* **2017**, *7*, 494. [CrossRef]
49. Rossi, A.; Orsini, F.; Scorza, A.; Botta, F.; Belfiore, N.P.; Sciuto, S.A. A review on parametric dynamic models of magnetorheological dampers and their characterization methods. *Actuators* **2018**, *7*, 16. [CrossRef]

50. Botta, F.; Marx, N.; Gentili, S.; Schwingshackl, C.W.; Di Mare, L.; Cerri, G.; Dini, D. Optimal placement of piezoelectric plates for active vibration control of gas turbine blades: Experimental results. In Proceedings of the SPIE - The International Society for Optical Engineering, San Diego, CA, USA, 11–15 March 2012; Volume 8345.
51. Botta, F.; Dini, D.; Schwingshackl, C.; Di Mare, L.; Cerri, G. Optimal placement of piezoelectric plates to control multimode vibrations of a beam. *Adv. Acoustics Vib.* **2013**. . [CrossRef]
52. Botta, F.; Rossi, A.; Schinaia, L.; Scorza, A.; Orsini, F.; Sciuto, S.A.; Belfiore, N.P. Experimental validation on optimal placement of pzt plates for active beam multimode vibrations reduction. In Proceedings of the 23rd Conference of the Italian Association of Theoretical and Applied Mechanics AIMETA 2017, Salerno, Italy, 4–7 September 2017; Volume 3, pp. 2258–2269.
53. Botta, F.; Toccaceli, F. Piezoelectric plates distribution for active control of torsional vibrations. *Actuators* **2018**, *7*, 23. [CrossRef]
54. Xiao, Y.; Wang, B.; Zhou, S. Pull-in voltage analysis of electrostatically actuated MEMS with piezoelectric layers: A size-dependent model. *Mech. Res. Commun.* **2015**, *66*, 7–14. [CrossRef]
55. Azizi, S.; Ghodsi, A.; Jafari, H.; Ghazavi, M.R. A conceptual study on the dynamics of a piezoelectric MEMS (Micro Electro Mechanical System) energy harvester. *Energy* **2016**, *96*, 495–506. [CrossRef]
56. Madinei, H.; Khodaparast, H.H.; Adhikari, S.; Friswell, M.I.; Fazeli, M. Adaptive tuned piezoelectric MEMS vibration energy harvester using an electrostatic device. *Eur. Phys. J. Spec. Top.* **2015**, *224*, 2703–2717. [CrossRef]
57. Kanno, I. Piezoelectric MEMS for energy harvesting. *J. Phys. Conf. Ser.* **2015**, *660*. [CrossRef]
58. Tian, W.; Ling, Z.; Yu, W.; Shi, J. A review of MEMS scale piezoelectric energy harvester. *Appl. Sci.* **2018**, *8*, 645. [CrossRef]
59. Nah, S.K.; Zhong, Z.W. A microgripper using piezoelectric actuation for micro-object manipulation. *Sens. Actuators A Phys.* **2007**, *133*, 218–224. [CrossRef]
60. Haddab, Y.; Chaillet, N.; Bourjault, A. A microgripper using smart piezoelectric actuators. In Proceedings of the 2000 IEEE/RSJ International Conference on Intelligent Robots and Systems, Takamatsu, Japan, 31 October–5 November 2000; Volume 1.
61. Wang, D.H.; Yang, Q.; Dong, H.M. A monolithic compliant piezoelectric-driven microgripper: Design, modeling, and testing. *IEEE/ASME Trans. Mechatron.* **2013**, *18*, 138–147. [CrossRef]
62. Loh, O.; Vaziri, A.; Espinosa, H.D. The potential of MEMS for advancing experiments and modeling in cell mechanics. *Exp. Mech.* **2009**, *49*, 105–124. [CrossRef]
63. Crawley, E.F.; Luis, J.D. Use of piezoelectric actuators as elements of intelligent structures. *AIAA J.* **1987**, *25*, 1373–1385. [CrossRef]
64. Eom, C.B.; Trolier-McKinstry, S. Thin-film piezoelectric MEMS. *MRS Bull.* **2012**, *37*, 1007–1017. [CrossRef]
65. Xu, R.; Lei, A.; Christiansen, T.L.; Hansen, K.; Guizzetti, M.; Birkelund, K.; Thomsen, E.V.; Hansen, O. Screen printed PZT/PZT thick film bimorph MEMS cantilever device for vibration energy harvesting. In Proceedings of the 2011 16th International Solid-State Sensors, Actuators and Microsystems Conference, TRANSDUCERS'11, Beijing, China, 5–9 June 2011; pp. 679–682.
66. Shen, D.; Park, J.H.; Ajitsaria, J.; Choe, S.Y.; Wikle, H.C.; Kim, D.J. The design, fabrication and evaluation of a MEMS PZT cantilever with an integrated Si proof mass for vibration energy harvesting. *J. Micromech. Microeng.* **2008**, *18*, 055017. [CrossRef]
67. Mayrhofer, P.M.; Wistrela, E.; Kucera, M.; Bittner, A.; Schmid, U. Fabrication and characterisation of ScAlN-based piezoelectric MEMS cantilevers. In Proceedings of the 2015 Transducers—2015 18th International Conference on Solid-State Sensors, Actuators and Microsystems, TRANSDUCERS 2015, Anchorage, AK, USA, 21–25 June 2015; pp. 2144–2147.
68. Nagano, T.; Nishigaki, M.; Abe, K.; Itaya, K.; Kawakubo, T. Fabrication and performance of piezoelectric MEMS tunable capacitors constructed with AlN bimorph structure. In Proceedings of the IEEE MTT-S International Microwave Symposium Digest, San Francisco, CA, USA, 11–16 June 2006; pp. 1285–1288.
69. Park, J.S.; Yang, S.J.; Kyung-Il, L.E.E.; Kang, S.G. Fabrication and electro-mechanical characteristics of piezoelectric micro bending actuators on silicon substrates. *J. Ceram. Soc. Jpn.* **2006**, *114*, 1089–1092. [CrossRef]
70. Yuan, Y.H.; Du, H.J.; Xia, X.; Wong, Y.R. Modeling, fabrication and characterization of piezoelectric ZnO-based micro-sensors and micro-actuators. *Appl. Mech. Mater.* **2014**, *444–445*, 1636–1643. [CrossRef]

71. Lou, L.; Yu, H.; Haw, M.T.X.; Zhang, S.; Gu, Y.A. Comparative characterization of bimorph and unimorph AlN piezoelectric micro-machined ultrasonic transducers. In Proceedings of the IEEE International Conference on Micro Electro Mechanical Systems (MEMS), Shanghai, China, 24–28 January 2016; Volume 2016-February, pp. 1090–1093.
72. Zeng, Y.; Groenesteijn, J.; Alveringh, D.; Steenwelle, R.J.A.; Ma, K.; Wiegerink, R.J.; Lotters, J.C. Micro Coriolis MASS flow sensor driven by integrated PZT thin film actuators. In Proceedings of the IEEE International Conference on Micro Electro Mechanical Systems (MEMS), Belfast, UK, 21–25 January 2018; Volume 2018-January, pp. 850–853.
73. Sindhanaiselvi, D.; Shanmuganantham, T. Investigation on performance of piezoelectric beam based MEMS actuator for focussing of micro lens in mobile application. In Proceedings of the IEEE International Conference on Circuits and Systems, ICCS 2017, Thiruvananthapuram, India, 20–21 December 2017; Volume 2018-January, pp. 398–403.
74. Chen, S.H.; Michael, A.; Kwok, C.Y. A Fast Response MEMS Piezoelectric Microlens Actuator with Large Stroke and Low Driving Voltage. In Proceedings of the NEMS 2018 - 3th Annual IEEE International Conference on Nano/Micro Engineered and Molecular Systems, Singapore, Singapore, 22–26 April 2018; pp. 199–203.
75. Tsaur, J.; Zhang, L.; Maeda, R.; Matsumoto, S.; Khumpuang, S.; Wan, J. Design and fabrication of 1D and 2D micro scanners actuated by double layered PZT bimorph beams. In Proceedings of the 2001 International Microprocesses and Nanotechnology Conference, MNC 2001, Shimane, Japan, 31 October–2 November 2001; pp. 204–205.
76. Tsaur, J.; Zhang, L.; Maeda, R.; Matsumoto, S.; Khumpuang, S. Design and Fabrication of 1D and 2D Micro Scanners Actuated by Double Layered Lead Zirconate Titanate (PZT) Bimorph Beams. *Jpn. J. Appl. Phys.* **2002**, *41*, 4321–4326. [CrossRef]
77. Kuo, C.L.; Lin, S.C.; Wu, W.J. Fabrication and performance evaluation of a metal-based bimorph piezoelectric MEMS generator for vibration energy harvesting. *Smart Mater. Struct.* **2016**, *25*, 1280–1284. [CrossRef]
78. Che, L.; Halvorsen, E.; Chen, X.; Yan, X. A micromachined piezoelectric PZT-based cantilever in d33 mode. In Proceedings of the 2010 IEEE 5th International Conference on Nano/Micro Engineered and Molecular Systems, NEMS 2010, Xiamen, China, 20–23 January 2010; pp. 785–788.
79. Kanno, I. Piezoelectric MEMS: Ferroelectric thin films for MEMS applications. *Jpn. J. Appl. Phys.* **2018**, *57*. [CrossRef]
80. Strambi, G.; Barboni, R.; Gaudenzi, P. Pin-force and Euler-Bernoulli models for analysis of intelligent structures. *AIAA J.* **1995**, *33*, 1746–1749. [CrossRef]
81. Waisman, H.; Abramovich, H. Active stiffening of laminated composite beams using piezoelectric actuators. *Compos. Struct.* **2002**, *58*, 109–120. [CrossRef]
82. Botta, F.; Scorza, A.; Rossi, A. Optimal piezoelectric potential distribution for controlling multimode vibrations. *Appl. Sci.* **2018**, *8*, 551. [CrossRef]
83. Wells, P.N.; Liang, H.D. Medical ultrasound: Imaging of soft tissue strain and elasticity. *J. R. Soc. Interface* **2011**, *8*, 1521–1549. [CrossRef]

Permissions

All chapters in this book were first published by MDPI; hereby published with permission under the Creative Commons Attribution License or equivalent. Every chapter published in this book has been scrutinized by our experts. Their significance has been extensively debated. The topics covered herein carry significant findings which will fuel the growth of the discipline. They may even be implemented as practical applications or may be referred to as a beginning point for another development.

he contributors of this book come from diverse backgrounds, making this book a truly international effort. This book will bring forth new frontiers with its revolutionizing research information and detailed analysis of the nascent developments around the world.

We would like to thank all the contributing authors for lending their expertise to make the book truly unique. They have played a crucial role in the development of this book. Without their invaluable contributions this book wouldn't have been possible. They have made vital efforts to compile up to date information on the varied aspects of this subject to make this book a valuable addition to the collection of many professionals and students.

This book was conceptualized with the vision of imparting up-to-date information and advanced data in this field. To ensure the same, a matchless editorial board was set up. Every individual on the board went through rigorous rounds of assessment to prove their worth. After which they invested a large part of their time researching and compiling the most relevant data for our readers.

The editorial board has been involved in producing this book since its inception. They have spent rigorous hours researching and exploring the diverse topics which have resulted in the successful publishing of this book. They have passed on their knowledge of decades through this book. To expedite this challenging task, the publisher supported the team at every step. A small team of assistant editors was also appointed to further simplify the editing procedure and attain best results for the readers.

Apart from the editorial board, the designing team has also invested a significant amount of their time in understanding the subject and creating the most relevant covers. They scrutinized every image to scout for the most suitable representation of the subject and create an appropriate cover for the book.

The publishing team has been an ardent support to the editorial, designing and production team. Their endless efforts to recruit the best for this project, has resulted in the accomplishment of this book. They are a veteran in the field of academics and their pool of knowledge is as vast as their experience in printing. Their expertise and guidance has proved useful at every step. Their uncompromising quality standards have made this book an exceptional effort. Their encouragement from time to time has been an inspiration for everyone.

The publisher and the editorial board hope that this book will prove to be a valuable piece of knowledge for researchers, students, practitioners and scholars across the globe.

List of Contributors

Yuichi Matsuzaki, Kelly John and Toshihiro Shoji
Center for Regenerative Medicine, Nationwide Children's Hospital, Columbus, OH 43205, USA

Toshiharu Shinoka
Center for Regenerative Medicine, Nationwide Children's Hospital, Columbus, OH 43205, USA
Department of Cardiothoracic Surgery, Nationwide Children's Hospital, Columbus, OH 43205, USA
Department of Surgery, The Ohio State UniversityWexner Medical Center, Columbus, OH 43210, USA

Ahmadreza Jahadakbar, Narges Shayesteh Moghaddam, Amirhesam Amerinatanzi and Mohammad Elahinia
Dynamic and Smart Systems Laboratory, The University of Toledo, Toledo, OH 43606, USA

David Dean
Department of Plastic Surgery, The Ohio State University, Columbus, OH 43212, USA

Haluk E. Karaca
Department of Mechanical Engineering, The University of Kentucky, Lexington, KY 40506, USA

Khaja Moiduddin, Syed Hammad Mian and Wadea Ameen
Advanced Manufacturing Institute, King Saud University, Riyadh 11421, Saudi Arabia

Mohammed Alkindi, Sundar Ramalingam and Osama Alghamdi
Department of Oral and Maxillofacial Surgery, College of Dentistry, King Saud University, Riyadh 11545, Saudi Arabia

Francesco Naddeo, Alessandro Naddeo and Nicola Cappetti
Department of Industrial Engineering, University of Salerno, Via Giovanni Paolo II, 132, 84084 Fisciano, SA, Italy

Emilio Cataldo
Techno DESIGN S.r.l., via Rosa Jemma, 2, 84091 Battipaglia, SA, Italy

Nicola Narciso
"San Giovanni di Dio e Ruggi d'Aragona" University Hospital, Largo Città di Ippocrate, 84131 Salerno, Italy

Warren A. Vieira and Catherine D. McCusker
Department of Biology, University of Massachusetts Boston, Boston, MA 02125, USA

Reto Allemann
Eye Clinic Orasis, Swiss Eye Research Foundation, 5734 Reinach AG, Switzerland

Zeljka Cvejic
Department of Physics, Faculty of sciences, University of Novi Sad, Trg Dositeja Obradovica 4, 21000 Novi Sad, Serbia

Bojan Pajic
Eye Clinic Orasis, Swiss Eye Research Foundation, 5734 Reinach AG, Switzerland
Department of Physics, Faculty of sciences, University of Novi Sad, Trg Dositeja Obradovica 4, 21000 Novi Sad, Serbia
Division of Ophthalmology, Department of Clinical Neurosciences, Geneva University Hospitals, 1205 Geneva, Switzerland
Faculty of Medicine of the Military Medical Academy, University of Defense, 11000 Belgrade, Serbia

Mirko Resan
Faculty of Medicine of the Military Medical Academy, University of Defense, 11000 Belgrade, Serbia

Kaweh Mansouri
Glaucoma Center, Montchoisi Clinic, 1000 Lausanne, Switzerland
Department of Ophthalmology, University of Colorado, Denver, CO 80014, USA

Pierbiagio Stilla
Department of Medical, Oral and Biotechnological Sciences and CeSI-Me, University of Chieti-Pescara, 3166100 Chieti, Italy

Antonio Scarano
Department of Medical, Oral and Biotechnological Sciences and CeSI-Me, University of Chieti-Pescara, 3166100 Chieti, Italy
Zirconia Implant Research Group (Z.I.R.G.), International Academy of Ceramic Implantology, Silver Spring, MD 20901, USA
Department of Oral Implantology, Dental Research Division, College Ingà, UNINGÁ, Cachoeiro de Itapemirim 29312, Brazil

Sammy Noumbissi
Zirconia Implant Research Group (Z.I.R.G.), International Academy of Ceramic Implantology, Silver Spring, MD 20901, USA
International Academy of Ceramic Implantology, Zirconia Implant Research Group (Z.I.R.G.), University of Chieti-Pescara, 3166100 Chieti, Italy

Saurabh Gupta
Zirconia Implant Research Group (Z.I.R.G.), International Academy of Ceramic Implantology, Silver Spring, MD 20901, USA
Private Practice Dentistry, Bangalore 560001, India

Francesco Inchingolo
Department of Interdisciplinary Medicine, University of Bari "Aldo Moro", 70121 Bari, Italy

Felice Lorusso
Department of Medical, Oral and Biotechnological Sciences, University of Chieti-Pescara, Via dei Vestini, 3166100 Chieti, Italy

Juan A. Sánchez-Margallo, J. Carlos Gómez-Blanco and J. Blas Pagador
Bioengineering and Health Technologies Unit, Jesús Usón Minimally Invasive Surgery Centre, 10071 Cáceres, Spain

Alfonso González González
Department of Mechanical, Energy and Materials Engineering, University of Extremadura, 06800 Mérida, Spain

Lorenzo García Moruno
Department of Graphical Expression, University of Extremadura, 06800 Mérida, Spain

Francisco M. Sánchez-Margallo
Scientific Direction, Jesús Usón Minimally Invasive Surgery Centre, 10071 Cáceres, Spain

Elena Carlotta Olivetti, Sara Nicotera, Federica Marcolin and Enrico Vezzetti
Department of Management and Production Engineering, Politecnico di Torino, corso Duca degli Abruzzi 24, 10129 Torino, Italy

Jacqueline P. A. Sotong, Emanuele Zavattero and Guglielmo Ramieri
Department of Maxillofacial unit, Città della Salute e della Scienza HOSPITAL, 10129 Torino, Italy

Brigitte Pajic-Eggspuehler
Eye Clinic Orasis, Swiss Eye Research Foundation, 5734 Reinach AG, Switzerland

Horace Massa
Division of Ophthalmology, Department of Clinical Neurosciences, Geneva University Hospitals, 1205 Geneva, Switzerland

Harald P. Studer
Eye Clinic Orasis, Swiss Eye Research Foundation, 5734 Reinach AG, Switzerland
OCTLab, Dept. of Ophthalmology, University of Basel, 4056 Basel, Switzerland

Deyuan Meng, Aimin Li, Jiang Yin and Qingyang Li
School of Mechatronic Engineering, China University of Mining and Technology, Xuzhou 221116, China

Bo Lu
National Quality Supervision and Inspection Centre of Pneumatic Products, Ningbo 315500, China

Federica Vurchio, Francesco Orsini, Andrea Scorza, Salvatore A. Sciuto and Nicola P. Belfiore
Department of Engineering, University of Roma Tre, via della Vasca Navale 79, 00146 Rome, Italy

Pietro Ursi
Department of General Surgery and Surgical Specialties "Paride Stefanini", Sapienza University of Rome, Viale del Policlinico 155, 00161 Rome, Italy

Rocco Crescenzi
Department of Information Engineering, Electronic and Telecommunications, Sapienza University of Rome, Via Eudossiana 18, 00184 Roma, Italy

Jianping Wang, Yongqiang Yang, Dong Guo, Shihua Wang, Long Fu and Yu Li
School of Mechanical and Power Engineering, Henan Polytechnic University, Jiaozuo 454000, China

Fabio Botta, Andrea Rossi and Nicola Pio Belfiore
Dipartimento di Ingegneria, Università degli Studi Roma Tre, Via della Vasca Navale, 79, 00146 Roma, Italy

Index

Printed in the USA
CPSIA information can be obtained
at www.ICGtesting.com
LVHW080042211023
761596LV00010BA/1872

9 781646 46557